T0344421

Dysphagia Evaluation and Management in Otolaryngology

Dysphagia Evaluation and Management in Otolaryngology

DINESH K. CHHETRI, MD
Professor
Department of Head and Neck Surgery
University of California, Los Angeles
Los Angeles, California, United States

KARUNA DEWAN, MD
Assistant Professor
Department of Otolaryngology - Head and Neck Surgery
Stanford University
Stanford, California, United States

ELSEVIER

ELSEVIER

3251 Riverport Lane
St. Louis, Missouri 63043

DYSPHAGIA EVALUATION AND MANAGEMENT IN OTOLARYNGOLOGY   ISBN: 978-0-323-56930-9

Content Strategist: Jessica McCool
Content Development Manager: Christine McElvenny
Content Development Specialist: Jennifer Horigan
Publishing Services Manager: Shereen Jameel
Project Manager: Nadhiya Sekar
Designer: Gopalakrishnan Venkatraman

Printed in United States of America

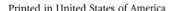

Last digit is the print number: 9 8 7 6 5 4 3 2 1

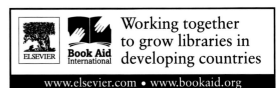

Working together
to grow libraries in
developing countries

www.elsevier.com • www.bookaid.org

List of Contributors

Jacqueline Allen, MBChB, FRACS ORL HNS
Laryngologist
Senior Lecturer
University of Auckland
Auckland, New Zealand

Kenneth W. Altman, MD, PhD
Professor and Vice Chair for Clinical Affairs
Director, The Institute for Voice and Swallowing
Bobby R. Alford Department of Otolaryngology - HNS
Baylor College of Medicine
Houston, TX, United States

David Chen, MD
Associate Professor of Clinical Surgery
Department of Surgery
University of California, Los Angeles
Los Angeles, CA, United States

Dinesh K. Chhetri, MD
Professor
Department of Head and Neck Surgery
University of California, Los Angeles
Los Angeles, CA, United States

Jeffrey L. Conklin, MD, FACG
Director
Center for Esophageal Diseases and GI Motility Lab
Division of Digestive Diseases
University of California, Los Angeles
Los Angeles, CA, United States

Karuna Dewan, MD
Assistant Professor
Department of Otolaryngology - Head and
   Neck Surgery
Stanford University
Stanford, CA, United States

Andrew Erman, MA, CCC-SLP
Speech Pathology Clinic Director
UCLA Medical System
Los Angeles, CA, United States

Aaron J. Feinstein, MD, MHS
Clinical Instructor
Department of Head and Neck Surgery
University of California, Los Angeles
Los Angeles, CA, United States

Kevin Ghassemi, MD
Assistant Clinical Professor
Vatche and Tamar Manoukian
   Division of Digestive Diseases
David Geffen School of Medicine at UCLA
Los Angeles, CA, United States

Alexander N. Goel, BA
Medical Student
David Geffen School of Medicine at UCLA
University of California, Los Angeles
Los Angeles, CA, United States

Jonathan Harounian, MD
Resident Physician
Department of Otolaryngology - Head and
   Neck Surgery
Lewis Katz School of Medicine at
   Temple University
Philadelphia, PA, United States

Langston T. Holly, MD
Professor and Vice Chair
Department of Neurosurgery
University of California, Los Angeles
Los Angeles, CA, United States

Nausheen Jamal, MD
Associate Professor of Surgery
Chief, Division of Otolaryngology
Associate Dean for Graduate
    Medical Education
University of Texas Rio Grande Valley
Edinburg, TX, United States

Jennifer L. Long, MD, PhD
Assistant Professor
Department of Head and Neck Surgery
University of California, Los Angeles
Los Angeles, CA, United States

Physician and Principal Investigator
Greater Los Angeles VA Health System
Los Angeles, CA, United States

Ian T. MacQueen, MD
Resident Physician
Department of General Surgery
University of California, Los Angeles
Los Angeles, CA, United States

Valeria Silva Merea, MD
Assistant Attending Surgeon
Head and Neck Service
Department of Surgery
Memorial Sloan Kettering Cancer Center
New York, NY, United States

Alexander Michael, BA
Medical Student
Lewis Katz School of Medicine at
    Temple University
Philadelphia, PA, United States

Michael I. Orestes, MD
Assistant Professor
Department of Surgery
Uniformed Services University
Bethesda, MD, United States

Pratik B. Patel, MD
Resident Physician
Department of Head and Neck Surgery
University of California, Los Angeles
Los Angeles, CA, United States

Michael J. Pitman, MD
Chief, Division of Laryngology
Columbia University Medical Center
New York, NY, United States

Steven S. Raman, MD
Professor
Department of Radiology
University of California, Los Angeles
Los Angeles, CA, United States

Siddharth U. Shetgeri, MD
Fellow in Spine Surgery
Department of Neurosurgery
University of California, Los Angeles
Los Angeles, CA, United States

Travis L. Shiba, MD
Assistant Clinical Professor
Department of Head and Neck Surgery
University of California, Los Angeles
Los Angeles, CA, United States

Resha Soni, MD
Laryngology Fellow
Division of Otolaryngology - Head and
    Neck Surgery
University of Wisconsin School of
    Medicine and Public Health
Madison, WI, United States

Heather Starmer, MA
Director - Head and Neck Speech and Swallowing
    Rehabilitation
Department of Otolaryngology - Head and
    Neck Surgery
Stanford University
Stanford, CA, United States

Andrew Vahabzadeh-Hagh, MD
Assistant Professor
Division of Head and Neck Surgery
University of California, San Diego
San Diego, CA, United States

Hilary Yankey, BS
Medical Student
Lewis Katz School of Medicine at Temple University
Philadelphia, PA, United States

Richard W. Thomas, MD, DDS, FACS
President of Uniformed Services
    University of the Health Sciences
Professor
Department of Emergency Medicine
Uniformed Services University
Besthesda, MD, United States

Preface

This book is edited by otolaryngologists with two decades of experience evaluating and treating patients with oropharyngeal dysphagia. It is intended to familiarize and update current clinicians who manage dysphagia, as well as students or clinicians who would like to obtain the relevant clinical knowledge to develop a dysphagia practice. All relevant topics for dysphagia evaluation and management in otolaryngology are covered. Until recently, dysphagia evaluation and management consisted of simple swallow assessments, such as an esophagram, and conservative management approaches, such as prescribing a nil per os status for any signs of aspiration. Significant developments in this field now facilitate a more comprehensive assessment, novel treatment options, and a patient-specific management approach. Advances and wider applications of fluoroscopic and endoscopic assessments of swallowing, combined with the ability to perform office-based endoscopy of the entire swallowing anatomy from the lips to the stomach, have led to more comprehensive understanding of swallow function and dysfunction, and how to manage dysphagia. Although otolaryngologists are positioned to play a central role in assessment and treatment of dysphagia due to their familiarity with the swallowing anatomy, a close collaboration with a speech language pathologist is essential for successful management of the dysphagic patient. Other clinicians such as gastroenterologists, general and thoracic surgeons, spine surgeons, and radiologists play important roles in evaluation and treatment. Thus, this book is a product of and relevant to this multidisciplinary team managing dysphagia.

This book is structured concisely and logically for dysphagia evaluation and management. In Section I, embryologic development, gross anatomy, and physiology of the swallowing apparatus from the oral cavity to the esophagus are comprehensively covered. An understanding of anatomy and physiology of the swallowing apparatus is critical to accurate assessment and optimal treatment of dysphagia. Section II follows by covering all contemporary and essential tools for assessment of swallowing function. Finally, in Section III, a practical clinical guide to evaluation and management of all major conditions and disease processes causing oropharyngeal and esophageal dysphagia is presented. Each section begins with a chapter that brings focus to the subsequent chapters of that section. Swallow therapy, an essential tool in managing dysphagia, is also covered. Future advances in dysphagia evaluation and management are needed and expected, as highlighted by the final chapter of the book.

Management of the dysphagic patient often brings great joy to the dysphagia specialist, by partaking in the improvement in quality of life and tremendous happiness brought to patients by advancing to a per oral diet and removing nonoral means of alimentation. We hope that all students and practitioners in the care of dysphagia patients find this book a valuable reference in their own endeavors managing patients with dysphagia.

Dinesh K. Chhetri, MD
Professor
Department of Head and Neck Surgery
University of California, Los Angeles
Los Angeles, California, United States

Karuna Dewan, MD
Assistant Professor
Department of Otolaryngology—Head and Neck Surgery
Stanford University
Stanford, California, United States

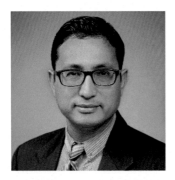

Dinesh K. Chhetri

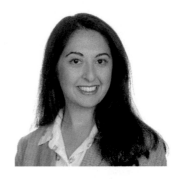

Karuna Dewan

Contents

CHAPTER 1

General Principles of Swallowing

DINESH K. CHHETRI, MD

INTRODUCTION

Normal swallowing plays a critical human function: safe ingestion of food and liquid is vital to our survival and comfort. Human physiology requires regular and frequent eating and drinking for nutrition, and it is imperative that swallowing is not a nuisance or a burden. The goal of swallowing is to safely and efficiently propel food and liquid from the mouth to the stomach. In addition to serving the nutritional function, normal swallowing is necessary to clear saliva and secretions from the oral cavity and pharynx. Adult humans produce over 2 L of saliva daily and spontaneously swallow on average one and a half times a minute (over 2000 times per day). When an individual has difficulty managing saliva due to dysphagia, drooling (sialorrhea) or aspiration may occur.

Normal swallowing is also critical for maintaining a satisfying human quality of life (QOL). We humans are a highly social species who find it pleasurable and desirable to eat, drink, and socialize with others. We design special rooms in our homes for cooking and eating. Outside our homes, we gather to barbecue, picnic, potluck, and party and even hunt for food. Family gatherings, celebrations, and rites of passages in all stages of human life nearly always include a moment of eating together in celebration of shared emotions. Religious gatherings often involve a component where food and liquid are consumed or shared. However, when a person has difficulty swallowing or is unable to swallow safely, the possibility of participating in many of these social interactions diminishes. This is psychologically and functionally devastating, bringing depression and anxiety, and significantly diminishing the human QOL. Although a person can certainly be fed and kept alive using a gastric tube, this is clearly neither considered pleasurable nor psychologically meaningful as

eating by mouth. Nonoral feeding is typically considered artificial rather than "human." In fact, it is not unusual in otolaryngology to encounter patients who would trade their voice for the opportunity to swallow normally again. Therefore, it is imperative that we understand the etiologies of dysphagia and how to manage them, not only to prevent morbidity and mortality but also to improve and maintain satisfying QOL.

Dysphagia practice is a relatively new clinical focus in otolaryngology. Currently, otolaryngologists often refer patients with dysphagia to other specialties such as gastroenterologists or speech and language pathologists for evaluation and management. I suggest that the otolaryngologist is the logical physician to manage patients' oropharyngeal dysphagia, given the field's extensive knowledge of head and neck anatomy. It is a reasonable extension for otolaryngologists to learn normal and abnormal swallow physiology, as well as how to assess and treat dysphagia. Successful assessment and management of dysphagia is a multidisciplinary endeavor. The otolaryngologist who is well versed in oropharyngeal dysphagia can make the appropriate referrals to gather the necessary data to understand how to help patients with swallow issues. Managing dysphagia is highly satisfying, once the clinician becomes familiar with contemporary assessment and management techniques and understands which patients may be helped. Thus, the purpose of this book is to make dysphagia evaluation and management accessible to all otolaryngologists.

BASIC CONCEPTS OF SWALLOWING

The human developmental anatomy that provides voice and speech also creates one major challenge to swallowing: humans must swallow without food or liquids accidentally spilling into the airways. At birth, the human larynx is at the level of the oropharynx and the epiglottis tip is positioned at the superior oropharynx at the level of the soft palate. This allows the neonate to breathe through the nose and at the same time swallow liquids via mouth and through the lateral oropharyngeal channels. The descent of the laryngopharynx occurring as early as 6 months after birth with postnatal growth suddenly brings the laryngeal inlet directly into the path of the food bolus. While postnatal descent of the larynx allows for the glottic larynx to modulate the pulmonary airflow to produce voice that is further manipulated by the oral and pharyngeal structures to produce speech sounds, the crossing of the airway and the food way places human species at risk for aspiration and death when food falls below the level of the vocal folds into the tracheobronchial airway. A complex laryngeal protective mechanism therefore must be activated during each swallow. When this protective mechanism fails, aspiration and its complications may ensue. The major adverse consequence of aspiration is pneumonia which may result in death. However, more commonly, chronic aspiration leads to debilitation, malnutrition, chronic lung infection, and morbidity and mortality of chronic lung disease.

What is dysphagia? Often it is simply described as subjective difficulty with swallowing. It is also the inability to swallow safely, or reduced intake such that the person has difficulty maintaining adequate nutrition and/or hydration. Dysphagia can also be an objective finding of dysfunction in the phases of swallowing. A complex swallowing mechanism controls sequential passage of food bolus from the mouth to the stomach. Functionally and anatomically, the swallowing apparatus can be separated into three sections: oral, pharyngeal, and esophageal. Each section can be conceptualized as a conduit with a pump and valves. Valves at either end of the section open and close to propel food bolus toward the stomach and prevent improper backward or sideway leakage. Pumps squeeze sequentially and generate the propulsive force that facilitates an anterograde movement of the food bolus toward the stomach. In the oral phase, the lips anteriorly and the oropharyngeal faucial arch and base of tongue posteriorly form valves that hold liquid in the oral cavity tube prior to swallow onset (the posterior oral valve may remain open during solid food mastication to allow aroma to reach the nasopharynx). The tongue pumps the food and liquids into the oropharynx at the onset of swallowing while the lips stay sealed and the posterior oral cavity valve opens. In the pharyngeal phase, the tongue base and velum

valves close and the upper esophageal sphincter (UES) valve opens while the pharyngeal muscle pump pushes the food toward the upper esophagus. The laryngeal protective valve is also activated during this phase. The pharyngeal phase is completed in 1 s, a testament to the highly coordinated neuromuscular control required to swallow without aspirating! Once food is in the esophagus, the UES closes and the esophageal pump propels the food bolus toward the lower esophageal sphincter, which opens to allow food into the stomach. Details of the swallowing events are described in detail in the following chapters.

The valves, pumps, and pipes paradigm obviously simplifies the swallowing mechanism which is complex anatomically and functionally in the three dimensions. In addition, the pump and the pipe are often the same and changes shape with swallowing. The central and peripheral neural control is complex. However, this concept illustrates normal swallow function and identifies areas of dysfunctions in evaluating and managing dysphagia. The next chapters of this book will present the developmental anatomy, functional anatomy, and physiology of the swallowing apparatus in great detail. Then the swallow assessment tools will be covered in detail. Lastly, the most common swallow dysfunctions encountered by the otolaryngologist and management of these disorders will be covered in detail.

ETIOLOGIES OF DYSPHAGIA

Conceptualization of the normal swallow anatomy and physiology as a biomechanical event lends itself to determining the etiologies and pathophysiology of dysphagia. There should be no defects in the walls of the pipe, the valves should close adequately and open sequentially, and the pumps should be intact in their muscular components and innervation. In regard to neural control, while motor nerves are critical to maintaining the compliance of the swallow compartments and pump function, afferent sensory system should be intact as well to act as a feedback system for controlled flow of food and liquids. One can witness the devastating consequence of neuromuscular dysfunction in patients with multiple cranial neuropathies. The glossopharyngeal (CN IX), vagus (CN X), and hypoglossal (CN XII) nerves are the critical cranial nerves for safe oropharyngeal swallowing. The trigeminal (CN V) and facial (CN VII) nerves play a crucial function as well, especially for oral phase swallowing. The importance of the afferent system is seen in the more severe swallow dysfunction seen in high vagal injury compared to recurrent laryngeal nerve injury, and challenges in swallow therapy training in patients with insensate laryngopharynx. Silent aspiration is often present in patients with injuries to the laryngopharyngeal sensory nerves.

Surgical and nonsurgical treatment of head and neck diseases can cause dysfunctions of the many valves in the swallowing system. Lip valve dysfunction leads to oral incompetence and external leakage of saliva and food, velopharynx valve dysfunction may lead to nasopharyngeal regurgitation of food, laryngeal valve dysfunction may lead to penetration and aspiration, upper esophageal valve dysfunction may lead to inefficient handover of food bolus from the oropharynx to esophagus, and lower esophageal valve dysfunction may lead to esophageal stasis. Valve dysfunction also may lead to decreased or absent bolus pressure and release of swallow pressure strength in the improper direction. Proper pump function is arguably the most important requirement of the normal swallow task—and the most difficult to treat when dysfunctional—and pump failure leads to food stasis and residue in the respective compartments. The tongue pump, pharyngeal muscle pump, and esophageal muscle pumps are all under voluntary and involuntary cortical neuromuscular control, and sequential activation of the pumps is another major requirement for normal swallowing function.

CONCLUSIONS

Eating and drinking are essential for human survival and should be pleasurable and effortless. Normal swallowing is a highly coordinated physiologic activity involving over 30 paired muscles and multiple cranial nerves under voluntary and involuntary control. Food and liquid are passed sequentially and seamlessly from the mouth to the stomach. For the purposes of assessment and treatment, the swallow process can be anatomically and functionally separated into three compartments, where each compartment consists of valves, pipe, and pump. This allows for manageable conceptualization of swallow function and assessment and treatment of dysphagia. Treatment of dysphagia can be is a highly satisfying clinical activity as you will help patients achieve their goal to restore a basic and essential function of normal human life.

CHAPTER 2

The Oral Cavity

ALEXANDER N. GOEL, BA • JENNIFER L. LONG, MD, PHD

INTRODUCTION

The oral cavity or mouth is bounded anteriorly by the lips, posteriorly by the faucial arches just anterior to the tonsils, laterally by the cheeks, superiorly by the palate, and inferiorly by the muscular floor (Fig. 2.1). The tongue occupies the floor of the oral cavity. The oral cavity can be divided into two parts: (1) the oral vestibule, which is the space between the lips or cheeks and the teeth and (2) the oral cavity proper, the region medial to the teeth. A mucous membrane of stratified squamous epithelium lines and protects the inside of the mouth. A multitude of minor and major salivary glands secrete viscous and mucoid fluid to moisten and lubricate the oral cavity. Functionally, the oral cavity comprises the first part of the digestive tract and is essential for the ingestion of nutrients. The oral stages of swallowing involve complex coordination within and among the several motor systems of the oral cavity.

EMBRYOLOGY

The embryologic development of the oral cavity is a complex process that involves the growth, migration, and fusion of a number of different embryologic tissues. The process is marked by the formation of the branchial arches which appear in the fourth to fifth week of development.[1] The branchial arches are derived from mesodermal tissue and are separated by external, ectoderm-derived branchial clefts and internal, endoderm-derived pharyngeal pouches.

The formation of the face and palate are based on the proliferation of the first branchial arch.[2] Early on, the first arch splits into mandibular and maxillary processes. By the fourth week, these portions develop into five distinct facial prominences: paired maxillary prominences, paired mandibular prominences, and the frontonasal prominence. The growth of these tissues is driven by neural crest cells that originate in the neuroectoderm and migrate ventrally into the branchial arches and rostrally to the facial region. During the fifth week of development, ectodermal thickenings from the

frontonasal prominence, called the nasal placodes, invaginate to form the nasal pits.[1] The raised margins of each nasal pit are divided into a medial and lateral nasal prominence. The upper lip forms from the fusion of the maxillary and medial nasal prominences. Failure of these prominences to properly fuse results in *cleft lip*. The lower lip and jaw form from the fusion of the mandibular prominences. Fusion of the medial nasal prominences results in the development of the intermaxillary segment which will form the *primary palate* and carries the four maxillary incisor teeth.[2] Separation of the oral cavity from the nasal cavity occurs during the seventh to eighth weeks of development. The palatine shelves arise from the maxillary prominences and initially are directed inferiorly toward the tongue until the seventh week of development when they rotate to a horizontal position above the tongue and fuse to form the *secondary palate*. Anteriorly, the secondary palate fuses with the primary palate. The tongue begins to develop in the fourth week and is formed from several local proliferations from the floor of mouth known as lingual swellings.[2] These swellings are derived from the first through fourth branchial arches. The anterior two-thirds of the tongue arise from the first and second arches, while the posterior third arises from the third and fourth arches (see Chapter 3 for more on tongue development). The composition of the tongue from different embryologic tissues accounts for the different sensory innervation to the anterior and posterior parts of the tongue, which is described in more detail below.

ANATOMY

Lips and Cheeks

The lips and cheeks comprise largely of mimetic muscle and surround the alveolar arches. Between the alveolar arches and lips and cheeks are sulci called the *anterior and lateral sulci*. The lamina propria (submucosal connective tissue) of both the lips and cheeks contain numerous small salivary glands which continually drain into the oral vestibule.[3] The orbicularis oris

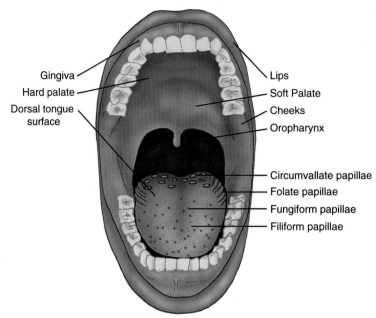

FIG. 2.1 Frontal view of the oral cavity. (From Cook S, Bull S, Metheven L, et al. Mucoadhesion: A Food Perspective. *Food Hydrocolloids.* 2017;72:281−296: with permission)

muscle forms the muscular framework of the lips and contraction of this muscle during swallowing ensures an adequate seal to prevent material from leaking from the oral cavity. The buccinator forms the muscular framework of the cheek. The parotid duct (Stensen's duct) runs through the buccinator muscle before opening into the mucosa of the cheek opposite the second upper molar tooth. Tension in the buccinator muscle during mastication closes off the lateral sulcus to prevent accumulation of food between the mandible and cheek.[4,5] The facial nerve (CN VII) provides motor innervation to the mimetic muscles including the orbicularis oris and buccinator. Injury to the marginal mandibular branch of the facial nerve may result from neck dissection surgery and can lead to *oral incompetence* with drooling of saliva and poor oral control of food bolus.

Palate

The hard palate separates the oral and nasal cavities. It is formed by the palatine processes of the maxilla anteriorly and horizontal plates of palatine bones posteriorly. The soft palate is located posterior to the hard palate and is formed by contributions from several muscles. The *palatoglossus* muscle runs in the anterior faucial arch, or palatoglossal arch, and the *palatopharyngeus* muscle runs in the posterial faucial arch, or palatopharyngeal arch of the tonsillar fossa. These muscles pull the back of the tongue upward toward the soft palate to

close off the oral cavity from the pharynx. Palatal muscles also include *tensor veli palatini* and *levator veli palatini* which tense and elevate the soft palate, respectively, during swallowing to prevent passage or regurgitation of food into the nose. The uvula also contains a small muscle, the *musculus uvulae.*[3]

Floor of the Mouth

The main support of the structures of the mouth is provided by the *mylohyoid muscle.* It is a flat triangular muscle just above the anterior belly of the digastric. It arises broadly from the mylohyoid line on the internal surface of the mandible. Its middle and anterior fibers are inserted into a median raphe while the posterior fibers attach to the front of the hyoid bone. The mylohyoid helps elevate the hyoid bone during swallowing and speech. Along with the mylohyoid, the geniohyoid and anterior belly of the digastric muscle comprise the muscular floor of the mouth (Fig. 2.2).

The paired *submandibular (submaxillary) glands* are located in the neck, beneath the mylohyoid in the submandibular triangle, bordered by the anterior belly of the digastric anteriorly, mandible laterally, and mylohyoid medially. The deep process of the gland extends behind the mylohyoid and extends internally deep to the mylohyoid muscle but lateral to the hyoglossus. The submandibular duct (Wharton's duct), which drains the saliva of the gland, runs along the floor of

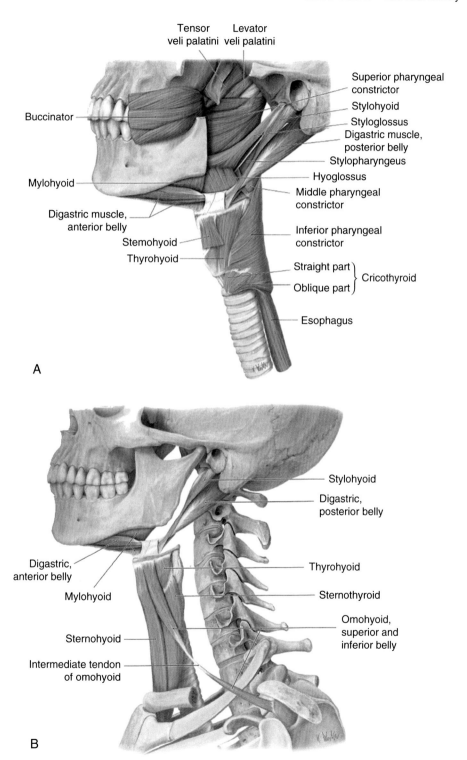

FIG. 2.2 **(A** and **B)** Lateral views of the head showing extrinsic tongue, suprahyoid, soft palate, and pharyngeal muscles. (From Shaw S, Martino R. The normal swallow: muscular and neurophysiological control. *Otolaryngol Clin N Am*. 2013;46(6):937−956; with permission.)

the mouth between the mylohyoid and the hyoglossus/genioglossus muscles then just medial to the sublingual gland to end in a small orifice at the base of the lingual frenulum. The smallest of the "major" salivary glands are the paired sublingual glands, which are also located within the floor of the mouth between the mandible and the submandibular ducts and lingual nerves. These drain through the small *ducts of Rivinus* that are generally not visible to the eye. These named salivary glands are strongly stimulated by food, aromas, and even mental suggestions of food via their parasympathetic efferent innervation.

Tongue

The tongue is a muscular structure that comprises the majority of the oral cavity and rests on the floor of mouth. It is comprised of intrinsic and extrinsic muscles. *Intrinsic muscles* originate and insert within the tongue and are directed vertically, longitudinally, and transversely; these muscles help alter the *shape* of the dorsal tongue. *Extrinsic muscles* originate from mandibular or hyoid bones and insert within the substance of the tongue. These include *genioglossus* arising from the mandible, *hyoglossus* from the hyoid bone, *styloglossus* from the styloid process, and *palatoglossus* from the palate (Fig. 2.2). The extrinsic muscles function to change the *position* of the tongue and protrude, retract, depress,

and elevate the tongue. Together, the intrinsic and extrinsic muscles facilitate the finely coordinated movements of the tongue during mastication, deglutition, and speech articulation.[6]

The anterior two-thirds of the tongue are developmentally separate from the posterior third and the two parts come together at the sulcus terminalis. The mucosa of the anterior part of the tongue is distinguished from the rest of the oral mucosa by the presence of papillae that cover its dorsal surface and give the tongue its characteristic rough texture. The lingual papillae are distinguished into four types—filiform, fungiform, foliate, and vallate—and are largely responsible for taste perception. The posterior third of the tongue (base of tongue) contains the lingual tonsils, collections of lymphoepithelial tissue, and is anatomically classified as part of the oropharynx rather than the oral cavity.

The tongue receives innervation in varying degrees from the cranial nerves V, VII, IX, X, and XII, as determined by the developmental origin of its different components (Fig. 2.3). Motor innervation to all intrinsic and extrinsic tongue muscles is supplied by the hypoglossal nerve (CN XII). This nerve runs between the mylohyoid and hyoglossus muscles in the posterior floor of the mouth then continues forward in the fibers of the genioglossus giving small branches until it

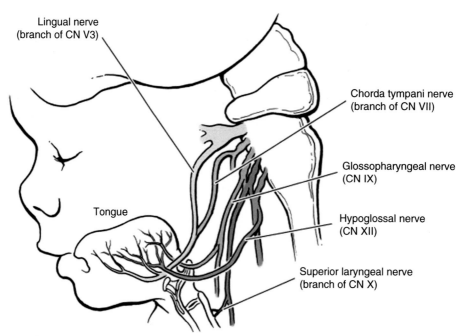

FIG. 2.3 Sensory and taste innervations of the tongue. *CN*, cranial nerve. (From Chen E, Sie K. Development anatomy. In: *Cummings Otolaryngology*, 6th ed. Elsevier; 2015:2821–2830; with permission.)

Labels in figure:
Lingual nerve (branch of CN V3)
Chorda tympani nerve (branch of CN VII)
Glossopharyngeal nerve (CN IX)
Tongue
Hypoglossal nerve (CN XII)
Superior laryngeal nerve (branch of CN X)

reaches the tip of the tongue. General sensation to the anterior two-thirds of the tongue is carried by the lingual nerve, which branches from the third division of the trigeminal nerve (CN V3) and travels through the floor of the mouth before entering the tongue posteriorly to its floor of mouth attachments. General sensation to the posterior third of the tongue is carried by the glossopharyngeal nerve (CN IX) and superior laryngeal branch of the vagus nerve (CN X). Taste sensation is carried from the anterior two-thirds of the tongue by the chorda tympani branch of the facial nerve (CN VII) and from the posterior third by the glosso-pharyngeal nerve (CN IX).

Masticatory Muscles

There are four muscles of mastication—*the masseter, temporalis, medial pterygoid, and lateral pterygoid.* They are embryologically derived from the first pharyngeal arch and, consequently, are all supplied by the third division of the trigeminal nerve (CN V3). The masseter, temporalis, medial pterygoid, and superior head of the lateral pterygoid primarily close the jaw by elevating the mandible, while contraction of the inferior head of the lateral pterygoid protrudes, lowers, and laterally displaces the mandible. Contraction of muscles attached to the hyoid bone, including the anterior belly of the digastric, mylohyoid, and geniohyoid, also depress the mandible.[7] Combined actions of these muscles result in a rotary motion of the mandible during mastication that facilitates efficient shearing and grinding of ingested food. Table 2.1 lists the innervation and actions of the muscles of mastication, as well as other major muscles involved in oropharyngeal swallowing.

TABLE 2.1
Innervation and Actions of Major Muscles Involved in the Oral Phases of Swallowing

Muscle Group	Muscle	Innervation	Function(s) in Swallowing
Masticatory	Masseter	Trigeminal Nerve Mandibular branch (V$_3$)	Elevate/protrude mandible
	Temporalis		Elevate/retrude mandible
	Lateral pterygoid		Concerted effort of both muscles depresses mandible Unilateral effort produces contralateral excursion
	Medial pterygoid		Elevate mandible Unilateral effort produces contralateral excursion
Facial	Orbicularis oris	Facial nerve (VII)	Seal lips/mouth
	Buccinator		Tense cheeks to aid positioning of food over the teeth; seal lateral sulci
Tongue	Intrinsic tongue muscles	Hypoglossal nerve (XII)	Alter tongue shape
	Genioglossus		Protrude/depress tongue
	Hyoglossus		Depress/retract back of tongue
	Styloglossus		Elevate/retract tongue
Palate	Tensor veli palatini	Mandibular branch (V$_3$)	Tense soft palate
	Levator veli palatini	Vagus nerve (X) via pharyngeal branch to pharyngeal plexus	Elevate soft palate, seal oropharynx from nasopharynx
	Palatopharyngeus		Depress soft palate Elevate pharynx
	Palatoglossus		Depress soft palate Elevate back of tongue
	Musculus uvulae		Elevate/retract uvula

Teeth

The teeth play a key role in mastication. Humans develop two sets of teeth. Deciduous teeth erupt between 6 months and 2 years of age and are replaced by permanent teeth beginning at about 6 years of age and continuing into adulthood. Each half of the adult mandible and maxilla contains a set of eight permanent teeth: two incisors, one canine, two premolars, and three molars. Incisors shear and cut ingested food, and the molars grind food.

PHYSIOLOGY

The physiology of swallowing involves a rapid yet complex sequence of movements traditionally divided into three stages: (1) the oral stage, (2) the pharyngeal stage, and (3) the esophageal stage. The oral stage of swallowing is often divided into two functional phases, the oral preparatory and the oral transport phases.

Oral Preparatory Phase

In the oral preparatory phase, material is ingested and prepared into a suitable bolus for swallowing. Ingestion of a bolus usually involves active lowering of the mandible, opening of the lips, and depression of the tongue to increase the volume of the oral cavity available to receive the ingested material. The masticatory muscles and orbicularis oris then contract to close the jaw and seal the lips, respectively, in order to prevent the spillage of food or liquid. Mastication is necessary in order to reduce solid food into a *bolus of an appropriate size, shape, and consistency* for swallowing. During this process, contraction of the muscles of mastication bring the upper and lower occlusal surfaces of the teeth together to tear and grind the food into smaller particles. Salivary secretions soften the bolus to help achieve optimal consistency. Cyclic movements of the jaw are coordinated with actions of the tongue, soft palate, and cheeks that lead to the rhythm of mastication.[8] The tongue generally moves forward as the jaw opens and backward as it closes, preventing tongue biting. As food is crushed between the teeth, it falls medially toward the tongue which moves laterally to reposition the food on the occlusal surface.[9] The buccinator contracts to apply counterpressure toward the jaw and tongue that aids this repositioning. Reduced lateral range of motion of the tongue or loss of proper tone in the buccinators, as may result from head and neck cancer surgery, may impair the patient's ability to position material over the teeth for adequate mastication.[10] Additionally, tension in the buccinators also acts to seal off the lateral sulci (between the cheeks and teeth) to prevent the accumulation of food in this space.[4,5]

Impairments in the oral preparatory phase can lengthen mealtimes, produce social embarrassment from food leakage, and cause downstream management challenges from inadequately prepared bolus.

The soft palate also moves in relation to the jaw during food processing, moving upward as the jaw opens and moving downward as it closes. The cyclical movements of the soft palate and tongue during this stage keep the faucial isthmus open, allowing communication between the oral cavity and oropharynx.[11,12] This is in contrast to the process of drinking in which the soft palate and tongue come together to form a seal to the posterior passage of liquid. The pumping of air through the faucial isthmus by jaw and tongue movements allows food aroma to reach chemoreceptors in the nasopharynx and nasal cavity.[13] Until swallowing is initiated, the airway remains open and nasal breathing may continue. Thus, if an individual loses control of the food bolus at this stage, it may pass into the pharynx and continue into the open airway.[14]

Oral Transport Phase

During the oral propulsive phase, the tongue initiates the posterior movement of the bolus. The anterior tongue contacts the hard palate just behind the upper teeth and the posterior tongue lowers to open the faucial isthmus.[15] The anterior two-thirds of the tongue then elevate to make peristaltic sequential contact with the hard palate from anterior to posterior. As the area of contact between the tongue and palate increases, the bolus is squeezed backward through the fauces and into oropharynx.[10] Concurrently, the soft palate is elevated by the contraction of the *tensor veli palatini* and *levator veli palatini* muscles into contact with the posterior pharyngeal wall to seal off the oropharynx from the nasopharynx, preventing nasal regurgitation.[16] The lateral walls of the nasopharynx, composed of the superior pharyngeal constrictors, also come together to reinforce this closure. The entry of the bolus into the oropharynx is further facilitated by the flattening and forward movement of the posterior tongue that results primarily from the contraction of the *hyoglossus* muscle. This expands the pharynx, effectively creating a chute, down which the bolus can more easily slide.[17] The transport of food from the oral cavity to oropharynx occurs intermittently during food processing cycles.[18] Transported food accumulates on the oropharyngeal surface of the tongue and the vallecula. Chewing of food remaining in the oral cavity continues, leading to progressive enlargement of the bolus in the oropharynx with subsequent oral transport cycles until the pharyngeal phase of swallowing is initiated with posterior movement of the base of tongue. Fig. 2.4

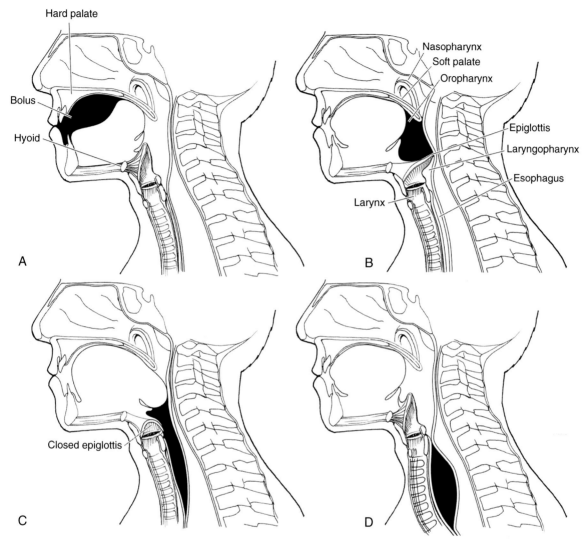

FIG. 2.4 Bolus propagation during swallowing. **(A)** Wave-like elevation of the tongue propels the bolus into the oropharynx. **(B)** Soft palate elevation closes the opening of the nasal cavity as the bolus passes into the pharynx. **(C)** Bolus is propelled through the pharynx past the closed epiglottis and enters the esophagus through the upper esophageal sphincter. **(D)** Bolus travels through the esophagus via peristaltic waves to the stomach. The soft palate and tongue relax, and the epiglottis opens to resume respiration. (From Hennessey M, Goldberg D. Surgical anatomy and physiology of swallowing. *Op Tech Otolaryngol Head Neck Surg.* 2016; 27(2):60–66; with permission.)

illustrates the progression of the bolus during swallowing. Impaired oral transport commonly results in premature and uncoordinated food dropping into the pharynx, thus risking entry into the unprotected glottis.

Role of Saliva in Swallowing

Saliva has several key functions during the oral phases of swallowing. Saliva solubilizes food particles to release substances responsible for the perception of taste and aroma. As ingested material is chewed, saliva also lubricates the food to facilitate the formation of a *cohesive bolus* before swallowing. Oral digestive enzymes in saliva, such as *amylase and lipase*, begin the breakdown of starches and lipids to aid digestion. Factors that affect salivary production can have significant consequences for oral health and swallowing. Salivary gland hypofunction and *xerostomia*, the sensation of dry mouth, may result from radiotherapy for head and neck cancer, medication side effects, or Sjogren's syndrome. Patients with xerostomia may have trouble eating due to the inability to lubricate food, with resulting difficulty in forming a cohesive bolus and sticking of food within the oral cavity. Altered taste sensation (*dysguesia*) and oral discomfort may diminish the enjoyment of eating. Treatments are currently limited to short-acting saliva substitutes, and cholinergic drugs which can have significant systemic side effects. *Sialorrhea*, or excess drooling, may be caused by neuromuscular dysfunction in patients with cerebral palsy, stroke, or Parkinson disease. Increased risk of aspiration may result as pooled saliva can flood the bolus and separate food particles, making oral control of ingested material difficult.[19] Common treatments aim to reduce saliva production with anticholinergic pharmaceuticals or by botulinum toxin injection that temporarily blocks transmission of parasympathetic nerve signals via acetylcholine. These approaches can be effective, even though the drooling is most often due to poor oral control of saliva, rather than hyperproduction.[20]

REFERENCES

1. Sadler TW. *Langman's Medical Embryology*. 12th ed. LWW; 2011.
2. Moore KL, Persaud TVN, Torchia MG. *The Developing Human: Clinically Oriented Embryology*. 10th ed. Saunders; 2016.
3. Netter F. *Atlas of Human Anatomy*. 6th ed. Saunders; 2014.
4. Dutra EH, Caria PHF, Rafferty KL, Herring SW. The buccinator during mastication: a functional and anatomical evaluation in minipigs. *Arch Oral Biol*. 2010;55(9):627–638.
5. Matsuo K, Palmer JB. Anatomy and physiology of feeding and swallowing – normal and abnormal. *Phys Med Rehabil Clin N Am*. 2008;19(4):691–707.
6. Fehrenbach MJ, Herring SW. *Illustrated Anatomy of the Head and Neck*. Saunders; 2011.
7. Hiatt JL, Gartner LP. *Textbook of Head and Neck Anatomy*. 4th ed. LWW; 2009.
8. Gay T, Rendell JK, Spiro J. Oral and laryngeal muscle coordination during swallowing. *Laryngoscope*. 1994;104(3 Pt 1):341–349.
9. Steele CM, Lieshout PV. Tongue movements during water swallowing in healthy young and older adults. *J Speech Lang Hear Res*. 2009;52(5):1255–1267.
10. Logemann JA. *Evaluation and Treatment of Swallowing Disorders*. 2nd ed. Austin, Texas: Pro Ed; 1998.
11. Palmer JB, Rudin NJ, Lara G, Crompton AW. Coordination of mastication and swallowing. *Dysphagia*. 1992;7(4):187–200.
12. Hiiemae KM, Palmer JB. Food transport and bolus formation during complete feeding sequences on foods of different initial consistency. *Dysphagia*. 1999;14(1):31–42.
13. Buettner A, Beer A, Hannig C, Settles M. Observation of the swallowing process by application of videofluoroscopy and real-time magnetic resonance imaging-consequences for retronasal aroma stimulation. *Chem Senses*. 2001;26(9):1211–1219.
14. Logemann JA, Rademaker AW, Pauloski BR, Ohmae Y, Kahrilas PJ. Normal swallowing physiology as viewed by videofluoroscopy and videoendoscopy. *Folia Phoniatr Logop*. 1998;50(6):311–319.
15. Jones B. *Normal and Abnormal Swallowing: Imaging in Diagnosis and Therapy*. 2nd ed. Springer Verlag; 2003.
16. Cook IJ, Dodds WJ, Dantas RO, et al. Timing of videofluoroscopic, manometric events, and bolus transit during the oral and pharyngeal phases of swallowing. *Dysphagia*. 1989;4(1):8–15.
17. Dodds WJ, Stewart ET, Logemann JA. Physiology and radiology of the normal oral and pharyngeal phases of swallowing. *AJR Am J Roentgenol*. 1990;154(5):953–963.
18. Matsuo K, Hiiemae KM. Cyclic motion of the soft palate in feeding. *J Dent Res*. 2005;84(1):39–42.
19. Nobrega AC, Rodrigues B, Melo A. Silent aspiration in Parkinson's disease patients with diurnal sialorrhea. *Clin Neurol Neurosurg*. 2008;110(2):117–119.
20. Lakraj AA, Moghimi N, Jabbari B. Sialorrhea: anatomy, pathophysiology and treatment with emphasis on the role of botulinum toxins. *Toxins*. 2013;5(5):1010–1031.

CHAPTER 3

Oropharynx

TRAVIS L. SHIBA, MD • DINESH K. CHHETRI, MD

INTRODUCTION

The oropharynx serves both the respiratory and digestive systems. The oropharynx is the critical region that joins the oral cavity and nasopharynx with the larynx and hypopharynx. The complexity of the swallowing process involves over 30 muscles, multiple motor and sensory nerves, and coordination by the brainstem, and cortex and subcortical structures. Much of this complexity is found within the oropharynx, where the primarily voluntary meet the largely reflexive portions of the swallowing mechanism. We will describe the embryology and anatomy of the oropharynx, followed by the physiology of the oropharyngeal swallow.

EMBRYOLOGY AND DEVELOPMENT

The head and neck structures develop primarily from the pharyngeal (branchial) arches, which are derived from neural crest cells and first appear in the developing embryo at 3–4 weeks of gestation. These transverse swellings of mesenchyme are labeled arches 1, 2, 3, 4, and 6 in mammals (arch 5 does not develop). The embryologic origin of the oropharynx includes components from several *branchial arches*, as well as *occipital somites*. The lateral aspect of the arches forms the lateral portions of the pharynx, while the ventral-medial aspect and the *occipital somites* form the basis for early tongue development.

The branchial arches develop around the fourth to fifth weeks of gestation and begin to differentiate. Each branchial arch comprises a mesenchymal core covered by a surface ectoderm on the outside and foregut-derived endoderm on the inside lumen. The arches have an arterial component and an associated cranial nerve (or branch) and give rise to the associated musculature and skeletal components that are served by that nerve and artery.[1–3] The arches create a series of ectodermal clefts and endodermal pouches. In fish, these arches lead to the formation of gills, from which the term "branchial" is derived, but no true gills are ever formed in mammals as the pouches and clefts do not connect.[2]

The oropharynx is derived from contributions of multiple pharyngeal arches. From the first arch, the muscles of mastication supplied by the mandibular branch of the trigeminal nerve (CN V3) are the *mylohyoid* muscle and the *tensor veli palatini*. From the second arch, the following skeletal structures are derived: the stylohyoid ligament, styloid process, and upper body and lesser horns of the hyoid. The facial nerve (CN VII) is associated with the second arch, and the muscles innervated by the facial nerve and relevant to the oropharyngeal swallow are the *stylohyoid* and *posterior belly of the digastric*. Arches 3, 4, and 6 are particularly important in the development of the oropharynx. Skeletal contributions from arch 3 include the greater horn and inferior part of the hyoid, while the associated glossopharyngeal nerve (CN IX) innervates the *stylopharyngeus* muscle. The fourth arch carries the superior laryngeal nerve from the vagus nerve (CN X), and the *palatoglossus, pharyngeal constrictors*, and *levator veli palatini* muscles are derived from the fourth arch. The sixth arch carries the recurrent laryngeal nerve (from CN X) and is also the origin of the *intrinsic laryngeal muscles*.[1–4]

Pharyngeal pouches develop on the endodermal side (inside of the lumen) between the pharyngeal arches. The first pharyngeal pouch forms the eustachian tube and is an attachment point for the tensor veli palatini muscle. The second pharyngeal pouch forms the tonsillar fossa. The endodermal lining forms buds and proliferates, mixing with the mesenchymal cells of the second arch and eventually forming the *palatine tonsils*. These structures will later be infiltrated by the cells of the lymphatic system to form the mature tonsils, which will expand in childhood, then regress with age.[2,3]

Tongue Development

Development of the tongue is complex in that the sensory innervation and connective tissue are derived from the branchial arches, while the skeletal muscle supplied by the hypoglossal nerve is derived from the *occipital somites*. Skeletal muscle throughout the human body is derived from the *paraxial mesoderm* that develops between the ectoderm and endoderm layers. From the occiput to the sacrum, the paraxial mesoderm forms distinct somites which develop into the skeletal muscle of the body. In the head and neck region, there are four occipital somites that form the tongue musculature. The occipital somites develop into two parts, a small dorsal *epimere* and a large ventral *hypomere* by around the fifth embryonic week. The hypomeres migrate to the developing floor of the oral cavity and form the tongue muscles except for the palatoglossus muscle, which is supplied by the vagus nerve via the *pharyngeal plexus*. The cervical hypomeres eventually become the prevertebral, scalene, geniohyoid, and infrahyoid *strap muscles*.

Three swellings from the first branchial arch fuse to become the oral tongue connective tissue and vasculature. Two lateral swellings (lingual) and one ventromedial swelling (tuberculum impar) form in the floor of the primordial pharynx around the fourth week. These swellings form the basis for development of the anterior two-thirds of the tongue (oral tongue). A v-shaped *sulcus terminalis* forms between the anterior two-thirds and posterior one-third of the tongue (base of the tongue). This is the line between the first and second arch derivatives), and at its center point is the *foramen cecum*. The foramen cecum is the site of origin of the thyroid gland and persistence of the thyroglossal duct or tract may lead to a *thyroglossal duct cyst*. Additional ventromedial swellings arise caudal to the foramen cecum and give rise to the base of the tongue mucosa, taste organs, and connective tissues. These include the copula from arch 2 and the hypobranchial eminence from arches 2 and 4. Some authors describe the copula and the hypobranchial eminence as synonymous, as the hypobranchial eminence likely overgrows the copula, and the second arch ultimately only supplies the taste buds of the oral tongue through the chorda tympani nerve. The ventromedial swellings eventually become the connective tissue and vasculature of the oropharyngeal tongue, or the base of the tongue. A ventromedial swelling (epiglottal swelling) from the fourth arch eventually forms the *epiglottis*.

While one would expect that the sensory nerve to the base of the tongue should be a combination of CN VII (second arch) and CN IX (third arch), in fact the glossopharyngeal (CN IX) and superior laryngeal nerves (CN X) provide the sensation, suggesting that the third and fourth arch (hypobranchial eminence) assumes the sensory development of the base of the tongue from the initial second branchial pouch swelling (copula). The second arch–derived CN VII only supplies the taste

buds to the oral tongue via the chorda tympani. Also interesting is the fact that the sulcus terminalis is supplied by the glossopharyngeal nerve, despite being part of the oral tongue. It is hypothesized that the posterior tongue is pulled slightly anteriorly with development.

The posterior border of the tongue base, at the *vallecula*, represents a junction of the hypobranchial eminence from the third and fourth arches and the epiglottal swelling from the fourth arch, and is innervated by sensory branches of the vagus nerve via the superior laryngeal nerve.[2-4] Taste to the tongue base is provided by the glossopharyngeal nerve with some overlap provided by the vagus nerve.[5] Taste buds develop on the dorsal tongue, palate, palatoglossal arches, and posterior oropharynx around weeks 8–11 and are supplied by the gustatory nerve cells effectively by week 26.

Palate Development

The first pharyngeal arch–derived maxillary prominences fuse to form the intermaxillary segment which gives rise to the following oral cavity structures: philtrum of the lip, the maxilla and incisors, and the primary palate. Behind the primary palate, additional outgrowths, the palatal shelves, form from the maxillary prominences. These appear around the sixth week and fuse at the midline palatine raphe around the eighth week. The secondary palate fuses with the primary palate and the descending nasal septum. Failure to fuse properly, leads to a variety of *cleft palate and uvula* combinations. Bone develops in the primary palate and anterior portion of the secondary palate, but not in the posterior aspect of the secondary palate. This line of ossification separates the hard and soft palates. Of the muscles associated with the palate, the Tensor veli palatini muscle is derived from the first arch, while the levator veli palatini, palatoglossus, palatopharyngeus, and musculus uvulae are derived from the fourth arch. As the secondary palate extends posteriorly, these muscles take their neonatal position.[2-4]

Postnatal Development

As the newborn ages, the oropharynx continues to enlarge, and the epiglottis and laryngeal complex descend. Around 6 months, the previous nasal obligate breathing infant thus develops the ability to improve transoral airflow and speech production, but at the cost of swallowed substances passing over the airway and thus exposure to the risk of aspiration. Interestingly, most mammals have a high larynx, whereby the epiglottis overlaps or apposes to the soft palate. This allows for separation of deglutitive and respiratory pathways, but significantly limits the supraglottic larynx and oropharynx resonators' ability to create different sounds required for speech.[1,4,6,7]

ANATOMY

The oropharynx starts where the oral cavity ends at the junction of the hard and soft palate superiorly and the circumvallate papillae inferiorly. It is composed of the *soft palate, tonsillar fossa, base of the tongue, posterior pharyngeal wall*, and the *lateral pharyngeal wall*. The *lingual tonsils* and *palatine tonsils* are present in the oropharynx, while the adenoid pad is primarily confined to the naso-pharynx. The oropharynx ends anteroinferiorly at the larynx where the base of the tongue meets the epiglottis and forms the vallecula, and posteroinferiorly at the level of the hyoid bone and pharyngoepiglottic folds. The pharynx below the oropharynx is labeled the hypo-pharynx, or laryngopharynx, and is composed posteri-orly of the inferior constrictor and anteriorly of the laryngeal cartilages. All muscles of deglutition in the oropharynx are striated. In the resting position of the adult, the oropharynx typically spans the level of cer-vical vertebrae 1−3. The lymphatic drainage is to cervi-cal node levels 2 through 4.[8−10]

Soft Palate

The muscles of the soft palate include the *paired tensor veli palatini* and *levator veli palatini*, and the *musculus uvu-lae*. The muscle attachments of the soft palate include the *palatoglossus* and *palatopharyngeus*. All of these mus-cles are innervated by the pharyngeal plexus and CN X, except the tensor veli palatini which is innervated by CN V3. The tensor veli palatini tenses the soft palate and opens the eustachian tube; the levator veli palatine elevates the soft palate; the musculus uvulae elevates and retracts the uvula; the palatoglossus brings the base of the tongue and soft palate together; and the pal-atopharyngeus shortens the pharynx.

Sensation is supplied by the branches of the maxil-lary division of the fifth cranial nerve (CN V2). The blood supply is from the branches of the external ca-rotid including the facial artery, ascending pharyngeal artery, and maxillary artery and is drained by the pharyngeal venous plexus.[3,8,9,11]

The mucosa is a nonkeratinized stratified squamous epithelium with a dense collection of elastic tissues and interspersed minor salivary gland tissue. The nasal mu-cosa of the soft palate anteriorly consists of pseudostra-tified ciliated columnar epithelium and posteriorly of stratified squamous epithelium.[12]

Tongue

The muscles of the tongue are typically divided into intrinsic and extrinsic. The *intrinsic muscles* are all supplied by the hypoglossal nerve. They have no attachments to skeletal structures, mostly consist of the dorsal tongue, and control the *shape* of the tongue. These include the transverse, superior longitudinal, inferior longitudinal, and vertical muscles. The *extrinsic muscles* are attached to bony structures and move the tongue as a whole and control its *position*. These include the palatoglossus, styloglossus, hyoglossus, and the genioglossus.

The *intrinsic muscles* of the tongue are layered. Start-ing from the overlying mucosa and proceeding deep, the first muscle encountered is the superior longitudi-nal. This is followed by the interwoven transverse and vertical muscle fibers, then the inferior longitudinal muscle. Laterally, the inferior longitudinal muscle inter-faces with the largest muscle of the tongue: the fan shaped genioglossus.

The *genioglossus* is a fan-shaped muscle that origi-nates at the anterior midline of the inner cortex of the mandible and forms the bulk of the tongue. It inserts posterior-inferiorly to the anterosuperior surface of the hyoid bone and superiorly to the ventral surface of the intrinsic tongue muscles to intermix with the transverse and vertical fibers. The left and right genio-glossus are separated by a connective tissue septum. The genioglossus can protrude the tongue, lower the tongue and make the dorsum concave, and can move the tongue laterally with unilateral action. The *hyoglossus* muscle runs lateral to the genioglossus, arising from the greater cornu and anterior body of the hyoid bone and inserting in the lateral tongue between the styloglossus and palatoglossus laterally, and the inferior longitudi-nal muscle medially. It depresses and retracts the tongue. The styloglossus and palatoglossus are superior to the genioglossus at the dorsolateral aspect of the tongue. The *styloglossus* originates at the styloid process and blends into the fibers of the inferior longitudinal tongue muscles and the hyoglossus, and elevates and re-tracts the tongue posteriorly and superiorly. The genio-glossus, hyoglossus, and styloglossus are all innervated by the hypoglossal nerve (CN XII). The *palatoglossus* originates on the inferior surface of the palatine aponeurosis and inserts on the posterolateral tongue to the dorsal tongue and fibers of the transverse muscle. The palatoglossus is innervated by the vagus nerve (CN X) via the pharyngeal plexus and helps to appose the tongue and soft palate. Beneath the genioglossus are the *geniohyoid* and then the *mylohyoid* muscles which connect the anterior mandible to the hyoid bone and form the floor of the mouth.

Blood supply to the tongue is primarily via the lingual artery, a branch of the external carotid artery, but there are also contributions from other external carotid artery branches: the facial and ascending pharyngeal arteries. Venous drainage is from the lingual vein and facial vein which then drain into the internal jugular vein. Taste and sensation are provided primarily by the glossopharyngeal nerve (CN IX) with some contribution from the superior laryngeal nerve; the latter is more prominent toward the epiglottis. The mucosa consists of keratinized stratified squamous epithelium with intermixed papilla to house the taste buds. The base of the tongue also has a variable amount of tonsillar tissue that changes with age, becoming more active than the palatine tonsils or adenoids by the fourth and fifth decades.[3,8–11,13,14]

Palatine Tonsils and Tonsillar Fossa

The palatine tonsils, in addition to the adenoids and lingual tonsils, are classified as mucosa-associated lymphoid tissue. They are housed in the tonsillar fossa, bordered by the palatoglossus anteriorly, palatopharyngeus posteriorly, superior constrictor laterally, and the base of the tongue inferiorly. The fossa and tonsil are lined by nonkeratinizing stratified squamous epithelium that on the tonsillar surface forms multiple crypts. A connective tissue "capsule," consisting of loose areolar tissue, separates the tonsil from the pharyngobasilar fascia and the superior constrictor muscle. Nerves and vessels pass through the fascia. The palatine tonsils are supplied by branches of the external carotid artery: the inferior tonsillar artery via the facial artery, the superior tonsillar artery via the greater palatine branch of the maxillary artery, the posterior tonsillar artery from the ascending pharyngeal arteries and the facial artery, and the anterior tonsillar artery from the dorsal lingual artery. The venous drainage is via the peritonsillar plexus, which drain to the pharyngeal plexus or facial vein and into the internal jugular vein. Sensation is provided via the tonsillar branches of the glossopharyngeal nerve and the lesser palatine branch of the maxillary division of the trigeminal nerve. Some taste is provided by the tonsillar pillars and that is supplied by the glossopharyngeal nerve.[3,8–11,13]

Pharyngeal Wall

The muscles of the pharynx are arranged with the longitudinal muscles on the interior and the circumferential muscles on the exterior, which is the opposite of most of the gastrointestinal tract. *The superior, middle, and inferior constrictor* muscles make up the outer circumferential layer and constrict the pharynx during swallowing. The superior constrictor is overlapped by the middle constrictor, and the middle constrictor is overlapped by the inferior constrictor analogous to a trio of stacked cups. The longitudinal muscles are the *stylopharyngeus*, *salpingopharyngeus*, and *palatopharyngeus* muscles, and they elevate and shorten the pharynx during swallowing. The stylopharyngeus is innervated by the glossopharyngeal nerve and enters the pharynx between the superior and middle constrictors and inserts just anterior to the palatopharyngeus. The salpingopharyngeus blends with the palatopharyngeus and is innervated by the vagus nerve via the pharyngeal plexus.

At the posterior midline, a fibrous pharyngeal raphe marks a longitudinal attachment point for the pharyngeal constrictors. From the pharyngeal raphe, the superior constrictor attaches to the medial plate of the pterygoid, the pterygomandibular raphe, and the mandible. The middle constrictor attaches to the hyoid bone and stylohyoid ligament. The transition of the oropharynx to the hypopharynx occurs here. The inferior constrictor attaches to the laryngeal cartilages. The suprahyoid muscles stylohyoid (innervated by CN VII), digastric (CN V and CN VII), geniohyoid (CN XII), and mylohyoid (CN V) move the hyoid and thus also affect the shape of the pharynx.

The mucosa of the pharynx is a nonkeratinized stratified squamous epithelium. Sensation and taste in the pharyngeal walls is provided by CN IX and CN X via the pharyngeal plexus. This plexus lies on the posterior surface of the middle constrictor. The blood supply is from the pharyngeal plexus which is primarily from the ascending pharyngeal artery (a branch of the external carotid artery) and also from the tonsillar branch of the facial artery. As the oropharynx becomes the hypopharynx, the inferior thyroid artery, from the thyrocervical trunk of the subclavian artery, increasingly contributes to the pharyngeal plexus in addition to the ascending pharyngeal artery.[4,8–11,13,15,16]

PHYSIOLOGY AND FUNCTION IN SWALLOW

The oropharynx plays a central and critical role in deglutition. It is at this stage that food has to pass safely from the oral cavity into the esophagus without falling into the endolarynx or trachea. The complex interplay between the oral cavity, nasopharynx, oropharynx, hypopharynx, larynx, and esophagus in normal swallowing involves multiple cranial and peripheral nerves, over 30 paired muscles (Table 3.1), and the coordination of the brainstem where sensory and motor information are networked.[11,17]

Various models exist to describe swallowing mechanics. Breaking the components of swallow into

TABLE 3.1
Innervation of Muscles and Their Function in the Oropharyngeal Swallow Phase

Muscle Group	Muscle (s)	Innervation	Function(s) in Swallowing
Tongue	Intrinsic muscles	Hypoglossal nerve (XII)	Alter tongue shape
	Genioglossus		Protrude/depress tongue; move tongue laterally with unilateral action
	Hyoglossus		Depress/retract the base of the tongue
	Styloglossus		Elevate tongue posteriorly; form a trough for bolus to pass
Palate	Tensor veli palatini	Mandibular branch (V3)	Tense soft palate
	Levator veli palatini	Vagus nerve (X) via pharyngeal plexus	Elevate soft palate; seal nasopharynx from oropharynx
	Palatopharyngeus		Depress soft palate/elevate pharynx
	Palatoglossus		Depress soft palate/elevate posterior tongue/appose soft palate and tongue
	Musculus uvulae		Elevate/retract uvula
Pharynx	Superior constrictor	Vagus nerve (X) via pharyngeal plexus	Constrict and narrow pharynx
	Middle constrictor		Constrict and narrow pharynx
	Salpingopharyngeus		Elevate and shorten pharynx
	Palatopharyngeus		Depress soft palate/elevate and shorten pharynx
	Stylopharyngeus	Glossopharyngeal (IX)	Elevate and shorten pharynx
Hyoid	Stylohyoid	Facial nerve (VII)	Elevate hyoid
	Digastric	Mandibular branch (V3)/facial nerve (VII)	Elevate hyoid
	Mylohyoid	Mandibular branch (V3)	Elevate hyoid
	Geniohyoid	Hypoglossal nerve (XII)/C1–C2	Pull hyoid anteriorly to mandible
	Omohyoid	Ansa cervicalis (C1–C3)	Depress and retract hyoid
	Sternohyoid		Depress hyoid
	Sternothyroid		Depress hyoid
	Thyrohyoid	C1 via hypoglossal nerve (XII)	Depress hyoid

subsegments based on anatomic location is the most common. However, it can be helpful to take into account the functional intent of swallowing. In this chapter, we will discuss two models: the four-stage model, that describes swallowing a liquid bolus, and the process model, that describes nonliquid boluses. Nonliquid boluses require more processing and space, thus limiting the value of pure anatomic descriptors.

The four-stage model has the following phases: oral preparatory, oral propulsive, pharyngeal, and esophageal. The first two phases are primarily under voluntary control, while the last two phases are primarily reflexive-like swallow events. In the oral preparatory phase of a liquid bolus swallow, the palate and tongue form a seal preventing the liquid bolus from entering the oropharynx. Next, in the oral propulsive stage, the tongue tip elevates, while the posterior tongue descends. The liquid bolus is moved from anterior to posterior as the tongue increases its contact with the palate and passes the bolus into the pharynx to start the pharyngeal stage.[15,18] Hyoglossal contraction depresses the central tongue, to allow easier passage into the oropharynx. Contraction of the suprahyoid muscles helps to keep the tongue and larynx stabilized.[11,19,20] Once the oropharyngeal and esophageal phases of swallow are initiated, there are not significant differences between how liquid and nonliquid boluses are handled.

With solid foods, the oral preparatory stage is not marked by sealing of the oral cavity by the tongue and soft palate. Instead the palate, tongue, mandible, and hyoid move cyclically. This allows food to accumulate in the oropharynx for a period of time before the pharyngeal phase is initiated.[15,18,19,21] In the process model, stage 1 describes transporting the food to the molar and premolars, lateral to the tongue. This is followed by food processing in which large food particles are reduced in size and mixed with saliva until the bolus is of the proper consistency. Then stage 2 transport describes movement of the bolus posteriorly into the oropharynx, similar to the oral propulsive stage described earlier.[15,18,19,21]

Food consistency, taste, size, and individual patient factors will alter the timing of the pharyngeal phase trigger after the oral transport stage. Classically, the pharyngeal phase is considered to be initiated by bolus contact at the anterior tonsillar pillars. The pharyngeal phase occurs quickly, typically in less than a second in normal adults. The common conduit shared by the airway and the digestive tract in the oropharynx makes accurate coordination of the pharyngeal phase (with laryngeal seal) essential for airway protection and the prevention of aspiration.[11,17,19,22] As the bolus is passed from the posterior oral cavity to the anterior

oropharynx, the soft palate elevates and seals the nasopharynx to prevent nasal regurgitation. The levator veli palatini and musculus uvulae muscles contract to elevate the palate. The levator veli palatini also will help to open the eustachian tube. The superior constrictor and part of the palatopharyngeus constrict and form a posterior pharyngeal bulge known as *Passavant's ridge*. This helps the elevated soft palate contact the posterior pharyngeal wall and seal off the nasopharynx to prevent regurgitation of food bolus into the nasopharynx.[1,3,15] The pharyngeal constrictor muscles squeeze from superior to inferior, as the base of the tongue retracts. The pharynx shortens as the hyolaryngeal complex elevates and moves anteriorly. This hyolaryngeal movement is controlled by the suprahyoid and infrahyoid muscles, while the pharyngeal shortening is accomplished with contraction of the palatopharyngeus, stylopharyngeus, and salpingopharyngeus muscles. In addition to elevating the pharynx, the stylopharyngeus widens the pharynx.[1,11,15,18,20,23]

The tongue base pushes posteriorly via contraction of the styloglossus and hyoglossus muscles.[23] This, combined with coordinated pharyngeal contraction from superiorly to inferiorly pushes the tail of the bolus through at a speed of about 10–25 cm/s and a pressure of about 20 mmHg.[11,24] Simultaneously, the epiglottis first retroflexes to horizontal at the epiglottis/thyroid cartilage junction. Then, as the bolus passes, the upper one-third of the epiglottis further retroflexes below horizontal. Finally, the epiglottis returns to its semivertical position as the hyolaryngeal complex descends and the pharynx relaxes after the bolus has passed though the upper esophageal sphincter (UES).[1,25]

During the oropharyngeal phase of the swallow, the airway is anatomically blocked at the nasopharynx (palate) and the larynx (glottis, supraglottis, epiglottis) and respiration is suppressed in the brainstem.[15,26] This pause typically lasts from 0.5 to 1.5 s, and respiration resumes with expiration first.[27] In states of hypoventilation, this suppression can be overridden or result in a delay of the swallow initiation.[16,28,29] Further airway protection mechanisms such as glottal closure and supraglottic squeeze will be discussed in other chapters. In the last stage of the pharyngeal swallow, the UES opens to allow food to pass into the esophagus and initiates the esophageal phase of swallowing. The inferior constrictor, cricopharyngeus, and upper esophageal muscles comprise the UES (see Chapter 5). Importantly, failure to open the UES due to insufficient relaxation, fibrosis, insufficient hyolaryngeal elevation to pull the UES open, or insufficient bolus pressure can all lead to UES dysfunction and residue in the hypopharynx and oropharynx. The residue then poses a risk for penetration and aspiration.[1,15,20]

Neurologic Control of Oropharyngeal Swallow

The cortex and subcortical structures involved in sensation and voluntary behaviors, such as chewing and bolus control, are more active in the oral preparatory and oral transit stages. They are also important for *pharyngeal swallow inhibition* so as to prevent premature swallows. The cortex and subcortical structures tend to be bilaterally involved and asymmetric, but without relation to the handedness of the patient. The medulla is more active in the pharyngeal and esophageal phases of swallow, where a central *swallowing pattern generator* consisting of sensory neurons, motor neurons, and interneurons coordinates this complex activity. The interaction of motor nuclei for C1, C3, and cranial nerves 5, 7, 9, 10, and 12, as well as afferent sensory input from cranial nerves 5, 7, 9, 10 constitute the swallowing central pattern generator. This is closely associated with respiratory drive centers as well. Input from the higher cortical centers helps to modulate the pattern.[11,16,30]

Variability in Swallow Initiation

The initiation of the pharyngeal swallow is more variable in both timing and initiating factors than previously believed. Direct stimulation of the solitary tract nucleus can stimulate a swallow, as can stimulation of the superior laryngeal nerve. Thus contact of the bolus within the sensory distribution of the superior laryngeal nerve corresponds to the initiation of the pharyngeal swallow via stimulation of the swallow pattern generator.[11,16,30,31] Thus, classically the swallow was thought to be elicited very shortly after the bolus reached the pharynx. On modified barium swallow study, this occurs when the head of the bolus crosses the shadow of the angle of the mandible at the pharyngeal surface of the tongue. Delayed initiation of swallow was noted if more than 1 second passed after the entry of the bolus into the pharynx. We now know that the complex input of sensory stimuli and cortical input significantly alter when the pharyngeal swallow is initiated. Normal healthy volunteers can demonstrate a "delayed initiation" of swallow with a bolus of liquids or solids entering the oropharynx, or even into the hypopharynx, before a swallow is initiated. This swallow initiation starting greater than one second after entry of bolus into the pharynx tends to become more prevalent in the elderly population. Pharyngeal swallow times were studied by Kendall et al. in healthy volunteers. Swallowing was broken down into discrete gestures

starting with soft palate elevation and ending with the return of the epiglottis to its native position. They also examined timing of the pharyngeal transit time (bolus passing into the oropharynx until it entered the hypopharynx and the upper esophagus) and hyolaryngeal elevation. They reported that about 1 in 5 healthy young volunteers had the bolus enter the vallecula before the arytenoid would elevate. They found the entire swallow from soft palate elevation to epiglottis return to take between 0.75 and 1.25 s. The oropharyngeal swallow from oropharynx to hypopharynx took on average about 0.25 s, while the pharyngeal phase (oropharynx to maximal UES opening) took between 0.3 and 0.75 s. They found variability in the sequences of events including when the arytenoids and hyoid would elevate relative to the bolus location. Interestingly, they found less variability with larger bolus volumes, which they hypothesized is related to the shorter transit time and thus less time for the creation of variability via volitional behavioral on lay.[32] Another study measured healthy oropharyngeal clearance (from bolus at the tonsillar fauces to UES opening), a mean of 0.5 s with a standard deviation of 0.27 ms.[33] There was also variability in swallow initiation from one swallow to the next within individuals, or with bolus characteristics. Our understanding of oropharyngeal is thus incomplete.[11,15,22,34,35]

Pharyngeal Manometry

One of the major challenges in dysphagia evaluation and management is objective measurement of pharyngeal strength. The measurement of pressures in the oropharynx is challenging due to its complex three-dimensional anatomy. Developments in high resolution manometry (HRM), including three-dimensional HRM for the pharynx, may be an important complement to video fluoroscopic and functional endoscopic evaluation of swallowing.[36,37] Studies continue to provide more information but current data on 10-mL liquid boluses suggests that most of the force on a bolus in the oropharynx is posteriorly generated, emphasizing the importance of the pharyngeal constrictor muscles in oropharyngeal swallow. The lateral pressure generation is measured as about half to one-third of the posterior pressure, likely because the rigid support of the spine and also the muscle mass of the posterior wall is lacking laterally. Even the anterior pressures coming from the base of the tongue were less than the posterior wall, though it was unclear if there is a small artifactual component to the force distribution as the tongue retracts. Certainly the base of the tongue is essential to producing an effective oropharyngeal swallow, but we still need to further understand the relative roles of pharyngeal pressure distribution during deglutition to guide therapy.[37]

SUMMARY

The oropharynx is a common conduit shared by the respiratory and digestive tracts. Precision in coordination and sensation while swallowing is critical to avoid the major consequences of aspiration into the lungs. The embryologic origins of the oropharynx help to explain the complex motor and sensory innervation; while the complex anatomy and physiology provide a background upon which we can understand normal and abnormal swallow conditions. More information is needed to fully understand the neural inputs involved in the transition from the voluntary oral propulsive stage to the reflexive pharyngeal phase of swallow. The precise functions and coordination of sensory output and motor input need continued study. High-resolution three-dimensional manometry and advanced neurologic imaging hold promise for future developments in understanding of oropharyngeal swallowing physiology.

REFERENCES

1. Leder SB, Neubauer PD. *The Yale Pharyngeal Residue Severity Rating Scale*. Cham: Springer International Publishing; 2016. https://doi.org/10.1007/978-3-319-29899-3.
2. Sadler TW. *Langman's Medical Embryology*. 10th ed. Philadelphia: Lippincott Williams & Wilkins; 2006.
3. Moore KL, Persaud TVN. *The Developing Human: Clinically Oriented Embryology*. 7th ed. Saunders; 2003.
4. German RZ, Palmer JB. *Anatomy and Development of Oral Cavity and Pharynx*. GI Motility Online. Nature Publishing Group; May 16, 2006. https://doi.org/10.1038/gimo5.
5. Purves Dale, Augustine GJ, Fitzpatrick D, et al. *The Organization of the Taste System*. Sinauer Associates; 2001. https://www.ncbi.nlm.nih.gov/books/NBK11018/.
6. Laitman JT, Reidenberg JS. The evolution and development of human swallowing: the most important function we least appreciate. *Otolaryngol Clin N Am*. 2013;46(6):923−935. https://doi.org/10.1016/j.otc.2013.09.005. Elsevier Inc.
7. Lieberman P, Laitman JT, Reidenberg JS, et al. The anatomy, physiology, acoustics and perception of speech: essential elements in analysis of the evolution of human speech. *J Hum Evol*. 1992;23:447−467.
8. Gray H. *Anatomy of the Human Body*. Bartleby.Com, May 2000; 1918. www.bartleby.com/107/.
9. Netter FH. Atlas of human anatomy, professional edition. *Netter Basic Sci*. 2011, 5th Edition. Section 1 Pages 1-148.
10. Moore KL, Dalley II AF, Agur AMR, D'Antoni AV. Clinically oriented anatomy, 7th ed. *Clin Anat*. 2014;27. https://doi.org/10.1002/ca.22316.
11. Shaw SM, Martino R. The normal swallow: muscular and neurophysiological control. *Otolaryngol Clin N Am*. 2013; 46. https://doi.org/10.1016/j.otc.2013.09.006.
12. Kuehn DP, Kahane JC. Histologic study of the normal human adult soft palate. *Cleft Palate Craniofac J*. 1990. https://doi.org/10.1597/1545-1569.
13. Brennan PA, Mahadevan V, Evans BT. *Clinical Head and Neck Anatomy for Surgeons*. CRC Press; 2015.
14. Kamata T. Histological study of human lingual tonsil, especially changes with aging. *J Otolaryngol Jpn*. 1992; 95(6):825−843. http://www.ncbi.nlm.nih.gov/pubmed/1634989.
15. Matsuo K, Palmer JB. Anatomy and physiology of feeding and swallowing-normal and abnormal. *Phys Med Rehabil Clin N Am*. 2009;19(4):691−707. https://doi.org/10.1016/j.pmr.2008.06.001.Anatomy.
16. Sasegbon A, Hamdy S. The anatomy and physiology of normal and abnormal swallowing in oropharyngeal dysphagia. *Neurogastroenterol Motil*. 2017:e13100. https://doi.org/10.1111/nmo.13100.
17. Dodds WJ, Stewart ET, Logemann JA. Physiology and radiology of the normal oral and pharyngeal phases of swallowing. *Am J Roentgenol*. 1990. https://doi.org/10.2214/ajr.154.5.2108569.
18. Hiiemae KM, Palmer JB. Food transport and bolus formation during complete feeding sequences on foods of different initial consistency. *Dysphagia*. 1999;14(1):31−42. https://doi.org/10.1007/PL00009582.
19. Palmer JB, J Rudin N, Lara G, Crompton AW. Coordination of mastication and swallowing. *Dysphagia*. 1992;7(4):187−200. http://www.ncbi.nlm.nih.gov/pubmed/1308667.
20. Massey BT. *Physiology of Oral Cavity, Pharynx and Upper Esophageal Sphincter*. GI Motility Online. Nature Publishing Group; May 2006. https://doi.org/10.1038/gimo2.
21. Dua KS, Ren J, Bardan E, Xie P, Shaker R. Coordination of deglutitive glottal function and pharyngeal bolus transit during normal eating. *Gastroenterology*. 1997;112(1):73−83. http://www.ncbi.nlm.nih.gov/pubmed/8978345.
22. Martin-Harris B, Brodsky MB, Michel Y, Lee FS, Walters B. Delayed initiation of the pharyngeal swallow: normal variability in adult swallows. *J Speech Lang Hear Res*. 2007; 50(3):585. https://doi.org/10.1044/1092-4388(2007/041).
23. McKeown MJ, Torpey DC, Gehm WC. Non-invasive monitoring of functionally distinct muscle activations during swallowing. *Clin Neurophysiol*. 2002;113(3):354−366. https://doi.org/10.1016/S1388-2457(02)00007-X.
24. Dodds WJ, J Hogan W, B Lydon S, T Stewart E, J Stef J, C Arndorfer R. Quantitation of pharyngeal motor function in normal human subjects. *J Appl Physiol*. 1975;39(4):692−696. http://www.ncbi.nlm.nih.gov/entrez/query.fcgi?cmd=Retrieve&db=PubMed&dopt=Citation&list_uids=1194163.
25. Vandaele DJ, Perlman AL, Cassell MD. Intrinsic fibre architecture and attachments of the human epiglottis and their contributions to the mechanism of deglutition. *J Anat*. 1995;186:1−15.

26. Nishino T, Hiraga K. Coordination of swallowing and respiration in unconscious subjects. *J Appl Physiol (Bethesda Md 1985)*. 1991;70(3):988−993. http://www.ncbi.nlm. nih.gov/pubmed/2033013.
27. Klahn MS, Perlman AL. Temporal and durational patterns associating respiration and swallowing. *Dysphagia*. 1999; 14(3):131−138. https://doi.org/10.1007/PL00009594.
28. Kobayashi S, Kubo H, Yanai M. Impairment of swallowing in COPD. *Am J Respir Crit Care Med*. 2009. https://doi.org/ 10.1164/ajrccm.180.5.481.
29. Sumi T. The activity of brain-stem respiratory neurons and spinal respiratory motoneurons during swallowing. *J Neurophysiol*. 1963;26:466−477.
30. Jean A. Brain stem control of swallowing: neuronal network and cellular mechanisms. *Physiol Rev*. 2001; 81(2):929−969. https://doi.org/10.1002/cne.902830207.
31. Miller AJ. Characteristics of the swallowing reflex induced by peripheral nerve and brain stem stimulation. *Exp Neurol*. 1972;34(2):210−222. https://doi.org/10.1016/0014-4886(72)90168-9.
32. Kendall KA. Oropharyngeal swallowing variability. *Laryngoscope*. 2002;112(3):547−551. https://doi.org/ 10.1097/00005537-200203000-00025.
33. Cassiani RA, Santos CM, Parreira LC, Dantas RO. The relationship between the oral and pharyngeal phases of swallowing. *Clinics*. 2011;66(8):1385−1388. https:// doi.org/10.1590/S1807-59322011000800013.
34. Inamoto Y, Saitoh E, Okada S, et al. The effect of bolus viscosity on laryngeal closure in swallowing: kinematic analysis using 320-row area detector CT. *Dysphagia*. 2013;28(1):33−42. https://doi.org/10.1007/s00455-012-9410-4.
35. Robbins J, Hamilton JW, Lof GL, Kempster GB. Oropharyngeal swallowing in normal adults of different ages. *Gastroenterology*. 1992;103(3):823−829. pii:S001650859 2003846.
36. Cock C, Omari T. Diagnosis of swallowing disorders: how we interpret pharyngeal manometry. *Curr Gastroenterol Rep*. 2017;19(3). https://doi.org/10.1007/s11894-017-0552-2.
37. Rosen SP, Jones CA, McCulloch TM. Pharyngeal swallowing pressures in the base-of-tongue and hypopharynx regions identified with three-dimensional manometry. *Laryngoscope*. 2017;127(9):1989−1995. https://doi.org/ 10.1002/lary.26483.

CHAPTER 4

Larynx

AARON J. FEINSTEIN, MD, MHS • KARUNA DEWAN, MD

INTRODUCTION

The larynx is a precisely arranged cartilaginous structure connected by ligaments and muscles and lined by mucous membrane. Situated between the trachea and oropharynx, the larynx has critical roles in respiration, speech, swallowing, and prevention of aspiration. Nine cartilages compose the larynx, including the single epiglottic, thyroid, and cricoid cartilages, and the paired corniculate, cuneiform, and arytenoid cartilages. During deglutition the hyolaryngeal complex moves anteriorly and superiorly, and not only prevents aspiration but also plays the critical role in opening the upper esophageal sphincter.

The most important function of the larynx in deglutition is prevention of aspiration of liquid or food bolus into the airway. Aspiration can lead to pneumonia and death, thus redundancies are built into the laryngeal airway protective mechanisms. Three layers of airway closure work together to occlude the endolarynx during swallowing and prevent aspiration: adduction of the true vocal folds, adduction of the false vocal folds, and purse string closure of the laryngeal aditus with contact of the base of the epiglottis to the arytenoids. The embryology, anatomy, and physiology of the larynx as it relates to deglutition is detailed in this chapter.

EMBRYOLOGY

The larynx begins to develop around the fourth week of gestation.[1,2] The respiratory primordium—predecessor of the larynx, trachea, bronchi, and lungs—arises from the ventromedial diverticulum of the foregut. The respiratory diverticulum develops two lateral furrows that deepen and later unite to create the vertical laryngotracheal tube. Toward the end of the fourth week, the lung bud begins to differentiate inferiorly.

As the embryo reaches the fifth week of gestation, there are three components to the primitive larynx: a single anterior primordium of the epiglottis (likely derived from the hypobranchial eminence from the second and fourth branchial arches), and paired lateral mesenchymal swellings that will become arytenoid cartilages (likely arising from the sixth arch). Continuing to the fifth-to-sixth fetal week, the three laryngeal components migrate toward the base of the tongue. At this time, the laryngeal surface area increases more horizontally than vertically, and thus transitions from a simple vertical tube shape to a complex "T"-shaped aditus. The tracheoesophageal septum becomes more defined. The glottis is completely occluded around week 8 due to epithelial proliferation, and ultimately opens (recanalizes) in the 10th fetal week.[1] Failure of recanalization may result in *congenital laryngeal web*.

The hyolaryngeal complex develops from the second, third, fourth, and sixth pharyngeal arch cartilages. The body of the hyoid bone is derived from the second and third pharyngeal arches; the second arch contributes to the upper portion of the hyoid bone, while the third arch contributes to the lower portion of the hyoid. Aberrations in the developmental process result in specific pathologies, such as hyoid bone variability most often manifested as a lack of symmetry in the greater and lesser horns.[3] Partial ossification of the stylohyoid ligament leads to elongation of the styloid process and *Eagle's syndrome*. When the hyoid is abnormal, the entire stylohyoid chain may be impacted.

The development of the thyroid cartilage is a joint contribution of the fourth and sixth pharyngeal arch cartilages, with the upper part of the thyroid cartilage deriving from the fourth arch, while the lower portion arises from the sixth arch. The cricoid cartilage is defined in the sixth-to-seventh fetal weeks. There are bilateral cartilaginous centers which unite to form the cricoid cartilage, first ventrally around week 6, and later dorsally around week seven. *Laryngeal clefts* develop when the posterior cricoid laminae fail to fuse, and this is accompanied by incomplete development of the tracheoesophageal septum. This developmental failure results in an abnormal communication between the posterior portion of the larynx and the esophagus, a *tracheoesophageal fistula*. Laryngeal clefts and congenital tracheoesophageal fistula are midline developmental abnormalities that cause dysphagia in newborns and infants.

The larynx continues to grow along with the developing embryo. The larynx of a neonate is approximately half the size of the adult larynx.[4] The infant larynx is more cephalad than the adult larynx. At birth, the larynx is located anterior to the first and second cervical vertebrae and the cricoid is anterior to C3. This relationship provides a functional separation between breathing and swallowing so that infants can suck, swallow, and breathe simultaneously without aspiration. By the time a child is 2 years old, the larynx has descended to the level of C3–C4. The infant and pediatric larynx is also more anteriorly positioned than the adult larynx. Therefore, the distances between the tongue, hyoid bone, and epiglottis are shorter than they are in the adult. In the adult, the laryngeal inlet is anterior to the C5–C6 interspace and the cricoid is located anterior to C7. This adult position is achieved by the eighth year. Male and female larynges are approximately the same size until puberty, but then the male larynx enlarges and on average becomes larger than the female larynx after puberty.[1]

ANATOMY
Cartilage and Ligaments

The larynx is composed of nine cartilages: the single epiglottic, thyroid, and cricoid cartilages, and the paired corniculate, cuneiform, and arytenoid cartilages. Among these, the thyroid, cricoid, and arytenoid cartilages each consists of hyaline cartilage. These structures undergo ossification, which typically begins at the age of 20 years, starting with the posterior-inferior margin of the thyroid and cricoid cartilage and progressing anterior-superiorly. The superior margin rarely ossifies. The remaining cartilages—corniculate, cuneiform, and epiglottic—consist of elastic cartilage and only rarely ossify.[1]

The hyolaryngeal complex includes the hyoid bone, the stylohyoid chain, and the thyroid cartilage. The stylohyoid chain consists of the styloid process, projecting down from the inferior surface of the temporal bone at the skull base, the stylohyoid ligament, and the lesser horn of the hyoid bone. The hyoid bone is a singular horseshoe-shaped bone in the anterior midline of the neck, just superior to the thyroid cartilage, with the following anatomic subsites: body, greater horns, and lesser horns. It is suspended from the styloid processes by the stylohyoid ligaments and connected to the thyroid cartilage by the medial and lateral thyrohyoid

ligaments. The hyoid bone aids in tongue movement and swallowing, and it maintains patency of the pharynx. It functions as an anchor for the suprahyoid and infrahyoid strap muscles.

The cricoid cartilage has a signet ring shape with a posterior lamina (signet) and an anterior arch (band). The cricoid is the only complete cartilaginous ring of the airway. The cricothyroid articulation is a small, round depression at the junction of the arch and lamina. These are synovial joints between the cricoid itself and the inferior horn of the thyroid cartilage, and each joint is surrounded and reinforced by fibrous tissue.

The arytenoid cartilages maintain a three-sided pyramidal shape and include an anterior vocal process, a posterolateral muscular process, and a superior apex. The vocal process connects to the vocal ligament, and movement of the vocal process is a key focus of any endoscopic examination. The apex supports the corniculate cartilage, and the overlying aryepiglottic fold. The muscular process serves as the site of insertion for the posterior cricoarytenoid (PCA) and lateral cricoarytenoid (LCA) muscles.

The cricoarytenoid (CA) joints are located posteriorly and laterally on the cricoid lamina, and these small, oval depressions are also synovial joints that interact with the base of the arytenoid cartilages.[1] The CA joints allow rotation, anterior and posterior tilt, and sliding motion of the arytenoids to and from each other. The complex motions arising from the CA joints allow for opening and closing the glottic inlet, as well as altering the tension of the vocal fold to control phonatory parameters.

The epiglottis is a thin cartilaginous structure comprising the most superior aspect of the larynx. It is covered by mucosa and has multiple ligamentous attachments to the laryngopharynx. The inferior tip of the epiglottis, known as the petiole, attaches to the thyroid cartilage's inner surface at the thyroid notch by the thyroepiglottic ligament. More superiorly, the hyoepiglottic ligament attaches the epiglottis to the hyoid bone's posterior surface. The anterior, or lingual, surface of the epiglottis is connected to the base of the tongue by the median and lateral glossoepiglottic folds. The vallecula is the open space between the epiglottis and base of the tongue and is a critical area for inspection during dysphagia evaluations. The *epiglottic tubercle* is the convexity at the lower part of the epiglottis over the upper part of the thyroepiglottic ligament and is the critical region of the epiglottis above the petiole which contacts the arytenoid cartilages during deglutition to prevent laryngeal penetration.

The *quadrangular membrane* extends from the epiglottis to the arytenoid and corniculate cartilages. The quadrangular membrane is covered with mucosa and is more commonly referred to as the aryepiglottic fold. This intrinsic ligament also provides the structure for the false vocal folds. The laryngeal introitus is the entrance to the larynx between the two aryepiglottic folds. Lateral to the quadrangular membrane/aryepiglottic fold is the *pyriform sinus*.

Inferiorly at the level of the vocal fold, the intrinsic ligament of the larynx is the conus elasticus, also known as the cricovocal membrane. This extends bilaterally from the vocal processes of the arytenoid cartilage posteriorly to the inner surface of the thyroid cartilage at the anterior midline, and extends inferiorly as a broad wall to insert on the cricoid cartilage. The thickening of this triangular ligament between the thyroid cartilage and the vocal process of the arytenoid is the *vocal ligament*, which is the main connective tissue support for the multilayered true vocal fold.

Muscles

The extrinsic and intrinsic muscles of the larynx control larynx position and function. The extrinsic muscles include the infrahyoid muscles that depress and the suprahyoid muscles that elevate the hyolaryngeal complex. The four infrahyoid muscles are the sternohyoid, omohyoid, sternothyroid, and thyrohyoid muscles. The four suprahyoid muscles are the mylohyoid, geniohyoid, stylohyoid, and digastric muscles. Action of the extrinsic muscles moves the entire larynx as a unit, and failure of these muscles may result in dysphagia from insufficient hyolaryngeal elevation.

Action of the intrinsic laryngeal muscles (ILMs) control abduction, adduction, and tensing of the vocal fold. The PCA muscles are the sole vocal fold abductors. As the PCA contracts, it moves the muscular process of the arytenoid posteriorly and inferiorly, which rotates the vocal process laterally and superiorly and thus opens the glottis. The LCA muscles have an opposite effect: as the LCA moves the muscular process of the arytenoid anteriorly, the vocal process rotates medially and inferiorly to narrow the glottis. The interarytenoid muscle (IA) connects each arytenoid medial body to the other and assists in adducting the arytenoid cartilages at the posterior commissure. The thyroarytenoid muscle (TA) acts to adduct the vocal folds, in concert with the action of the LCA and IA muscles. The TA has a primary adductor effect on the mid-membranous vocal fold, as compared to the role of the LCA and IA on adducting the posterior cartilaginous region. The cricothyroid muscle (CT) brings the anterior aspect of the cricoid and thyroid cartilages closer together, tilting the arytenoid posteriorly, and thus increasing tension on the vocal folds. The CT also acts synergistically with the PCA muscle to widen the anteroposterior dimension of the glottis during vigorous inspiration.[5]

Three muscles attach to the outer thyroid cartilage at its oblique line: inferior pharyngeal constrictor, sternothyroid, and thyrohyoid. Laryngeal framework or reinnervation surgery may disrupt these muscles or their motor innervation, and surgeons should be aware of the potential effects on swallowing.

Innervation

The ILMs, including the TA, LCA, IA, and PCA, are each innervated by branches of the recurrent laryngeal nerve (RLN). The CT muscle, however, is innervated by the external branch of the superior laryngeal nerve (eSLN). Sensory innervation is also provided by the RLN, in addition to the internal branch of the superior laryngeal nerve (iSLN); the RLN innervates the mucosa of the vocal folds and subglottis, while the iSLN innervates the supraglottic mucosa above the vocal folds. The ILMs each receive ipsilateral innervation; however, the IA muscle, which is a midline structure, does have bilateral innervation.[6]

Sensory nerves have their greatest density within the supraglottic mucosa, and there is a relative paucity of sensory innervation of the true vocal folds.[6] The *laryngeal adductor reflex* (LAR), also known as the glottic closure reflex, is a critical airway protective response, and also activated during swallowing. Touch, chemical, or thermal stimulation of the supraglottis activates the iSLN (afferent limb). The iSLN projects to the ipsilateral nucleus tractus solitarius which then transmits to the nucleus ambiguus. The nucleus ambiguus then activates the vagus and RLN (efferent limb) resulting in vocal fold adduction. Unilateral stimulation is known to result in bilateral response. Disruption can occur at any point on this pathway, including the lack of sensation from iSLN damage, or motor failure from RLN paralysis. The impact of sensory denervation can be profound, with studies in the porcine model demonstrating that unilateral section of the iSLN resulted in a reduction of glottal closing force to only 54% of normal, as compared to RLN section (unilateral paralysis) which resulted in a reduction to 24% of normal.[7]

Vascular Supply

The arterial supply of the larynx is principally from the paired superior and inferior laryngeal arteries. The superior laryngeal artery arises from the superior thyroid artery, itself a branch of the external carotid artery. The superior laryngeal artery passes between the middle and inferior pharyngeal constrictor muscles, and most commonly enters the larynx through the thyrohyoid membrane; however, it may pass through an opening in the thyroid lamina in patients with absent superior cornu and may rarely enter through the cricothyroid ligament.[4] This artery typically gives off a branch to the small cricothyroid artery at the level of the cricothyroid membrane.

The inferior laryngeal artery arises from the inferior thyroid artery, itself a branch of the thyrocervical trunk. This artery travels along the same course as the RLN. The inferior laryngeal artery passes posterior to the cricothyroid joint and passes between the inferior pharyngeal constrictor muscle and cricopharyngeus muscle before entering the larynx. The venous outflow parallels the course of the superior and inferior arterial supply.

Lymphatic

The supraglottic and subglottic larynx frequently have bilateral lymphatic drainage, while the glottis itself has quite minimal lymphatic supply that mainly passes to the subglottic region. The supraglottic larynx drains to the deep cervical nodal chain, while the subglottis drains to the prelaryngeal and pretracheal nodal chain. The posterior and lateral subglottis may also drain to the deep jugular or supraclavicular region.[4]

PHYSIOLOGY AND FUNCTION IN SWALLOWING

The larynx has redundant airway protective mechanisms to prevent foreign materials from entering the airway during the swallow.[8] As the food bolus passes into the oropharynx, the true vocal folds adduct to close the airway.[9] Next, the false vocal folds contract causing the arytenoids to tilt forward to close the supraglottis. The action of the suprahyoid musculature results in hyolaryngeal elevation and the epiglottis retroflexes with the arytenoids touching the epiglottic tubercle at this time for an additional layer of airway protection. In a feline model, it was determined that vocal fold closure was the principal mechanism for airway protection; unilateral vocal fold resection resulted in the most aspiration, followed by transection of the suprahyoid musculature, while epiglottidectomy did not result in aspiration at all.[10]

The laryngeal closure mechanism is felt to be a reflexive action, corresponding to subcortical neural activation.[11] Electromyographic (EMG) studies of swallowing support this theoretical model. In healthy subjects performing a swallow, while undergoing fine-wire EMG measurement, the TA, LCA, and CT muscles were found to activate simultaneously at the initiation of the swallow.[12] The IA muscle was activated after a 20-ms delay. The PCA muscles had no activity during the swallow, and then activated after completion of the swallow.

The third layer of closure—contact of the arytenoids and epiglottic base—is under both neural control and also significantly subject to biomechanical forces without volitional control. Investigation of healthy adult subjects demonstrated that there is predictable variability in the timing of epiglottic movement in relation to the bolus size, with increasing bolus sizes associated with earlier time of closure in relation to laryngeal elevation as well as longer closure time.[13] This closure is related to the anterior tilt of the arytenoids, which is caused by thyroarytenoid and supraglottic muscular contraction. In contrast, the descent of the epiglottis is related to biomechanical forces acting upon the epiglottis, including hyolaryngeal elevation, tongue base retraction, and bolus movement.

During active deglutition, central respiratory neurons are inhibited, respiratory muscle activity ceases, and positive subglottic air pressure develops below the adducted vocal folds.[14] Each deglutitive event involves an apneic period of approximately 0.75 s.[15] The most common respiratory pattern involves expiratory breathing occurring both before and after the apneic period; one study found that respiratory activity prior to the apneic period was expiratory in 93% of trials while that following the apneic period was expiratory in 100%[15]; another found that up to 18%–21% of deglutitive events were preceded by inspiration, while all were followed by expiration.[16] Inspiration after deglutitive apnea is quite rare.[17] Although apnea always occurs before initiation of the swallow, expiration has been found to occur after or even during the pharyngeal phase of swallowing. This suggests a role for expelling any food particles that may have passed into the glottis during the preceding deglutitive event.[17]

As laryngeal closure is critical to prevention of aspiration, laryngeal motor dysfunction can result in dysphagia. For example, the probability of aspiration is greatly increased in the setting of unilateral vocal fold paralysis (UVFP). Aspiration rates in patients with UVFP vary from 35% to 50% of patients depending upon etiology, RLN versus vagal nerve injury, and timing of the evaluation.[18–23] Laryngeal penetration without aspiration can be identified in up to 12% of patients.[24] UVFP is not an uncommon finding in patients referred for dysphagia evaluation in the acute care setting, with one study identifying UVFP in 5.6% of

1452 consecutive patients.[18] Vocal fold closure works in concert with the base of tongue propulsive force, pharyngeal stripping wave, hyolaryngeal elevation, and UES opening to produce an efficient swallow. Aspiration in patients with UVFP results from a malfunction in one or more of these steps, particularly laryngeal incompetence, impaired airway protection, and sensory deficits. Vagal paralysis results in increased pharyngeal dysfunction and increased aspiration, as both motor and sensory function are compromised. A protective cough reflex is the final safeguard against tracheal aspiration, and this can be impaired or absent in the setting of vagal injury. Functional outcomes are better for patients with unilateral RLN paralysis as compared to those with unilateral vagal paralysis. Restoring laryngeal competence is a critical intervention in patients with dysphagia due to UVFP (see Chapter 18).

Sensation of the laryngeal and pharyngeal mucosa also plays a vital role in safe deglutition, and patients with impaired sensation after partial laryngeal surgery develop significant dysphagia. Supraglottic laryngectomy encompasses a variety of techniques wherein structures above the true vocal folds—including the false vocal fold, aryepiglottic folds, epiglottis, and/or hyoid bone—may be resected. Open transcervical surgery entails resection of one or both superior laryngeal nerves with subsequent loss of sensation to the remaining supraglottic structures. This loss of sensation affects the patient's ability to recognize that penetration or aspiration occurs, and also impairs the patient's protective cough reflex. Aspiration following supraglottic laryngectomy may occur in 50%–97% of patients and may occur both during and after the deglutitive event.[25] Endoscopic supraglottic laryngectomy has improved swallowing outcomes compared to open procedures, with nearly normal diet in 60 of 75 patients within 1 month of surgery,[26] and 18 of 18 patients tolerating unrestricted diet within 45 days of transoral robotic surgery.[27] In contrast to supraglottic laryngectomy, swallowing outcomes are much better in patients undergoing vertical partial laryngectomy.[28] These patients generally have both aryepiglottic folds and the epiglottis maintained intact, and sensation is typically preserved. Patients undergoing vertical partial laryngectomy achieved swallowing outcomes including resuming preoperative diet and normal swallow function in 86% of cases, as compared to only 57% of patients undergoing supraglottic laryngectomy.[29] Postpartial laryngectomy patients require specialized swallowing therapy, including techniques such as the supraglottic swallow and chin tuck maneuver. This topic is explored in greater detail in Chapters 21 and 24.

CONCLUSIONS

The larynx is a trifunctional organ, playing a key role in phonation, respiration, and deglutition. Any alteration in the development or structure of the larynx can have significant impact on these important functions. Dysphagia results when structure or function of the larynx is changed such that glottal competence and/or normal sensation is lost. The inability to protect the airway through closure of the glottis and elevation of the hyolaryngeal complex is central to the development of dysphagia. Swallowing therapy and surgical intervention are the two mainstays of treatment and are discussed further in the following chapters.

REFERENCES

1. Janfaza P, Nadol Jr JB, Galla RJ, Fabian RL, Montgomery WW. *Surgical Anatomy of the Head and Neck*. Cambridge, Massachusetts: Harvard University Press; 2011.
2. Som PM, Smoker WRK, Reidenberg JS, Bergemann AD, Hudgins PA, Laitman J. Embryology and anatomy of the neck. In: Som PM, Curtin HD, eds. *Head and Neck Imaging*. 5 ed. St. Louis, Missouri; 2011.
3. de Bakker BS, de Bakker HM, Soerdjbalie-Maikoe V, Dikkers FG. The development of the human hyoid-larynx complex revisited. *Laryngoscope*. 2017;295(6):742.
4. Krmpotić-Nemanić J, Draf W, Helms J. *Surgical Anatomy of Head and Neck*. Springer; 1988.
5. Suzuki M, Kirchner JA, Murakami Y. The cricothyroid as a respiratory muscle. Its characteristics in bilateral recurrent laryngeal nerve paralysis. *Ann Otol Rhinol Laryngol*. 1970; 79(5):976–983.
6. Sasaki CT. Anatomy and development and physiology of the larynx. In: *GI Motility Online PART 1 Oral Cavity, Pharynx and Esophagus*. Nature Publishing Group; 2006.
7. Sasaki CT, Hundal JS, Kim Y-H. Protective glottic closure: biomechanical effects of selective laryngeal denervation. *Ann Otol Rhinol Laryngol*. 2005;114(4):271–275.
8. Pressman JJ. Sphincters of the larynx. *AMA Arch Otolaryngol*. 1954;59(2):221–236.
9. Doty RW, Bosma JF. An electromyographic analysis of reflex deglutition. *J Neurophysiol*. 1956;19(1):44–60.
10. Medda BK, Kern M, Ren J, et al. Relative contribution of various airway protective mechanisms to prevention of aspiration during swallowing. *Am J Physiol Gastrointest Liver Physiol*. 2003;284(6):G933–G939.
11. Malandraki GA, Sutton BP, Perlman AL, Karampinos DC, Conway C. Neural activation of swallowing and swallowing-related tasks in healthy young adults: an attempt to separate the components of deglutition. *Hum Brain Mapp*. 2009;30(10):3209–3226.
12. Hillel AD. The study of laryngeal muscle activity in normal human subjects and in patients with laryngeal dystonia using multiple fine-wire electromyography. *Laryngoscope*. 2001;111(4 Pt 2 suppl 97):1–47.

13. Logemann JA, Kahrilas PJ, Cheng J, et al. Closure mechanisms of laryngeal vestibule during swallow. *Am J Physiol.* 1992;262(2 Pt 1):G338–G344.
14. Gross RD, Steinhauer KM, Zajac DJ, Weissler MC. Direct measurement of subglottic air pressure while swallowing. *Laryngoscope.* 2006;116(5):753–761.
15. Klahn MS, Perlman AL. Temporal and durational patterns associating respiration and swallowing. *Dysphagia.* 1999;14(3):131–138.
16. Martin-Harris B, Brodsky MB, Price CC, Michel Y, Walters B. Temporal coordination of pharyngeal and laryngeal dynamics with breathing during swallowing: single liquid swallows. *J Appl Physiol.* 2003;94(5):1735–1743.
17. Martin-Harris B, Brodsky MB, Michel Y, Ford CL, Walters B, Heffner J. Breathing and swallowing dynamics across the adult lifespan. *Arch Otolaryngol Head Neck Surg.* 2005;131(9):762–770.
18. Leder SB, Ross DA. Incidence of vocal fold immobility in patients with dysphagia. *Dysphagia.* 2005;20(2):163–167; discussion 168–9.
19. Tabaee A, Murry T, Zschommler A, Desloge RB. Flexible endoscopic evaluation of swallowing with sensory testing in patients with unilateral vocal fold immobility: incidence and pathophysiology of aspiration. *Laryngoscope.* 2005;115(4):565–569.
20. Domer AS, Leonard R, Belafsky PC. Pharyngeal weakness and upper esophageal sphincter opening in patients with unilateral vocal fold immobility. *Laryngoscope.* 2014;124(10):2371–2374.
21. Kraus DH, Ali MK, Ginsberg RJ, et al. Vocal cord medialization for unilateral paralysis associated with intrathoracic malignancies. *J Thorac Cardiovasc Surg.* 1996;111(2):334–339; discussion 339–41.
22. Bhattacharyya N, Kotz T, Shapiro J. Dysphagia and aspiration with unilateral vocal cord immobility: incidence, characterization, and response to surgical treatment. *Ann Otol Rhinol Laryngol.* 2002;111(8):672–679.
23. Morpeth JF, Williams MF. Vocal fold paralysis after anterior cervical diskectomy and fusion. *Laryngoscope.* 2000;110(1):43–46.
24. Heitmiller RF, Tseng E, Jones B. Prevalence of aspiration and laryngeal penetration in patients with unilateral vocal fold motion impairment. *Dysphagia.* 2000;15(4):184–187.
25. Kreuzer SH, Schima W, Schober E, et al. Complications after laryngeal surgery: videofluoroscopic evaluation of 120 patients. *Clin Radiol.* 2000;55(10):775–781.
26. Bron LP, Soldati D, Monod M-L, et al. Horizontal partial laryngectomy for supraglottic squamous cell carcinoma. *Eur Arch Otorhinolaryngol.* 2005;262(4):302–306.
27. Mendelsohn AH, Remacle M, Van Der Vorst S, Bachy V, Lawson G. Outcomes following transoral robotic surgery: supraglottic laryngectomy. *Laryngoscope.* 2013;123(1):208–214.
28. Pauloski BR. Rehabilitation of dysphagia following head and neck cancer. *Phys Med Rehabil Clin N Am.* 2008;19(4):889–928, x.
29. Rademaker AW, Logemann JA, Pauloski BR, et al. Recovery of postoperative swallowing in patients undergoing partial laryngectomy. *Head Neck.* 1993;15(4):325–334.

Anatomy and Physiology of the Upper Esophageal Sphincter

VALERIA SILVA MEREA, MD • MICHAEL J. PITMAN, MD

INTRODUCTION

The upper esophageal sphincter (UES) is a high-pressure zone that forms a barrier between the pharynx and the esophagus. When closed, the UES prevents aerophagia or possible aspiration of refluxate. When it opens, it allows for swallowing, belching, or vomiting.

EMBRYOLOGY

The striated muscle of the UES is derived from mesenchyme of the branchial arches 4 and 6.[1] Studies of preterm infants performed at 33 weeks postgestational age have shown that the UES is already well developed at this age but continues to mature postnatally.[2]

ANATOMY

Upper Esophageal Sphincter Closing Muscles

Cricopharyngeus

The cricopharyngeus (CP) is the principal component of the UES, but it does not account for the entire high-pressure zone, which also encompasses the distal inferior pharyngeal constrictor (IPC) and the uppermost portion of the esophagus, and spans for 4 cm (range 3.0–4.5 cm).[3] The CP arises bilaterally from the lateral aspect of the cricoid cartilage and forms a posterior C-shaped band at the level of the junction of the pharynx and esophagus. It is formed by two sets of muscle fibers. The pars oblique (CP_O) is composed of obliquely oriented fibers that extend from the lateral cricoid cartilage on either side to a median raphe.[4,5] The pars fundiformis (CP_F) has horizontally oriented fibers originating from the cricoid cartilage, posteroinferior to the attachment of the CP_O. They extend to the opposite side of the cricoid cartilage, without forming a median raphe.[4,5] The CP is composed of small striated muscle fibers with an average diameter between 25 and 35 μm, which are not strictly parallel,[4,5] and contains a large amount of endomysial connective tissue at about 40%.[4] The CP has both slow-twitch (type 1, oxidative) and fast-twitch (type 2, glycolytic) muscle fibers, with slow twitch being predominant.[4–6] Furthermore, the CP is composed of two layers of muscle which also exhibit differences in fiber-type distribution, the inner layer containing significantly more slow-twitch fibers than the outer layer.[6] The CP muscle fiber composition is thought to be consistent with its function, requiring the generation of tone with periods of rapid relaxation followed by contraction in response to swallowing, vomiting, or belching.[4,5,7]

The CP achieves maximal active tension at approximately 1.7 times its resting length,[8] while for most striated muscles, the maximum tension develops at resting length itself.[9] This results in an elasticity that allows the UES to be opened by increased intraluminal pressure (by a bolus), or active distraction (by movement of the hyoid), without active relaxation or inhibition of the CP.[8] It also makes it unlikely that the diameter of the UES during a swallow of maximal volume would exceed the optimal length of the CP.[8] Similar to Starling's law of the cardiac muscle, the UES tension increases throughout its range of distension.[8] Thus, as a bolus passes the UES, the tension of the sphincter increases, which allows for a greater force to be exerted by the UES behind the bolus, resulting in propulsion of the bolus and rapid closure of the UES.[8]

Innervation

CP innervation in humans has not been fully elucidated.[10] Anatomical dissection suggests it is innervated by the pharyngeal plexus from above and the recurrent laryngeal nerve from below.[11] The pharyngeal plexus is supplied by three nerves: the vagus nerve by way of the pharyngoesophageal nerve and superior laryngeal nerve, the glossopharyngeal nerve, and sympathetic fibers. Physiologic testing using intraoperative electromyography (EMG) showed contraction of the ipsilateral CP with stimulation of the recurrent laryngeal nerve, while stimulation of the pharyngeal plexus did not lead to a contraction in all patients.[12] In contrast, a retrospective review of EMG studies of clinical cases showed a higher correlation between CP and IPC innervation than that of CP and the laryngeal musculature, suggesting that the pharyngeal plexus plays a more important role than the recurrent laryngeal nerve in CP innervation.[13] The sympathetic nerves have not been shown to have a role in CP motor innervation.[14] Motor neurons of the CP are located in the nucleus ambiguus.[15]

Sensory innervation of the pharyngeal epithelium is supplied by branches of the glossopharyngeal nerve, superior laryngeal nerve, and vagus nerve.[16–18] Afferents mediating UES reflexes stimulate the nucleus tractus solitarius.[19]

Inferior pharyngeal constrictor
The IPC originates on either side of the thyroid cartilage and inserts into the median raphe in the posterior pharynx.[20] It is compartmentalized and like the CP, it has a differential distribution of muscle fiber types, with increasing slow-twitch (type 1) fibers in a rostral to caudal direction.[20] Moreover, similar to the CP, the IPC also has two layers: an inner layer of type 1 fibers and an outer layer of type 2 fibers.[21]

Innervation
Studies tracing nerves using Sihler's stain have shown that the IPC is supplied by the dense pharyngeal plexus.[11] Notably, motor innervation of IPC appears to be layer dependent and nerve specific: the fast-twitch outer layer is innervated by the pharyngeal branch of the vagus nerve, while the slow-twitch inner layer is innervated by the pharyngeal branch of the glossopharyngeal nerve.[21] No physiologic studies have been conducted to correlate these findings. Branches of the glossopharyngeal nerve, superior laryngeal nerve, and vagus nerve provide sensory innervation to the pharyngeal epithelium.[16–18]

Cervical esophagus
The proximal 5% of the esophagus is exclusively composed of striated muscle, and muscle fibers are arranged in a horizontal fashion.[22] The predominant muscle fiber type in animals is type II or fast twitch,[23–25] but muscle fiber composition in humans has not been definitively established.[23,26,27] Muscle fiber type distribution in the esophagus does not show regional differences, in contrast to CP and IPC muscles.[26]

Innervation
The recurrent laryngeal nerve provides motor innervation to the cervical esophagus in a circular fashion around the muscle.[27] The superior laryngeal nerve mediates afferent fibers of many physiological responses like swallowing and belching, and reflexes such as the esophago-UES contractile reflex and esophago-lower esophageal sphincter relaxation reflex, both activated from the cervical esophagus.[28]

Upper Esophageal Sphincter Opening Muscles
The UES opening muscles are histologically similar to limb muscles, with uniformly sized fibers which are parallel, predominantly type II fibers, and a small amount of connective tissue.[29–31] Opening muscles can be divided into two groups: anterior and posterior muscles.

Anterior muscles
Among the anterior opening muscles, there are supra- and infrahyoid muscles. The suprahyoid musculature includes the geniohyoid, mylohyoid, stylohyoid, hyoglossus, and the anterior belly of the digastric muscle. These muscles attach to the superior aspect of the hyoid bone, and their main combined function is to elevate the hyoid and larynx and move them superiorly and anteriorly. The thyrohyoid, sternohyoid, sternothyroid, and omohyoid muscles, also referred to as strap muscles, are part of the infrahyoid musculature. They insert on the inferior aspect of the hyoid bone and their contraction pulls the hyoid bone inferiorly.[32] In addition, the thyrohyoid muscle moves the thyroid ala superiorly and anteriorly, while the sternothyroid depresses the larynx.[32] The individual anterior muscles have different motor innervations which are listed along with their motor nuclei on Table 5.1.[3]

Posterior muscles
The posterior pharyngeal muscles involved in UES opening include the stylopharyngeus, palatopharyngeus, and salpingopharyngeus, all named according to their site of origin: styloid process, soft palate, and pharyngotympanic or Eustachian tube, respectively.[32] Their main function is to elevate the pharynx. The palatopharyngeus also participates in the closure of the oropharyngeal isthmus, and the salpingopharyngeus opens the pharyngotympanic tube.[32] Table 5.2 lists the posterior UES opening muscles with their respective motor innervation and motor nuclei.[32]

TABLE 5.1
Anterior Opening Muscles

Muscle	Motor Innervation	Motor Nucleus
SUPRAHYOID		
Geniohyoid	C1 (carried along CN XII)	C1
Mylohyoid	Trigeminal nerve (CN V)	Trigeminal nucleus (CN V)
Stylohyoid	Facial nerve (CN VII)	Facial nucleus (CN VII)
Hyoglossus	Hypoglossal nerve (CN XII)	Hypoglossal nucleus (CN XII)
Anterior belly of digastric	Trigeminal nerve (CN V)	Trigeminal nucleus (CN V)
INFRAHYOID		
Thyrohyoid	C1 (carried along CN XII)	C1
Sternohyoid	Ansa cervicalis (C1–C3)	C1–C3
Sternothyroid	Ansa cervicalis (C1–C3)	C1–C3
Omohyoid	Ansa cervicalis (C1–C3)	C1–C3

TABLE 5.2
Posterior Opening Muscles

Muscle	Motor Innervation	Motor Nucleus
Stylopharyngeus	Glossopharyngeal nerve (CN IX)	Nucleus ambiguus
Palatopharyngeus	Vagus nerve (CN X)	Nucleus ambiguus
Salpingopharyngeus	Vagus nerve (CN X)	Nucleus ambiguus

PHYSIOLOGY
Generation of Tone
Basal UES pressure or tone is the result of active muscle contraction and passive mechanical factors.[33] Given that the UES is composed of striated muscle exclusively, it has no intrinsic tone-generating mechanism as is seen in smooth muscles.[10] Evidence suggests that the UES basal tone is not constant but fluctuating, set by many reflex functions.[7,10]

Manometry studies have shown normal UES pressure to range from 30 to 175 mmHg.[34] There is an inverse relationship between age and resting UES pressure,[35] and women have a higher UES resting pressure than men.[35] UES pressure drops to very low levels during sleep[36] or general anesthesia,[37] and it has been found to increase to very high levels during acute stress.[38] EMG studies have also shown increased UES activity during changes in posture.[37,39]

The UES shows radial and axial asymmetry in pressure with a sharp ascent in its upper part and a more gradual decline in its lower part.[40,41] The pressures are higher in the anterior–posterior than the lateral dimensions.[40] Moreover, in humans, peak pressures occur 1 cm below the upper border of the high-pressure zone anteriorly but 2 cm below the upper portion of the high-pressure zone posteriorly.[40] These asymmetries are not observed after laryngectomy, suggesting that the rigid cartilage forming the anterior wall of the UES plays a role in these asymmetries.[40,42]

Swallowing
During swallowing, the CP relaxes first.[43] During this relaxation, the hyoid moves superiorly, then anteriorly, and 0.15 s after initial UES relaxation, the UES opens.[43] During the swallow, the UES elevates along with the larynx. Overall, the CP relaxes only for about 0.5 s during swallowing.[44,45] Superior movement of the hyoid is achieved by contraction of the suprahyoid musculature and complete relaxation of the infrahyoid musculature.[39,43,46] Anterior hyoid and laryngeal excursion have been correlated with maximal activation of the geniohyoid muscle and concomitant activity of the stylopharyngeus.[39,46]

The dynamics of the UES function are dependent on the volume of the bolus.[44,47] For instance, graded increases in bolus volume lead to increases in UES dimension, with only minimal increases in intrabolus pressure.[43] In addition, there is modulation of suprahyoid opening muscles to maintain the opening at greater aperture for longer.[47]

Belching
UES opening with eructation differs significantly from swallowing. During belching, there is no associated primary peristalsis,[48] the decrease in UES pressure persists for significantly longer than that in swallowing[48] and the hyoid excursion is mainly anterior compared to anterosuperior during swallowing.[49] When gas escapes the stomach and stimulates esophageal

receptors, it leads to opening of the UES and protection of the airway, shortly followed by contraction of the diaphragm and retrograde contraction of the esophagus.[50] During eructation, the UES is opened by the complete relaxation of the CP and IPC, and a constant low-level contraction of the thyrohyoid, stylopharyngeus, hyoglossus, and hyopharyngeus muscles.[51]

Vomiting

Three distinct stages have been described during the retching and vomiting sequence: pre-retch, retch, and vomit.[46] Just before the first retch, the tone of the CP, cervical esophagus, and hyoid musculature increases in phase with the diaphragm allowing for full lung inflation without aerophagia.[46] Retching then involves a rhythmically alternating elevation and descent of the entire pharyngolaryngoesophagogastric apparatus in synchrony with diaphragmatic movement.[46] Glottal closure during retches and contraction of the three closing muscles of the UES between retches are the principal mechanisms of airway protection.[46] During vomitus expulsion, all of the UES closing muscles relax. The UES is maximally opened by contraction of both anterior and posterior UES opening muscles.[46]

REFLEXES

Esophago-Upper Esophageal Sphincter Relaxation Reflex

Rapid distension of the esophagus causes relaxation of the CP, activation of the laryngeal and hyoid musculature, and decreased UES pressure.[52] This reflex is thought to be part of the belch response, as it shares the stimulus, and the muscular activation in the pharynx and larynx is identical.[52] It has been hypothesized that the receptors for this reflex must be rapidly adapting mucosal mechanoreceptors, and the afferent limb of this reflex is the vagus nerve.[52]

Pharyngo-Upper Esophageal Sphincter Contractile Reflex

Pharyngeal stimulation with amounts of water significantly lower than those required to stimulate a swallow leads to increased resting UES tone.[53] It has been suggested that this reflex may be activated during pharyngeal reflux of esophageal contents, leading to an increase in UES pressure and thereby possibly preventing further regurgitation into the pharynx; thus, it may function as an airway protective mechanism.[54]

In the feline model of this reflex, the afferent limb was found to be the glossopharyngeal nerve, while the efferent limb was the pharyngeal branch of the vagus nerve.[55] Deterioration of this reflex has been described in the elderly, and it is attributed abnormalities of the afferent limb.[56]

Esophago-Upper Esophageal Sphincter Contractile Reflex

Slow esophageal distension leads to an increase in tone of the UES or CP.[52,57] This reflex is not only triggered by distension but also by esophageal peristalsis. The closer the contraction is to the UES, the stronger the increase in CP activation.[52] Thus, it has been hypothesized that the function of this reflex is to prevent esophagopharyngeal reflux during propagation of peristalsis.[52] The afferent limb of this reflex is the vagus nerve in the thoracic esophagus[52] and the recurrent laryngeal nerve in the cervical esophagus.[57] The efferent route is the motor nerves to the CP, including the pharyngeal plexus and likely the recurrent laryngeal nerve.[10]

Other Contractile Reflexes

During respiration, there are variations in UES pressure, CP tone, and EMG activity.[37,58] Both tone and activity increase with each inspiration, particularly during vigorous breathing,[37] hyperinflation, and rapid deflation.[58] This has been referred to as the "lung-UES contractile reflex."[10] These findings support the idea that one of the functions of the UES is to prevent aerophagia.[37] An increase in UES tone during phonation[37,59] and coughing[60] has also been noted.

Finally, experiments in dogs have shown an increase in UES tone and EMG activity, primarily in the CP, with changes in head position.[37,39] It has been hypothesized this may be due to activation of the vestibular system and may serve to prevent reflux of esophageal contents when the direction of peristalsis is opposite to that of gravity.[10] This reflex has been referred to as the "vestibulo-UES contractile reflex."[10]

ABBREVIATIONS

CN	Cranial nerve
CP	Cricopharyngeus
CP_F	Cricopharyngeus pars fundiformis
CP_O	Cricopharyngeus pars oblique
EMG	Electromyography
IPC	Inferior pharyngeal constrictor
UES	Upper esophageal sphincter

REFERENCES

1. Kuo B, Urma D. Esophagus — anatomy and development. GI Motility online. In: *PART 1 Oral Cavity, Pharynx and Esophagus.* 2006.
2. Jadcherla SR, Duong HQ, Hofman C, Hoffmann R, Shaker R. Characteristics of upper oesophageal sphincter and oesophageal body during maturation in healthy human neonates compared with adults. *Neurogastroenterol Motil.* 2005;17:663—670.
3. Hernandez LV, Dua KS, Surapeni SN, Rittman T, Shaker R. Anatomic-manometric correlation of the upper esophageal sphincter: a concurrent US and manometry study. *Gastrointest Endosc.* 2010;72:587—592.
4. Bonington A, Mahon M, Whitmore I. A histological and histochemical study of the cricopharyngeus muscle in man. *J Anat.* 1988;156:27—37.
5. Brownlow H, Whitmore I, Willan P. A quantitative study of the histochemical and morphometric characteristics of the human cricopharyngeus muscle. *J Anat.* 1989;166:67—75.
6. Mu L, Sanders I. Muscle fiber-type distribution pattern in the human cricopharyngeus muscle. *Dysphagia.* 2002;17:87—96.
7. Lang IM, Shaker R. Anatomy and physiology of the upper esophageal sphincter. *Am J Med.* 1997;103(5A):50S—55S.
8. Medda BK, Lang IM, Dodds WJ, et al. Correlation of electrical and contractile activities of the cricopharyngeus muscle in the cat. *Am J Physiol.* 1997;273:G470—G479.
9. Wilkie DR. The mechanical properties of muscle. *Br Med Bull.* 1956;12:177—182.
10. Lang IM. Development, anatomy, and physiology of the upper esophageal sphincter and pharyngoesophageal junction. In: Shaker R, Belafsky PC, Postma GM, Easterling C, eds. *Principles of Deglutition: A Multidisciplinary Text for Swallowing and Its Disorders.* New York: Springer; 2013:235—255.
11. Mu L, Sanders I. The innervation of the human upper esophageal sphincter. *Dysphagia.* 1996;11:234—238.
12. Brok HA, Copper MP, Stroeve RJ, Ongerboers de Visser BW, Venker-van Haagen AJ, Schouwendburg PF. Evidence for recurrent laryngeal nerve contribution in motor innervation the human cricopharyngeal muscle. *Laryngoscope.* 1999;109:705—708.
13. Halum SL, Shemirani NL, Merati AL, Jaradeh S, Toohill RJ. Electromyography findings of the cricopharyngeus in association with ipsilateral pharyngeal and laryngeal muscles. *Ann Otol Rhinol Laryngol.* 2006;115:312—314.
14. Sasaki CT, Kim YH, Sims HS, Czibulka A. Motor innervation of the human cricopharyngeus muscle. *Ann Otol Rhinol Laryngol.* 1999;108:1132—1139.
15. Holstege G, Graveland G, Bijker-Biemond C, Schuddeboom I. Location of motoneurons innervating soft palate, pharynx and upper esophagus. Anatomical evidence for a possible swallowing center in the pontine reticular formation. An HRP autoradiographic tracing study. *Brain Behav Evol.* 1983;23:47—62.
16. Maeyama T, Miyasaki J, Tsuda K, Shin T. Distribution and origin of the intraepithelial nerve fibers in the feline pharyngeal mucosa. *Acta Otolaryngol Suppl.* 1998;539:87—90.
17. Miyasaki J, Shin T, Murata Y, Masuko S. Pharyngeal branch of the vagus nerve carries intraepithelial afferent fibers in the cat pharynx: an elucidation of the origin and central and peripheral distribution of these components. *Otolaryngol Head Neck Surg.* 1999;120:905—913.
18. Yoshida Y, Tanaka Y, Hirano M, Morimoto M, Nakashima T. Sensory innervation of the pharynx and larynx. *Am J Med.* 2000;108:51S—61S.
19. Altschuler SM, Bao X, Bieger D, Hopkins DA, Miselis RR. Viscerotopic representation of the upper alimentary tract in the rat: sensory ganglia and nuclei of the solitary tract and spinal trigeminal tracts. *J Comp Neurol.* 1989;283:248—268.
20. Mu L, Sanders I. Neuromuscular compartments and fiber-type regionalization in the human inferior pharyngeal constrictor muscle. *Anat Rec.* 2001;264:367—377.
21. Mu L, Sanders I. Neuromuscular specialization within the human pharyngeal constrictor muscles. *Ann Otol Rhinol Larygol.* 2007;116:604—617.
22. Meyer GW, Austin RM, Brady CE, Castell DO. Muscle anatomy of the human esophagus. *J Clin Gastroenterol.* 1986;8:131—134.
23. Shedlofsky-Deschamps G, Krasue WJ, Cutts JH, Hansen S. Histochemistry of the striated musculature in the opossum and human oesophagus. 1982;134:407—414.
24. Mascarello F, Rowlerson A, Scapolo PA. The fibre type composition of the striated uscle of the oesophagus in ruminants and carnivores. *Histochemistry.* 1984;80:277—288.
25. Hudson LC. Histochemical identification of the striated muscle of the canine esophagus. *Anat Histol Embryol.* 1993;22:101—104.
26. Leese G, Hopwood D. Muscle fibre typing in the human pharyngeal constrictors and oesohagus: the effect of aging. *Acta Anat.* 1986;127:77—80.
27. Mu L, Sanders I. Neuromuscular organization of the human upper esophageal sphincter. *Ann Otol Rhinol Laryngol.* 1998;107:370—377.
28. Lang IM, Medda BK, Jadcherla S, Shaker R. The role of the superior laryngeal nerve in esophageal reflexes. *Am J Physiol Gastrointest Liver Physiol.* 2012;302:G1445—G1457.
29. Dick TE, Van Lunteren E. Fiber subtype distribution of pharyngeal dilator muscles and diaphragm in the cat. *J Appl Physiol.* 1990;687:2237—2240.
30. Hisa Y, Malmgren LT, Lyon MJ. Quantitative histochemical studies on the cat infrahyoid muscles. *Otolaryngol Head Neck Surg.* 1990;103:723—732.
31. Cobos AR, Segade LA, Fuentes I. Muscle fibre types in the suprahyoid muscles of the rat. *J Anat.* 2001;198:283—294.
32. Drake RL, Vogl W, Mitchell AWM, eds. *Gray's Anatomy for Students.* Philadelphia: Elsevier Churchill Livingstone; 2005.
33. Sivarao DV, Goyal RK. Functional anatomy and physiology of the upper esophageal sphincter. *Am J Med.* 2000;108(4A):27S—37S.
34. Castell JA, Dalton CB, Castell DO. Pharyngeal and upper esophageal sphincter manometry in humans. *Am J Physiol.* 1990;258:G173—G178.

35. van Herwaarden MA, Katz PO, Gideon RM, et al. Are manometric parameters of the upper esophageal sphincter and pharynx affected by age and gender? *Dysphagia*. 2003: 211−217.

36. Kahrilas PJ, Dodds WJ, Dent J, Haeberle B, Hogan WJ, Arndorfer RC. Effect of sleep, spontaneous gastroesophageal reflux, and a meal on upper esophageal sphincter pressure in normal human volunteers. *Gastroenterology*. 1987;92:466−471.

37. Jacob P, Kahrilas PJ, Herzon G, McLaughlin B. Determinants of upper esophageal sphincter pressure in dogs. *Am J Physiol*. 1990;259:G245−G251.

38. Cook IJ, Dent J, Shannon S, Collins SM. Measurement of upper esophageal sphincter pressure. Effect of acute emotional stress. *Gastroenterology*. 1987;93: 526−532.

39. Lang IM, Dantas RO, Cook IJ, Dodds WJ. Videoradiographic, manometric and electromyographic analysis of canine upper esophageal sphincter. *Am J Physiol*. 1991; 260:G911−G919.

40. Welch RW, Luckmann K, Ricks PM, Drake ST, Gates GA. Manometry of the normal upper esophageal sphincter and its alterations in laryngectomy. *J Clin Investig*. 1979; 63:1036−1041.

41. Castell JA, Castell DO. Modern solid state computerized manometry of the pharyngoesophageal segment. *Dysphagia*. 1993;8:270−275.

42. Welch RW, Gates GA, Luckmann KF, Ricks PM, Drake ST. Change in the force-sumed pressure measurements of the upper esophageal sphincter prelaryngectomy and postlaryngectomy. *Ann Otol Rhinol Laryngol*. 1979;88: 804−808.

43. Cook IJ, Dodds WJ, Dantas RO, et al. Opening mechanisms of the upper esophageal sphincter. *Am J Physiol*. 1989;257:G748−G759.

44. Kahrilas PJ, Dodds WJ, Dent J, Logemann JA, Shaker R. Upper esophageal sphincter function during deglutition. *Gastroenterology*. 1988;95:52−62.

45. Goyal RK, Martin SB, Shapiro J, Spechler SJ. The role of cricopharyngeus muscle in pharyngoesophageal disorders. *Dysphagia*. 1993;8:253−258.

46. Lang IM, Dana N, Medda BK, Shaker R. Mechanisms of airway protection during retching, vomiting, and swallowing. *Am J Physiol*. 2002;283:G963−G972.

47. Cock C, Jones CA, Hammer MJ, Omari TI, McCulloch TM. Modulation of upper esophageal sphincter (UES) relaxation and opening during volume swallowing. *Dysphagia*. 2017;32:216−224.

48. Kahrilas PJ, Dodds WJ, Dent J, Wyman JB, Hogan WJ, Amdorfer RC. Upper esophageal sphincter function during belching. *Gastroenterology*. 1986;91:133−140.

49. Shaker R, Ren J, Kern M, Dodds WJ, Hogan WJ, Li Q. Mechanisms of airway protection and upper esophageal sphincter opening during belching. *Am J Physiol*. 1992; 262:G621−G628.

50. Lang IM. The physiology of eructation. *Dysphagia*. 2016; 31:121−133.

51. Lang IM, Medda BK, Shaker R. Digestive and respiratory tract motor responses associated with eructation. *Am J Physiol*. 2013;304:G1044−G1053.

52. Lang IM, Medda BK, Shaker R. Mechanisms of reflexes induced by esophageal distension. *Am J Physiol Gastrointest Liver Physiol*. 2001;281:G1246−G1263.

53. Shaker R, Ren J, Xie P, Lang IM, Bardan E, Sui Z. Characterization of the pharyngo-UES contractile reflex in humans. *Am J Physiol*. 1997;273:G854−G858.

54. Shaker R. Airway protective mechanisms: current concepts. *Dysphagia*. 1995;10:216−227.

55. Medda BK, Lang IM, Layman R, Hogan WJ, Dodds WJ, Shaker R. Characterization and quantification of a pharyngo-UES contractile reflex in cats. *Am J Physiol*. 1994;267:G972−G983.

56. Ren J, Xie P, Lang IM, Bardan E, Sui Z, Shaker R. Deterioration of the pharyngo-UES contractile reflex in the elderly. *Laryngoscope*. 2000;110:1563−1566.

57. Freiman JM, El-Sharkaway TY, Diamant NE. Effect of bilateral vagosympathetic nerve blockade on response of the dog upper esophageal sphincter (UES) to intraesophageal distention and acid. *Gastroenterology*. 1981;81:78−84.

58. Lang IM, Medda BK, Shaker R. Mechanism of the ventilator cycle fluctuations in UES tone. *Gastroenterology*. 2000;118: A133.

59. Perera L, Kern M, Hofmann C, et al. Manometric evidence for a phonation-induced UES contractile reflex. *Am J Physiol Gastrointest Liver Physiol*. 2008;294:G885−G891.

60. Amaris M, Dua KS, Naini SR, Samuel E, Shaker R. Characterization of the upper esophageal sphincter response during cough. *Chest*. 2012;142:1229−1236.

CHAPTER 6

The Esophagus

KARUNA DEWAN, MD • DINESH K. CHHETRI, MD

INTRODUCTION

The primary function of the esophagus is to transport food and liquids from the oropharynx through the thoracic cavity into the stomach. It is the only part of the gastrointestinal (GI) tract that lacks any metabolic, digestive, or absorptive function. However, it is a dynamic tube with unique neuromuscular anatomy and peristaltic mechanism to effectively propel food to the stomach. It also serves as a passageway for food and refluxate during vomiting and release of gastric pressure. The esophagus is innervated by the vagus nerve (CN X) and is also implicated in a variety of disorders in otolaryngology, including chronic cough, globus sensation, and referred oropharyngeal dysphagia. In this chapter, the developmental origins, anatomy, and physiology of the esophagus are explored.

EMBRYOLOGY

Esophageal embryonic development and anatomic features play important roles in both normal function and common pathology of the esophagus. During the first 4 weeks of gestation, the flat disc-shaped human embryo folds into a "body cylinder" to develop a basic body shape. The yolk sac, composed of endoderm, invaginates into the lateral plate mesoderm to become the embryonic gut tube, which can be divided into the foregut, midgut, and hindgut. The esophagus develops from the foregut immediately behind the pharynx. Development of the GI system takes place along four major patterned axes: anterior–posterior, dorsal–ventral, left–right, and craniocaudal. Each axis development is based on the epithelial–mesenchymal interactions and mediated by specific molecular pathways. Growth factors and endodermal proteins control esophageal development in the anterior–posterior axis. These factors influence both the esophageal environment and make the environment more permissive for neural crest cells to migrate into the gut. The neural crest cells originate between the neural plate and the ectoderm. They migrate ventrally toward the gut during the 5th and 12th weeks of gestation—eventually forming the *enteric nervous system.*

The airway separates from the esophagus by a process of elongation and septation. During the fourth embryonic week, the foregut develops a small ventral diverticulum below the pharynx. This *tracheobronchial diverticulum* subsequently elongates and separates gradually from the dorsal foregut through the formation of the *tracheoesophageal septum* to become the primitive respiratory tract. Anomalies of this separation process result in the various congenital esophageal atresia with concurrent *congenital tracheoesophageal fistula* malformations. The esophagus and trachea show distinct endodermal and mesenchymal development. The trachea develops pseudostratified columnar epithelium and is enveloped in cartilage rings ventrally. The esophagus forms multilayered squamous epithelium, and the esophageal mesenchyme develops the smooth muscle layer required for esophageal motility and propulsion of food.

The remaining portion of the foregut rapidly elongates with the continued growth of the embryonic body. During the seventh week, blood vessels enter the submucosa, and in the subsequent weeks, the luminal epithelium proliferates, almost completely occluding the foregut. By the 10th week, the foregut is recanalized, forming a single esophageal lumen with a superficial layer of ciliated epithelial cells. Anomalies of this recanalizing process leads to the formation of *congenital esophageal atresia. Congenital hiatal hernia* occurs when the esophagus fails to grow adequately in length. As a result, it is too short and pulls the cardiac stomach into the esophageal hiatus in the diaphragm. During the fourth gestational month, a stratified squamous epithelium begins to replace the ciliated epithelium at the proximal and distal ends of the esophagus. This process continues until birth. Small residual islands of ciliated epithelium eventually give rise to the esophageal submucosal glands. These submucosal glands provide a protective function, participating in luminal acid clearance.

The striated muscles of the UES and upper esophagus derive from the mesenchyme of branchial arches 4 through 6. This includes the muscularis propria of the upper part of the esophagus. The smooth muscle of the lower esophagus and lower esophageal sphincter (LES) are derived from the splanchnic mesenchyme of the somites surrounding the foregut. Mucosa and glandular structures are derived from the primitive endodermal layer. The embryologic origin of the gastroesophageal junction (GEJ) is still controversial, but gastric rotation together with augmentation of the fundus of the stomach is believed to determine its function. The middle third of the esophagus consists of a mixture of smooth and skeletal muscle. The origin of this mixture is controversial, with somites and endoderm influencing each other by molecular mechanisms. It appears that the two different muscle types may arise from two distinct differentiation pathways. The development of the concentric layers of smooth muscle, neural crest cells, and myenteric plexus is a coordinated process, controlled by numerous genes and signaling molecules.

The differentiation of the circular layer of smooth muscle begins after the neural crest cells have migrated to the gut and begun maturation. This maturation occurs in a rostrocaudal direction and is complete by week 9. The myenteric plexus demonstrates cholinesterase activity by week 10 and the ganglion cells are differentiated by week 13. Therefore, the esophagus is likely capable of peristalsis as early as the end of the first trimester. In the second trimester, three different patterns of motility have been observed. Opening of the esophageal lumen from the LES to the oropharynx, propulsive peristaltic contractions, and lastly, reflux from the stomach into the esophagus. At birth, the propagation of peristalsis along the esophagus and opening of the LES is immature, resulting in frequent regurgitation during the newborn period. The pressure at the LES reaches that of the adult at approximately 3–6 weeks after birth.

Aberrations in vascular development may cause congenital dysphagia. For example, the aortic arch arteries and dorsal aorta initially form a vascular ring that completely encircles the pharyngeal foregut. In normal development, the right dorsal aorta regresses, so that the esophagus is no longer completely encircled by vascular structures. However, occasionally the right dorsal aorta persists and maintains its connection with the left dorsal aorta, resulting in a *double aortic arch* forming a vascular ring around the trachea and esophagus. This ring may cause both dysphagia and dyspnea. Another example of a vascular malformation-causing dysphagia results from the abnormal disappearance of the right fourth aortic arch artery. This leaves an aberrant right subclavian artery, crossing over the midline, posterior to the esophagus. While often asymptomatic, in some patients, the aberrant subclavian artery compresses the esophagus causing dysphagia *(dysphagia lusoria)*, and the esophagus may also compress the right subclavian artery, reducing blood pressure in the right upper extremity.

ANATOMY

The esophagus originates at the level of the sixth cervical vertebrae (C6), approximately 18 cm from the incisors, posterior to the cricoid cartilage. From the pharyngoesophageal junction, the esophagus passes through the mediastinum and diaphragm and connects to the cardia of the stomach. It descends anterior to the vertebral column, through the mediastinum, and traverses the diaphragm at the diaphragmatic hiatus around the 11th thoracic vertebra (T11), and ends at its connection at the orifice of the cardia of the stomach. Three anatomically narrow points along its course can be appreciated on endoscopy or barium esophagram. The first is at the level of the cricoid cartilage. The second is at the level of the left main bronchus and aortic arch. The third is at the esophageal hiatus of the diaphragm. At rest, the adult esophagus is a collapsed muscular tube 18–22 cm. It can expand up to 2 cm in the anterior–posterior direction and 3 cm in the lateral direction.

The esophagus can be divided into three anatomic segments: cervical, thoracic, and abdominal. The cervical esophagus rests slightly to the left of midline, posterior to the larynx and trachea, and anterior to the prevertebral layer of the cervical fascia from the pharyngoesophageal junction to the suprasternal notch—about 4–5 cm. The blood supply is from the branches of the inferior thyroid arteries. The proximity of the esophagus to the vertebral column in this location creates a special opportunity for *cervical osteophytes*, either in isolation or as part of a systemic disease, to impinge upon the laryngopharynx and cervical esophagus causing dysphagia and possible aspiration (see Chapter 17).

The thoracic esophagus extends from the suprasternal notch at T1 to the diaphragmatic hiatus at T10. During its course, it curves slightly to the right in the region of the tracheal bifurcation, around the T4 level. It continues behind the pericardium and left atrium and enters the abdomen through the diaphragmatic hiatus, which is also the location of the LES. From the level of T8 until the diaphragmatic hiatus, the esophagus lies anteriorly and medial to the aorta. The most superior portion of the thoracic esophagus receives its blood supply from the bronchial arteries. The middle section is supplied by the esophageal branches that originate from the aorta. Besides dysphagia lusoria from an aberrant right subclavian artery, other vascular anomalies may cause dysphagia. In the setting of mitral stenosis and consequential right atrial hypertrophy, the esophagus may be obstructed secondary to the enlarged right atrium and result in dysphagia. The esophagus also runs between the aorta and left main bronchus in this region, creating the potential for narrowing of the esophageal lumen. This is the most common area for *pill-induced esophagitis* and *strictures*. The thoracic esophagus lies within a defined fascial compartment, allowing infections from the anterior esophageal wall to easily spread through the peritracheal space down to the pericardium. *Perforation of the esophagus* can lead to necrotizing mediastinitis with rapid and dissemination of infection with high mortality.

The abdominal esophagus is the shortest segment, 2−4 cm in length and extends from the diaphragmatic hiatus (T10) to the orifice of the cardia of the stomach (T11). The base of the esophagus transitions into the cardia of the stomach—this area forms a cone 1 cm in length. The high-pressure zone where the esophagus merges with the stomach is called the LES. The blood supply to the abdominal esophagus includes the left inferior phrenic artery and the esophageal branches of the left gastric artery. The anatomic relationship between the esophagus and the diaphragm is clinically important. The phrenoesophageal membrane, which serves as an anchor for the distal esophagus, loses its elasticity with aging. The loss of elasticity in combination with a wide diaphragmatic hiatus can result in herniation of the GEJ and cardia into the thorax. This is the pathophysiology of a *hiatal hernia*.

The venous drainage of the esophagus is a portal—caval connection and thus highly susceptible to *portal hypertension*. Esophageal varices are found in the lamina propria of the lower esophageal sphincter. Normally, the pressure in the small vessels in the LES is greater than normal portal pressure. However, factors reducing LES pressure promote the development of varices and enlargement of these small vessels. Development of esophageal varices depends on local esophageal factors and portal gradient, vascular resistance in the azygos vein, or the presence of other portosystemic collaterals. Contraction of the LES leads to reduction of the variceal and azygos vein flow. There is a resultant decrease in the pressure gradient across the varix wall and reduction of the varices.

The layers of the esophagus from inside out include the mucosa, submucosa, muscularis propria, and adventitia. The muscularis propria has two layers of muscle cells, an outer longitudinal layer and an inner circular layer. The longitudinal layer is continuous throughout the length of the esophagus, forming a uniform layer that covers the esophageal outer surface. The inner circular layer is arranged in concentric circles and responsible for the sequential peristaltic contractions that propel the food bolus toward the stomach. The UES (see Chapter 5) and the proximal one-third of the esophagus (roughly 5 cm in adults) are both composed of striated muscle. This area is followed by a 4-cm long *transition zone* where striated and smooth muscles are both present. Smooth muscle then comprises the remaining of the esophagus. Inferiorly, the inner thicker layer of the circular muscle layer comprises the intrinsic component of the LES.

The UES is formed by the cricopharyngeus (CP) muscle as well as fibers from the upper esophageal wall and the inferior pharyngeal constrictor (IPC) muscle of the pharynx on either side of the CP muscle (see Chapter 5). The LES is a poorly defined anatomic structure, consisting of a thickening of the circular esophageal musculature at the entrance of the stomach, and manometrically defined as a high-pressure zone located at the GEJ. It has both an intrinsic and an extrinsic component. The intrinsic component is made of semicircular layers of smooth esophageal muscle fibers as well as sling-like oblique gastric muscle fibers. The semicircular smooth muscles at the LES are thicker than in the rest of the esophagus and have significant tone but do not respond strongly to cholinergic stimulation. In contrast, the oblique gastric fibers have little resting tone but contract strongly to cholinergic stimulation. The extrinsic component is the crural diaphragm muscle, forming the esophageal hiatus, and functions as an adjunctive external sphincter that raises the pressure at the end of the esophagus in coordination with respiratory motion. Both sphincters are closed except during swallowing to assure a unidirectional flow of esophageal content toward the stomach and to prevent reflux of gastric contents into the esophagus or pharynx.

Several areas of the esophagus are prone to developing diverticula. A *Zenker's diverticulum* is the most frequent type of pharyngoesophageal diverticula. It originates in an anatomically weak posterior area called Killian's triangle between the CP and the IPC muscles. A functional obstruction, such as a hypertensive UES or a lack of coordination between the pharyngeal contraction and the UES, is thought to cause the formation of this mucosal outpouching through the muscular wall (see Chapter 20). A *Killian–Jamison* (KJ) diverticulum is less common and develops in the Killian–Jamison area, which is in the anterolateral wall of the cervical esophagus just below the CP muscle at the site where the recurrent laryngeal nerve enters the larynx. Finally, a diverticulum may develop at the Laimer's area, the posterior esophageal wall just below the CP muscle where the outer longitudinal muscle layer is deficient. This is a very rare entity with fewer than four reported cases.[2] Traction diverticula may form in the mid-esophagus. Adhesions between inflamed mediastinal lymph nodes and the esophagus may lead to traction of the esophagus wall and eventually a localized diverticulum. Finally, diverticula may form near the diaphragm (*epiphrenic diverticula*). These are pulsion diverticulum that form in the distal 10 cm of the esophagus due to motility disorders and/or increased esophageal pressure from outflow obstruction.

Often systemic diseases can have manifestations within the esophagus, impacting motility and function. *Scleroderma* is a systemic disorder characterized by functional and structural abnormalities of small blood vessels leading to fibrosis of the skin and internal organs. In the esophagus, there is a progressive fibrosis of smooth muscle resulting in decreased peristalsis to aperistalsis. The LES can become atonic, facilitating severe *gastroesophageal reflux* and the resultant development of strictures.

HISTOLOGY

The esophageal wall is composed of four layers: mucosa, submucosa, muscularis propria, and adventitia. The mucosa has three layers: epithelium, lamina propria, and muscularis mucosa. The squamous epithelium overlies the lamina propria and the muscularis mucosa. The muscularis mucosa separates the mucosa from the submucosa and is comprised of a thin layer of longitudinal muscle fibers. The simple histology of the esophageal mucosa provides a protective layer for food bolus that remains unmodified enroute to the stomach. The squamous epithelium joins the junctional columnar epithelium of the gastric cardia at the GEJ. In cases of severe gastroesophageal reflux, the GEJ can become irregular, and *Barrett's esophagus* may develop. It is characterized by displacement of the squamocolumnar junction proximal to the anatomic GEJ with the presence of intestinal metaplasia.

The submucosal layer contains elastic and fibrous tissue and is the strongest layer of the esophageal wall. The muscular layer has inner circular muscle fibers and outer longitudinal muscle fibers. The thickness of this muscular layer is 1.5–2 mm. The outer longitudinal layer is slightly thicker than the inner circular layer. Unlike the rest of the GI tract, the esophagus is not covered by a smooth serosal layer. The lack of serosal layer makes esophageal tears or luminal injuries more difficult to repair.

The muscularis propria layer is responsible for the esophageal peristaltic force and motor function. The upper one-third is composed exclusively of striated muscle while the distal one-third is composed entirely of smooth muscle. In-between these is a transition zone where there is a mixture of both kinds of muscles. Despite the presence of two different muscle types, they function as one unit. The *myenteric plexus* (Auerbach's plexus) is located between the two muscle layers. Some pathologic conditions affect only one layer. Scleroderma and achalasia impair function of only the circular muscle layer.

The adventitia is the external fibrous layer that covers the esophagus and connects it to the neighboring structures. It consists of loose connective tissue, small vessels, lymphatic channels, and nerve fibers.

INNERVATION

Innervation of the esophagus is from visceral afferents and efferents of the vagus nerve (CX). The vagus nerves run along each side of the neck until they reach the thoracic esophagus where they form an extensive plexus. There are also adrenergic receptors, autonomic fibers, and nonadrenergic noncholinergic nerves. It is surmised that nitric oxide (NO) is a possible mediator for this system. The esophagus is richly supplied with autonomic fibers derived from parasympathetic fibers and sympathetic chains. The striated muscle of the pharynx and upper esophagus receive nerve fibers that originate in the brain stem at the level of the nucleus ambiguus. The distal esophagus and LES are innervated by nerves that originate in the dorsal motor nucleus of the vagus and end in ganglia in the myenteric plexus. The myenteric plexus is located between the longitudinal and circular muscle layers and receives efferent impulses from the brain stem and afferent impulses from the esophagus. There are two main types of neurons found in this plexus: excitatory neurons and inhibitory neurons. They mediate contraction of the musculature via cholinergic receptors, vasoactive intestinal polypeptide (VIP), and NO. Branches of the superior and inferior cervical ganglia in the neck, the splanchnic nerves and the celiac plexus in the chest and abdomen provide the sympathetic innervation. These nerves modulate the activity of other nerves and do not serve a motor function.

The afferent nervous system collects information from the wall of the esophagus using a variety of receptors, including osmoreceptors, chemoreceptors, thermoreceptors, and mechanoreceptors. The afferent fibers are dendrites of the unipolar neurons located in the dorsal root ganglion in the thoracic spine (T1—T10). These neurons synapse with preganglionic neurons in the laterointermedial grey horns from the thoracic spine. The sensory information from the esophageal wall is transmitted ascending toward supraspinal and cortical centers, where sensory information is interpreted. The pain, temperature, and viseroceptive information is transmitted to the thalamus. Local stimulation of viscerosensory receptors in the esophageal body elicits a peristaltic wave at the point of stimulation that moves distally. The parasympathetic system at the esophageal level is represented by fibers of the vagus nerve. The afferent innervation of the muscularis propria originates in the nodose ganglion while the fibers supplying the mucosal layer originate from the petrosal and jugular ganglions. The vagal afferents respond to mechanical distension, while afferents in the mucosa respond to chemical intraluminal stimulus. The afferent innervation of the muscularis propria originates in the nodose ganglion. These respond primarily to mechanical distension. The parasympathetic afferents from the esophagus on their way to the sensory ganglion join the SLN. The axons of the neurons supplying sensation to the esophagus end in different nuclei of the brainstem. The afferents from the smooth muscle of the esophagus project to the central subnucleus, whereas the afferents from the striated muscle of the esophagus terminate in the medial aspect of the nucleus tractus solitarius.

At the proximal part of the esophagus, the pharyngeal—esophageal junction, the efferent innervation is supplied with fibers from the recurrent laryngeal nerves. These nerves originate from the vagus nerve curving backward and upward around the subclavian artery on the right side, around the aortic arch on the left side. The nerves travel in the groove between the trachea and the esophagus, giving off esophageal branches that participate in the esophageal plexus. The parasympathetic efferent fibers regulate the activity of the esophageal muscle by increasing the peristalsis, decreasing the pressure in the LES, and increasing the secretory activity.[1]

PHYSIOLOGY AND FUNCTION IN SWALLOWING

The coordinated activity of the UES, the esophageal body, and the LES is responsible for the motor function of the esophagus and the delivery of the bolus from the pharynx to the stomach. The UES receives motor innervation directly from the nucleus ambiguus. The sphincter is tonically contracted at rest and prevents passage of air from the pharynx into the esophagus as well as esophagopharyngeal reflux. During a swallow, the tongue and IPC move a bolus through the pharynx, which contracts while the UES relaxes. In addition to the biomechanical forces involved in opening the UES, relaxation of the CP muscle facilitates UES opening.[3] Relaxation lasts for approximately 0.5—1.2 s,[4] just enough time for the food to pass through the UES into the esophagus.

Once the bolus has successfully entered the esophagus, the CP muscle returns to its contracted state, thereby sealing off the esophagus and preventing any retrograde bolus entry into the hypopharynx. At that point, esophageal peristalsis begins, and the bolus is propelled toward the LES and stomach.[5] This esophageal peristaltic wave travels inferiorly at a rate of 3—4 cm/s at amplitudes of 60—140 mmHg and sequentially squeezes the bolus through the esophagus toward the stomach. This is called *primary peristalsis*. Transit times during the phase vary with age, bolus size, and bolus texture. However, in healthy adults, esophageal transit times should be between 8 and 13 s.[6]

Several secondary peristaltic waves may occur up to an hour after the swallow. The aim of *secondary peristalsis* is to improve esophageal emptying when the lumen is not completely cleared of ingested food by the primary peristalsis, or when gastric contents reflux into the esophagus. Secondary peristalsis is not accompanied by UES relaxation. *Tertiary waves* are nonpropulsive contractions. They are considered abnormal and are frequently diagnosed in asymptomatic elderly people or in patients with esophageal motility disorders.

Approximately 0.5—1.4 s after the hypopharyngeal pressure peaks, the LES is triggered to relax.[7] The primary function of the LES is to prevent reflux of gastric contents into the esophagus. The LES is 3—4 cm long. Its pressure profile, as determined through manometry, is asymmetric, and the resting pressure ranges from 15 to 35 mmHg. When a swallow occurs, the LES relaxes for 5—10 s to allow the bolus to enter the stomach, and then it returns to its resting tone. LES relaxation is mediated by nonadrenergic, noncholinergic neurotransmitters, such as vasoactive intestinal peptide and NO. The resting tone depends on the intrinsic myogenic activity. During fasting, the LES experiences cyclic phasic contractile activity. The LES also has periodic relaxations independent of swallowing called *transient lower esophageal sphincter relaxations*. The cause of these relaxations is unknown, but they are thought to be triggered by gastric distention. They are responsible for physiologic gastroesophageal reflux. When they occur too frequently or for too long a duration, this can result in gastroesophageal reflux disease (GERD). Decreased LES length or pressure can also be responsible for pathologic reflux in patients with GERD. The crus of the diaphragm at the level of the esophageal hiatus also contributes to the LES resting pressure. The pinching action of the diaphragm protects against reflux caused by a sudden increase in intraabdominal pressure. In a sliding hiatal hernia, this protective measure is lost, when the GEJ is located above the diaphragm.

CONCLUSIONS

The esophagus is a conduit for the transport of all oral intake from the pharynx through the thoracic cavity to the stomach. While it does not have any absorptive functions, normal actions of its upper and lower sphincters and propulsive motor function are essential for normal swallowing. Structural and functional aberrations of the esophagus may occur, both congenital and acquired, and result in dysphagia.

REFERENCES

1. Gray H, Williams PL, Bannister LH. *Gray's Anatomy: The Anatomical Basis of Medicine and Surgery*. New York: Churchill Livingstone; 1995.
2. Kumoi K, Ohtsuki N, Teramoto Y. Pharyngo-esophageal diverticulum arising from Laimer's triangle. *Eur Arch Otorhinolaryngol*. 2001;258:184−187.
3. Ertekin C, Aydogdu I. Electromyography of human cricopharyngeal muscle of the upper esophageal sphincter. *Muscle Nerve*. 2002;26:729−739.
4. Ingelfinger FJ. Esophageal motility. *Physiol Rev*. 1958;38:533−584.
5. Miller AJ. Swallowing: neurophysiologic control of the esophageal phase. *Dysphagia*. 1987;2:72−82.
6. De Vincentis N, Lenti R, Pona C, et al. Scintigraphic evaluation of the esophageal transit time for the noninvasive assessment of esophageal motor disorders. *J Nucl Med Allied Sci*. 1984;28:137−142.
7. Holloway RH, Penagini R, Ireland AC. Criteria for objective definition of transient lower esophageal sphincter relaxation. *Am J Physiol*. 1995;268:G128−G133.

CHAPTER 7

Dysphagia Evaluation

DINESH K. CHHETRI, MD • KARUNA DEWAN, MD

INTRODUCTION

What is the purpose of dysphagia evaluation? First, the clinician must gain an understanding of the nature of the swallowing problem and how it affects the patient's daily function and quality of life. Second, the patient's subjective symptoms should be evaluated and corroborated objectively with physical exam and appropriate swallow tests. Third, based on the combination of history, physical exam, and swallow tests, the anatomic and physiologic causes of dysphagia should be determined. Finally, treatment plans are developed that address the following: what diet should the patient be on right now? What are the medical or surgical options to improve the swallowing dysfunction? What are the risks and benefits of the proposed treatment approach? What is the expected course of dysphagia if no intervention is offered?

Most patients with dysphagia require an "instrumental swallow exam" to fully characterize the swallow dysfunction. Instrumental swallow exams such as flexible endoscopic evaluation of swallowing (FEES; see Chapter 8) and modified barium swallow study (MBSS; see Chapter 10) visualize the swallowing anatomy and function and provide objective, semiquantifiable assessments of swallow function. Instrumental exams are distinguished from noninstrumental exams such as the bedside clinical swallow evaluation.

Clinical swallow evaluation is a cognitive and behavioral screening assessment of dysphagia designed to answer the following questions *without* visualization of swallowing anatomy and function: (1) does the patient appear safe for oral intake, and if so what diet, and (2) is an instrumental assessment indicated, and if so, which one? A screening examination is performed of oral structural integrity, cranial nerve function, and trial swallowing. Six clinical features are assessed: dysphonia, dysarthria, abnormal volitional cough,

abnormal gag reflex, cough on trial swallow, and voice change on trial swallow. The clinical swallow assessment is considered a weak test because it can miss silent aspiration, a condition where aspiration does not elicit a cough.[1] Nevertheless, it has its role as a quick screening tool because the presence of any two of the six clinical features has a 92% accuracy in predicting risk for aspiration.[2]

In addition to FEES and MBSS, which primarily focus on the oropharyngeal swallow, other tests of swallowing function have unique roles in evaluation of esophageal dysphagia. These tests include transnasal esophagoscopy (TNE; see Chapter 9), barium esophagram (see Chapter 11), and high-resolution manometry of the esophagus (see Chapter 12).

HISTORY TAKING

Obtaining details of the symptoms and conditions affecting the patient is the cornerstone of all medical encounters. It sets the tone and the agenda for the patient-physician partnership. The primary objective is to discover the details about the patient's concerns, display genuine interest and curiosity, explore expectations of the clinical encounter and treatment goals, and develop a mutually agreeable plan toward evaluation and treatment of dysphagia.

A chronological history of dysphagia is generally useful. Was there a particular event such as surgery or stroke that precipitated the dysphagia? The duration of dysphagia, acute versus chronic, should be documented as it is relevant to the etiologies, treatment, prognosis, as well as expectations for response to treatment. How has dysphagia evolved over time? What is the current diet? Is the swallowing difficulty to solids, liquids, or both? If patient is Nil Oer Os (NPO) and has a gastric tube (G-tube), what is the duration of the G-tube and when was it placed in relation to the disease process that caused dysphagia (e.g., in a patient with history of head and neck cancer treatment, what was the timing of G-tube placement in regard to chemoradiation therapy?).

Some patients have difficulty describing their dysphagia symptoms and directed question can be asked: what food do you avoid? Is the swallowing problem constant or intermittent? Has the weight been stable? Is there a history of pneumonia, if so when was the last episode? How long does it take to eat meals? Is there pain with swallowing and if so where is it located?

Patients can often point to the location of dysphagia that can guide the clinical focus of examinations. For example, if dysphagia is felt in the chest area, then esophageal dysphagia is likely. Associated dysphagia symptoms such as coughing, nasal regurgitation, drooling, and odynophagia should be documented. Other important coincident and serious symptoms include difficulty in breathing and changes in voice quality. A validated dysphagia questionnaire should also be administered at each visit to document and follow up patient-reported dysphagia outcomes before and after intervention.

After a focused dysphagia history is obtained, all other pertinent medical and surgical history that could contribute to dysphagia should be documented. History of stroke, other neuropathies or neurodegenerative disease, myopathies and muscular dystrophy, head and neck surgery, congenital defects involving the head and neck, and recent endotracheal intubation are all relevant. Neurodegenerative diseases such as Parkinson's disease and amyotrophic lateral sclerosis cause varied degrees of dysphagia. There are many systemic conditions that may contribute to dysphagia. These include scleroderma, autoimmune diseases, and Sjogren's disease. Common iatrogenic etiologies of dysphagia include history of radiation therapy and cervical spine surgery. Dental issues, tobacco use, and alcohol use are documented. Medications can cause dysphagia by decreasing salivation. These include anticholinergics, diuretics, antihypertensive, antihistamines, antispasmodics, antidepressants, and tranquilizers. It is important to carefully review the patient's medication list for these and other mediations that may cause dysphagia.

PHYSICAL EXAMINATION

Dysphagia evaluation requires systematic assessment of the entire swallowing apparatus from the lips to the stomach. Physical examination of the patient with dysphagia thus begins with inspection of the lips and oral cavity and may end with an endoscopic assessment all the way to the gastroesophageal junction.

A general otolaryngologic examination is performed first with particular attention to swallowing structures. The clinician should stand directly in front of the seated patient and use a headlight or head-mounted reflective mirror so that both hands are free to examine the mouth and oral cavity. Facial nerve function, especially the ability to purse/pucker the lips and close the mouth to prevent leakage of food and saliva, is assessed. Have the patient open the mouth to check for trismus. The distance between the incisors should be about 35 mm or accommodate about three fingerbreadths. Next, inspect the teeth for occlusion, dental condition, and signs of jaw osteoradionecrosis in patients with a history of radiation therapy. Poorly fitting dentures can affect mastication and should be checked.

Oral cavity exam should proceed to visualization and palpation of the buccal mucosa, tongue, and floor of the mouth. Look for mucosal ulcerations, leukoplakia, and other masses. Bimanual palpation of the floor of the mouth and tongue base is often needed to detect lesions in these areas. Tongue function is assessed by asking the patient to protrude the tongue out of the oral cavity. Deviation of the tongue from midline during protrusion implicates hypoglossal nerve (CN XII) palsy. The tongue deviates ipsilateral to the side of CN XII palsy because the normal contralateral hemitongue "pushes" the paralyzed tongue toward the side of the lesion. The dorsal tongue musculature is also observed for fasciculations, which is generally a sign of motor neuron disease such as amyotrophic lateral sclerosis.

Salivary gland function can be inspected while examining the oral cavity as well. The ductal orifices of the parotid glands and the submandibular glands should be visualized. The condition of the papillae should be inspected including salivary flow from the ducts as the saliva glands are gently massaged.

To visualize the palate and the oropharynx adequately, the examiner must utilize a tongue depressor such as a wooden tongue blade. The patient is asked to open the mouth widely and breathe through the mouth. The tongue may be gently protruded but often leaving the tongue in the mouth and gently pressing the ventral tongue with tongue blades provides better visibility. Here again, use of a headlight frees the two hands for inspection with a tongue blade in each hand. The tongue blade should be placed around the middle third of the tongue. If the tongue depressor is placed too anteriorly, the tongue base will mound up, and if placed too posteriorly, the gag reflex may be stimulated, and both of these events will make it difficult to inspect the oropharynx. If there is history of tongue surgery then the extent of resection must be noted.

The palatine tonsils are inspected and their size documented. The posterior pharyngeal wall is examined for discharge, masses, ulcerations, and signs of infection. Palatal and velopharyngeal examination should focus on defects, symmetric elevation, and adequate velopharyngeal closure. Palatal elevation is noted as the patient phonates an "ah." The gag reflex is tested by gently touching the tongue base or the tonsillar arches. Velopharyngeal sufficiency (VPI) can be assessed by asking the patient to alternately say "bye bye" and "my my." Both utterances will sound nasal (i.e., "my my") if VPI is significant. In addition to oropharyngeal examination, nasopharyngeal endoscopy is also very useful to assess velopharyngeal closure.

The external neck should be inspected for any scars indicating previous surgical procedures or tracheostomy placement. In addition, any lymphadenopathy, enlargement of the thyroid gland, and deviation of the trachea are noted. The neck should be examined for suppleness, especially in those with a history of surgery or radiation therapy. Hyolaryngeal excursion during swallow should be palpated.

INSTRUMENTAL EXAMS

An instrumental exam of swallowing is essential to fully evaluate swallowing dysfunction. These tests are covered in detail in the following chapters of this book and will be mentioned only briefly here. Often, several instrumental exams are needed to fully assess the entire swallow anatomy and physiology.

The otolaryngologist has many options for instrumental assessment of swallowing. The typical office or clinic has video laryngoscopy readily available. A transnasal flexible laryngoscopy is necessary to leisurely examine the swallowing anatomy and function. The video laryngoscope can be easily adapted to perform FEES. FEES is the first swallow test to be performed in the office setting and immediately answers the following important questions: what are the anatomic and functional deviations contributing to dysphagia (scars, stenosis, masses, vocal fold paralysis, etc.), how severe is the dysphagia, and what is being swallowed safely? If FEES is normal but the patient has significant dysphagia complaints then dysphagia symptoms arise from elsewhere, typically the esophagus.

FEES has advantages of revealing anatomic details of pharyngeal swallowing apparatus and is invaluable for initial assessment and follow-up. Often, this is the only test that is needed to determine if the patient is currently on a safe diet. An MBSS can be subsequently obtained to assess UES function, swallow efficiency and safety, and overall coordination and efficiency of swallowing.

An office TNE is indicated if oropharyngeal swallow is normal on FEES but patient reports a strong dysphagia history, especially if pointing toward the sternal area or chest area as the site of dysphagia. Patients with severe pooling of secretions in the piriform sinuses or on G-tube feeding should also have a TNE performed to evaluate for stricture. Other situations where TNE is helpful is in patients with heartburn, regurgitation, or suggestion of a stricture on esophagram or MBSS.

High-resolution manometry and barium esophagram are ordered as indicated based on the initial findings. For example, if esophageal dysmotility is suspected, then high-resolution esophageal manometry or esophagram may reveal the functional nature and severity of disorder.

CONCLUSIONS

The overall goals of dysphagia evaluation are to evaluate the anatomy and physiology of swallowing and determine the dysfunctions contributing to dysphagia symptoms. Swallowing starts at the lips and ends in the stomach. Thus, the dysphagia clinician should approach assessment in a systematic fashion starting from the lips and ending at the lower esophageal sphincter. A combination of history and physical exam, and endoscopic, radiologic, and manometric evaluations of swallowing are required to generate a complete picture of swallowing dysfunction and the optimal individualized treatment plan. The subsequent chapters of this book will describe these tests of swallowing function in great detail.

REFERENCES

1. Smith CH, Logemann JA, Colangelo LA, Rademaker AW, Pauloski BR. Incidence and patient characteristics associated with silent aspiration in the acute care setting. *Dysphagia*. Winter; 1999;14(1):1—7.
2. Daniels SK, Brailey K, Priestly DH, Herrington LR, Weisberg LA, Foundas AL. Aspiration in patients with acute stroke. *Arch Phys Med Rehabil*. 1998;79(1):14—19.

CHAPTER 8

Flexible Endoscopic Evaluation of Swallowing

DINESH K. CHHETRI, MD • KARUNA DEWAN, MD

INTRODUCTION

Most individuals with dysphagia symptoms require an instrumental assessment to understand the specific nature of their swallowing problem. Understanding the underlying anatomic and physiologic etiology for dysphagia allows clinicians to make appropriate rehabilitation and/or management recommendations. The flexible endoscopic evaluation of swallowing (FEES) was introduced in the late 1980s to detect aspiration and to determine the safety of oral feeding in patients for whom the traditional videofluoroscopic evaluation may be difficult or impossible to perform.[1] FEES is an instrumental test for swallowing assessment that combines the traditional transnasal flexible laryngoscopy, to visualize the pharyngeal and laryngeal anatomy, while feeding food boluses of various consistencies, to assess the dynamics and safety of swallow function. The equipment to perform this test is routinely available in the otolaryngologists' office. Like the modified barium swallow study (MBSS), FEES can be used to assess swallow function and response to compensatory techniques for swallowing, and to recommend a safe diet. It has the following main advantages over the limitations of the MBSS: (1) no need for fluoroscopy or the radiology suite, (2) ability to be performed at the hospital bedside or in the clinic or office-based outpatient setting, and (3) ability to directly visualize the anatomy of the pharyngeal swallowing mechanism with the potential to directly visualize abnormalities that may not be apparent or can only be inferred based on a radiologic test.

The precursor to FEES was the MBSS, a videofluoroscopic swallow evaluation technique (see Chapter 10). MBSS has traditionally been performed in the fluoroscopy suites in radiology departments of large, tertiary care hospitals. Prior to FEES, the bedside clinical swallow evaluation, a noninstrumental assessment, was typically performed in smaller hospitals, outpatient clinics, and in nursing homes due to lack of videofluoroscopic equipment to perform swallow study. The disadvantage of relying just on bedside clinical evaluation is that not only the specific details of the swallowing dysfunction remain unclear but also silent aspiration is missed. Logemann et al. reported that nearly 40% of patients who silently aspirated may be missed by clinical swallow evaluation alone.[2] Even in hospitals where videofluoroscopic equipment is available, patients and circumstances preclude access to the videofluoroscopic suite. These situations include patients who may not be moved from the intensive care unit or those who cannot be adequately positioned sitting upright for the MBSS. On the other hand, FEES can be performed expeditiously in the outpatient or office-based setting, not only saving the patient the scheduling and wait required for MBSS but also providing an immediate answer to the swallow dysfunction present and the safety of a per oral diet. Thus, FEES has become a game changer in the ability of the otolaryngologist to assess the etiology and severity of swallow dysfunction and to develop a dysphagia practice. Comparison of the advantages and disadvantages of FEES versus MBSS are listed in Table 8.1.

While the focus of FEES is primarily limited to the pharyngeal phase of swallowing, pharyngeal dysfunction is the most important predictor for aspiration and thus the most critical phase to evaluate.[3] The most important information provided by FEES are (1) delay of swallowing initiation, (2) pharyngeal residue, (3) laryngeal penetration, and (4) aspiration. FEES is at least or more sensitive than MBSS for these four swallowing variables.[4,5] The food used in FEES can be mixed with food dye to provide contrast against the mucosa of the pharynx and larynx and improve visualization of pharyngeal residue, penetration, and aspiration.

TABLE 8.1
Comparison of the Advantages and Disadvantages of Flexible Endoscopic Evaluation of Swallowing (FEES) Versus Modified Barium Swallow Study (MBSS)

FEES	MBSS
No radiation (videoendoscopic procedure)	Radiation (videofluoroscopic procedure)
Test time limited only by tolerance to endoscope	Test time limited due to radiation exposure
Can't see oral cavity; can see the pharynx before and after the swallow but not during swallow	Can see the entire oropharyngeal swallow and the UES region; aspiration is easy to see
Superior to inferior view	Lateral and anteroposterior view
Can miss trace aspiration through posterior larynx	Can see all aspiration (but may be less sensitive)
FEES is invasive (endoscope)	MBSS is non-invasive (no endoscope)
Can be done at bedside or in clinic	Must be done in radiology suite
Patient does not have to sit up	Better if the patient can sit up
Risk of epistaxis	No risk of bleeding
Accurate anatomical info for velum/pharynx/larynx	Sketchy info of anatomy of oropharyngeal structures
Can diagnose vocal fold paralysis better than MBSS	Not as easy to diagnose vocal fold paralysis
Can assess velopharyngeal closure better than MBSS	Poorer at assessing velopharyngeal closure
Endoscopy can be uncomfortable/stressful	MBSS is comfortable if the patient can sit upright
Can be recorded	Can be recorded
FEES can be used for biofeedback	MBSS is not used for biofeedback due to radiation

UES, upper esophageal sphincter.

The green dye enhances the detection of residue/penetration/aspiration during FEES quite well and is use in the authors' practice.

In light of the relationship between laryngopharyngeal sensation, dysphagia, and aspiration pneumonia, Aviv and colleagues proposed combining FEES with sensory testing (FEEST).[6] One of the shortcomings of FEES and MBSS is that they primarily analyze the motor component of swallowing and only indirectly address the sensory component. Unrecognized, or insufficiently recognized, sensory deficits in the laryngopharynx can lead to dysphagia and aspiration, as it can be surmised that without adequate sensation of the food bolus, the normal laryngopharyngeal protective reflexes will not be properly initiated, and secretions and food debris will penetrate into the endolarynx and become aspirated. In sensory testing, laryngopharyngeal sensory discrimination threshold is measured by endoscopically delivering discrete levels of air pressure stimuli to the supraglottic laryngeal mucosa and observing the pressure required for the onset of laryngeal adductor reflex (LAR). However, the use of FEEST has fallen out of favor due to concerns about poor interobserver reliability of the test.[7]

TECHNOLOGY

The specific advantages of FEES are that it can be performed at the bedside even in bedridden, medically unstable, or weak patients, without the need for transfer to a fluoroscopy suite, special positioning, or concerns for radiation exposure. The equipment is readily available in the otolaryngologist's office, and immediate assessment of swallowing and diet recommendation can be performed. The equipment includes a transnasal flexible laryngoscope and a light source to allow visualization of the swallowing anatomy and function. The patient is seated upright in an exam chair. The exam is best observed on a video monitor, thus a charge-coupled device camera attached to a fiberoptic laryngoscope or a distal chip endoscope is typically used. The video recording system is critical for review and documentation of the exam. Additional items needed are food of various consistencies and green dye. The FEES equipment can also be made portable for use in inpatient settings such as hospitals and nursing facilities by placing the equipment on a portable cart that can easily be moved from room to room. Thus, this instrumental swallow assessment may be performed virtually anywhere. In addition, the patient does not need to be fully upright for the exam, thus making FEES a more versatile swallow test compared to an MBSS.

TECHNIQUE

FEES relies on adequate endoscopic visualization of the swallowed food bolus in the oropharynx, hypopharynx, and subglottic airway to accurately assess dysphagia characteristics and safety of the oral intake. The clinician performs flexible laryngoscopy, while an assistant feeds the patient food and liquid of various consistencies and assesses the effectiveness of oropharyngeal swallowing mechanism.

Patient Positioning

Posture may have notable effects on swallowing abilities. Therefore, FEES is performed with patients in their typical eating positions. Ambulatory patients are seated upright on the exam chair. Patients on wheelchair may remain on the wheelchair. Bedridden patients are examined in the bed, but the head of the bed is elevated to at least 45 degrees. Other adjustments may be performed to replicate a sitting eating posture.

Nasal Anesthesia

The appropriateness of topical anesthetic for the nasal cavity during the procedure has been debated since the introduction of FEES. Application of topical anesthetic increases tolerance of the transnasal endoscope but concerns remain that some topical anesthetic reaches the lower pharyngeal mucosa and may reduce sensation in the oropharynx and hypopharynx during swallowing. Sider et al. noted a reduction in both the urge and ability to swallow following the application of lidocaine in the pharynx.[8] However, it is not clearly understood if there is an optimal dose of topical anesthetic that would improve patient comfort but not alter swallowing/pharyngeal sensation.[9] Studies in normal volunteers showed only occasional trace aspiration with lidocaine anesthesia of the larynx and hypopharynx[10] but no change on LAR with topical nasal anesthesia alone using 4% cocaine.[11] It is the authors' practice to judiciously apply topical nasal anesthesia for FEES. We also apply lidocaine gel lubricant to the

flexible scope to allow easy passage of the scope through the nasal cavity.

Observation of Swallowing Anatomy

The endoscope is first used to screen the patency of both nasal cavities and the more open nasal cavity is chosen to introduce the scope. The scope is passed along the floor of the nose or through the middle meatus. With the scope in the nasopharynx, the velopharyngeal closure is visualized. Phonatory maneuvers such as "bye bye" and "my my" allow assessment of velopharyngeal closure. The patient is then asked to breathe through the nose while the scope is passed into the oropharynx. The base of the tongue, epiglottis, laryngopharynx, and hypopharynx are observed for any abnormal growths or shape (e.g., scarring, edema, tumor). The location and presence of any pooling of secretions is noted in the vallecula, endolarynx, and the hypopharynx. The laterality of secretions and the degree of pooling is noted. The presence of saliva or the pooling of secretions in the pharynx almost always indicates swallow dysfunction, even in patients who do not complain of swallowing problems. Laryngeal function, especially vocal fold paresis and paralysis and glottal closure is noted. Phonation of "e" followed by the sniff maneuver is most effective for the assessment of gross laryngeal function.

Observation of Swallowing Function

Assessment of laryngopharyngeal anatomy is followed by the most important portion of the procedure, during which measured quantities of foods and liquids are given to the patient to swallow. Five-milliliter and 10-mL boluses of water and pureed consistency are fed to the patient. Solids are fed in small bites. We typically feed apple sauce to test pureed consistency and pieces of Lorna Doone cookies to test for solid food consistency. Other quantities and consistencies such as nectar thick liquids and gelcaps to test for pill dysphagia may be given, depending on the objectives of the particular exam and the patient's swallowing status.

While the clinician performs endoscopy and visualizes the swallowing, an assistant feeds the patient using a teaspoon or straw. The food and liquid are mixed with green food dye to provide adequate contrast against the mucosa. Although the sequence of food consistency tested is not fixed, we typically start with pureed consistency followed by liquid consistency, as liquids are often more difficult to swallow than pureed in the presence of laryngeal weakness. On the other hand, with pharyngeal dysfunction but intact larynx, liquids are often less difficult to swallow than pureed or solid consistency.

Each consistency is tested at least twice to test for consistency of findings. Prior to the initiation of swallow, any premature spillage of food from the oral cavity is noted. Once the oropharyngeal swallowing phase is initiated, the actual dynamics of swallowing *during the swallow* cannot be assessed by FEES because the sequential closure of the velopharynx, oropharynx, hyolaryngeal elevation, and laryngeal closure squeeze the pharyngeal lumen and obscure the endoscopic view. This brief "white out" of endoscopic visualization occurs during the height of the oropharyngeal swallow phase. Prior to the "white out" on FEES, the posterior motion of the tongue base and inward movement of the lateral pharyngeal walls can be visualized on a normal examination. However, during the white out period, the retraction of the tongue, contraction of the pharyngeal walls, elevation of the larynx, and opening of the upper esophageal sphincter (UES) cannot be seen. Thus, the assessment of swallowing efficacy and safety is based on the clearance (or presence of residue) of food from the pharyngeal cavity as observed *after the swallow*. On the other hand, the lack of this white out signifies significant pharyngeal weakness and swallow dysfunction.

The video recording of the entire exam allows closer review of the exam. The exam can also be reviewed in slow motion for more detailed analysis. Still images of relevant findings are taken for documentation. The video and the stills may also be reviewed with the patient for education and demonstration. Assessments before the swallow include premature spillage, oral bolus control, penetration, and aspiration before the swallow. Assessments after the swallow include vallecular residue, piriform sinus residue, laryngeal penetration, and aspiration. These findings are reported in a semiquantitative manner. The patient's response to penetration and aspiration is also noted (cough, repeat swallow, throat clearing, ejection, and clearance of aspirated food, etc.). The exam is continued until all boluses have been assessed or significant aspiration occurs. If significant aspiration occurs during the examination, the patient is asked to hock and spit out the aspirated material and the test aborted. If a patient is not aspirating but has other notable findings such as excessive pharyngeal residue, minimal alertness, or premature spilling, the examination will continue to determine the patient's swallowing safety. Patients with

significant pharyngeal residue should be observed continuously for 1–2 min after the swallow to document any potential spillage into the laryngeal ventricle, penetration, or aspiration.

Pharyngeal residue, defined as preswallow secretions and postswallow food residue in the pharynx not entirely cleared by a swallow, is a clinical predictor of postswallow aspiration. Pharyngeal residue suggests an underlying impairment of oropharyngeal bolus driving forces and reduced swallowing efficiency. Clinical judgments of how efficiently the swallow mechanism moves the bolus through the pharynx and of aspiration risk are influenced by pharyngeal residue seen during instrumental swallowing examinations like the FEES. An accurate description of pharyngeal residue severity is important but difficult clinical challenge as the depth of residue is hard to judge. Pharyngeal residue occurs most commonly in either the vallecula or the pyriform sinuses. The valleculas are the spaces between the base of the tongue and the epiglottis. The pyriform sinuses are the hypopharyngeal spaces bordered by thyroid cartilage laterally and post-cricoid area medially.

Pharyngeal residue can also occur in a variety of areas including the lateral channels, epiglottis, pharyngeal walls, laryngeal inlet, interarytenoid space, post-cricoid region, along the true and false vocal folds, and laryngeal surface of the aryepiglottic folds. Since pharyngeal residue is an important predictor of swallowing success, it is important to ascertain residue severity in the valleculae and pyriform sinuses. The presence of preswallowed pooled secretions and postswallow food residue in the laryngeal vestibule is an important sign of dysphagia severity.

Assessment of Compensatory Swallowing Techniques

Another notable advantage of the FEES as compared to MBSS is the ability to try compensatory mechanisms during the test without concern for timing due to radiation exposure. The clinician can provide real-time feedback for the patient and determine their efficiency for remediation purposes. Postural changes that alter the pharyngeal dimensions or gravity's impact on bolus movement include the chin tuck, head rotation, and head tilt. Therapeutic swallow maneuvers can also be employed to improve airway protection, increase laryngeal elevation, and increase pharyngeal peristalsis. These maneuvers include supraglottic swallow, super-supraglottic swallow, effortful swallow, and Mendelsohn maneuver (see Chapter 24). These can all be employed with the transnasal flexible laryngoscope in place. Repeated boluses of various food consistencies can be administered. However, because FEES does not provide quantitative assessment of aspiration and airway clearance as it only provides limited view of the subglottic airway, certain swallow maneuvers (such as the "chug-a-lug") that require clear assessment of the degree of aspiration and the ability to clear the aspiration after the swallow are best assessed with MBSS rather than FEES.

The FEES procedure may be contraindicated for some patients who are extremely agitated. On rare occasions, patients do not tolerate the introduction of the endoscope or the amount of pharyngeal secretions makes it impossible to reliably perform the swallow assessment. It is an excellent adjunct to the MBSS and is the method of choice for many patients when prompt, reliable information is needed to assess for the presence of oropharyngeal swallowing dysfunction and to recommend a safe diet.

COMMON FINDINGS

Premature Spillage

Before the swallow, the tip of the endoscope remains at the level of the palate so the vallecula is visible to detect premature spillage: food and liquid falling and spilling into the vallecula and piriform sinus from the oral cavity with delayed onset of oropharyngeal swallow. An impression of the efficiency of the oral phase swallow can be made while waiting for the bolus to arrive at the pharynx. Watch for penetration and aspiration (Fig. 8.1).

Vallecular Residue

Food residue remaining in the valleculae, between the tongue base and epiglottis, after the swallow. Isolated finding signifies pharyngeal weakness and/or epiglottic dysfunction. Can also often be seen after anterior neck surgery (e.g., thyroidectomy and radioactive iodine therapy), anterior cervical spine surgery, and postradiation therapy for head and neck cancer (Fig. 8.2).

Piriform Sinus Residue

Food residue in the post-cricoid and piriform sinus (Fig. 8.3) after the swallow is seen with UES dysfunction (Fig. 8.4). However, pharyngeal weakness contributes to this as well. Occasionally, this residue is actually vallecular residue that falls to the piriform sinus during or just at the end of the "white-out" period and may not be apparent on FEES.

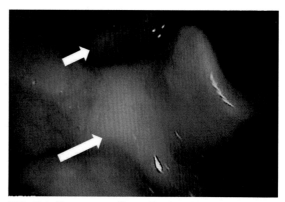

FIG. 8.1 Premature spillage. Food and liquid has entered and is filling the vallecula and piriform sinus (arrows), but the oropharyngeal swallow phase has not been triggered yet.

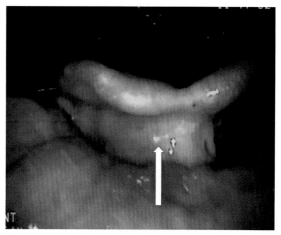

FIG. 8.2 Vallecular residue (arrow). Residue remains in the vallecular space between the base of the tongue and the epiglottis after the swallow (arrow).

Nasal Regurgitation

Nasal regurgitation is typically due to velopharyngeal insufficiency and/or distal obstruction such as epiglottic dysfunction and occasionally UES dysfunction.

Combined Vallecular and Piriform Sinus Residue

Residue in both the vallecula and piriform sinus indicates a more severe swallowing dysfunction due to combined pharyngeal weakness and obstruction. Typical clinical scenarios include history of chemoradiation therapy for pharyngeal cancer, tight upper esophageal stenosis, or severe pharyngeal weakness due to

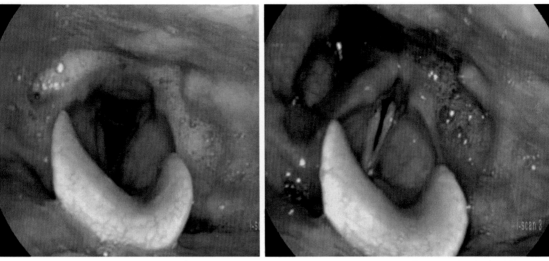

FIG. 8.3 Piriform sinus residue. Secretions in the oropharynx are highly predictive of swallowing dysfunction. Pooling of saliva is seen prior to feeding (*left panel*). Piriform sinus residue collects during flexible endoscopic evaluation of swallowing (*right panel*).

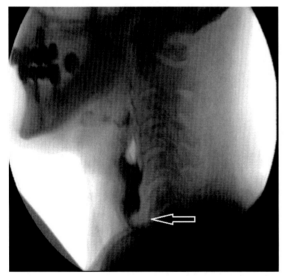

FIG. 8.4 A modified barium swallow study from the patient in Fig. 8.3 demonstrates upper esophageal sphincter dysfunction as the cause of piriform sinus pooling and residue (*arrow*).

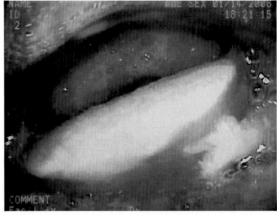

FIG. 8.5 Combined vallecular and piriform sinus residue is seen in this patient from complications of radiation therapy for oropharyngeal cancer. The severe dysfunction was due to a tight esophageal stricture. The epiglottis is also thickened and does not evert during swallowing.

neurologic dysphagia (e.g., oculopharyngeal muscular dystrophy) (Fig. 8.5).

Penetration

Penetration is defined as food or liquid bolus entering the endolarynx but not extending below the glottic level. Penetration can be mild (just entering the endolarynx but staying above the false vocal folds), moderate (extending up to the false vocal folds), or severe (extending up to the true vocal folds). Penetration signifies laryngeal incompetence due to weak, absent, or dysfunctional laryngeal valving mechanism (Fig. 8.6).

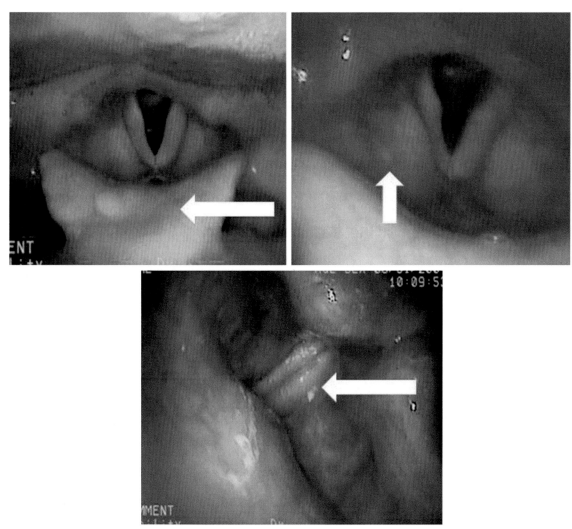

FIG. 8.6 Penetration. Various levels of residue in the larynx are seen after the swallow (arrows). Mild, just entering the endolarynx (*top left panel*); moderate, to the level of the false vocal folds (*top middle panel*); and severe, to the true vocal folds (*bottom panel*).

Aspiration

Aspiration is defined as food or liquid entering the subglottis and below into the trachea. It signifies severe laryngeal incompetence, and typically accompanies significant pharyngeal weakness and/or sensory deficit. Aspiration down the posterior wall of the trachea can be missed on FEES.

Esophagopharyngeal reflux

Previously swallowed food from the pharynx to the esophagus refluxing back to the pharynx is termed esophagopharyngeal reflux (EPR). This is typically seen with a Zenker's diverticulum (ZD). However, this may also occur with severe mid-to-distal esophageal stenosis or esophageal dysmotility. The EPR

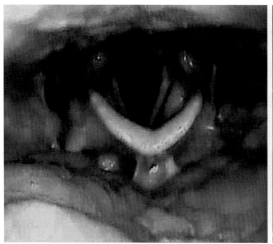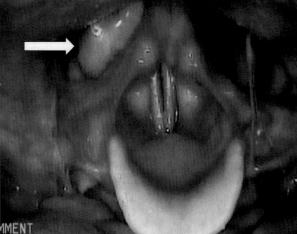

FIG. 8.7 Esophagopharyngeal reflux (EPR). *Left panel* shows findings immediately after the oropharyngeal swallow. The patient is subsequently asked to phonate, and food regurgitates in the right piriform sinus (*arrow*) during phonation (right panel). This is a typical finding in Zenker's diverticulum. EPR may also be elicited by pressing the lower neck around the site of the diverticulum.

associated with ZD is a "slow ooze" compared to "fast regurgitation" associated with the latter entities (Fig. 8.7).

SUMMARY

FEES has resulted in a paradigm shift in dysphagia management for the otolaryngologist. The otolaryngologist now has an excellent instrumental exam to assess the patient with dysphagia at the same clinic or office visit. The advantage to FEES is that it provides direct endoscopic visualization of the swallowing anatomy and function. Most studies have found FEES an equivalent, if not better, test than the MBSS for assessment of pharyngeal swallowing.[12-15] In reality, FEES and MBSS are complementary tests. Oral and esophageal phases are best assessed using MBSS. However, FEES will remain an important part of our armamentarium in the evaluation of dysphagia.

REFERENCES

1. Langmore SE. History of fiberoptic endoscopic evaluation of swallowing for evaluation and management of pharyngeal dysphagia: changes over the years. *Dysphagia*. 2017; 32:27–38.
2. Logemann JA, Rademaker AW, Pauloski BR, Ohmae Y, Kahrilas PJ. Normal swallowing physiology as viewed by videofluoroscopy and videoendoscopy. *Folia Phoniatr Logop*. 1998;50:311–319.
3. Ramsey D, Smithard D, Kalra L. Silent aspiration: what do we know? *Dysphagia*. 2005;20:218–225.
4. Park WY, Lee TH, Ham NS, et al. Adding endoscopist-directed flexible endoscopic evaluation of swallowing to the videofluoroscopic swallowing study increased the detection rates of penetration, aspiration, and pharyngeal residue. *Gut Liver*. 2015;9:623–628.
5. Kelly AM, Leslie P, Beale T, Payten C, Drinnan MJ. Fibreoptic endoscopic evaluation of swallowing and videofluoroscopy: does examination type influence perception of pharyngeal residue severity? *Clin Otolaryngol*. 2006;31:425–432.
6. Aviv JE, Kim T, Sacco RL, et al. FEESST: a new bedside endoscopic test of the motor and sensory components of swallowing. *Ann Otol Rhinol Laryngol*. 1998;107:378–387.
7. Cunningham JJ, Halum SL, Butler SG, Postma GN. Intraobserver and interobserver reliability in laryngopharyngeal sensory discrimination thresholds: a pilot study. *Ann Otol Rhinol Laryngol*. 2007;116:582–588.
8. Sider L, Mintzer RA, Deschler TW, Kim KS, Weinberg PE. Control of swallowing by use of topical anesthesia during digital subtraction angiography. *Radiology*. 1983;148:563–564.
9. O'Dea MB, Langmore SE, Krisciunas GP, et al. Effect of lidocaine on swallowing during FEES in patients with dysphagia. *Ann Otol Rhinol Laryngol*. 2015;124:537–544.

10. Bastian RW, Riggs LC. Role of sensation in swallowing function. *Laryngoscope.* 1999;109:1974–1977.

11. Johnson PE, Belafsky PC, Postma GN. Topical nasal anesthesia for transnasal fiberoptic laryngoscopy: a prospective, double-blind, cross-over study. *Otolaryngol Head Neck Surg.* 2003;128:452–454.

12. Brady S, Donzelli J. The modified barium swallow and the functional endoscopic evaluation of swallowing. *Otolaryngol Clin N Am.* 2013;46:1009–1022.

13. Leder SB, Sasaki CT, Burrell MI. Fiberoptic endoscopic evaluation of dysphagia to identify silent aspiration. *Dysphagia.* 1998;13:19–21.

14. Lim SH, Lieu PK, Phua SY, et al. Accuracy of bedside clinical methods compared with fiberoptic endoscopic examination of swallowing (FEES) in determining the risk of aspiration in acute stroke patients. *Dysphagia.* 2001;16:1–6.

15. Wu CH, Hsiao TY, Chen JC, Chang YC, Lee SY. Evaluation of swallowing safety with fiberoptic endoscope: comparison with videofluoroscopic technique. *Laryngoscope.* 1997;107:396–401.

CHAPTER 9

Transnasal Esophagoscopy

JACQUELINE ALLEN, MBCHB, FRACS ORL HNS

INTRODUCTION

As dysphagia is a symptom, it requires investigation to identify the cause and contributing factors. Causes for swallowing impairment may be considered by anatomic site of impairment, e.g., oropharyngeal versus esophageal, or by etiology, e.g., mechanical versus functional. In many cases, there is a combination of factors contributing to swallowing dysfunction and each must be identified and addressed to achieve the best possible outcomes. A multidisciplinary team (MDT) approach, therefore, enables contribution from several clinicians and promotes coordinated care that may include anything from dental remediation to exercise therapy or compensatory maneuvres, through to medical treatments or surgical procedures. Functional assessment offers the best chance of identifying real-life deficits and developing strategies that may be employed to assist with symptomatic swallow dysfunction. The more closely the assessment resembles real-life situations of ingesting food or fluid, the more tailored recommendations we can make.

History and examination are crucial and will quickly suggest potential pathologies related to the presenting complaint. Complete examination and assessment though requires visualization of the lumen and intraluminal structures of the pharyngolarynx and esophagus. To do this, specialized tools are needed. Whilst imaging provides excellent dynamic information as well as some structural information, it is endoscopy that allows us to establish sided-ness, reveals mucosal abnormalities (including malignancy), and detects subtle rings, strictures, and sphincter dysfunction. Endoscopic techniques have developed radically over the last 20 years with the advent of microchip technology and narrow caliber endoscopes. This has afforded us better access to the aerodigestive tract than ever before. Couple this with a magnified view, a working channel, and recording software, and we now have the ability to undertake diagnostic and therapeutic procedures in a single sitting. Even more important, most of these procedures may be undertaken using local anesthetic alone in the clinic, obviating the need for general anesthesia and its concomitant risks, particularly in the older adult population. Transnasal esophagoscopy (TNE) has developed in this setting[1] and provides the clinician with the ability to evaluate the larynx and pharynx as might be undertaken with a small flexible transnasal endoscope, but in addition, the channeled, longer flexible esophagoscope also enables examination of the esophagus and stomach (through insufflation), plus procedural intervention to occur such as biopsy, injection, laser application, or balloon dilatation. Now the otolaryngologist can truly evaluate the whole upper aerodigestive tract in the office!

In addition to the clinical advantages that channeled endoscopy offers us in management of aerodigestive tract and pharyngolaryngeal disease, there are also societal benefits through better resource utilization. As the bulk of transnasal endoscopic evaluations can be performed under local anesthesia alone, they are short, are less costly, and enable easier screening of disorders. This approach has now begun to change treatment paradigms in some disorders, e.g., recurrent respiratory papillomatosis, where earlier treatment of lesser disease bulk is possible without resecting tissue, risking voice damage, and with avoidance of multiple general anesthetics. Better for the patient, and faster and cheaper for the service.

We are now able to push further the utility and applicability of this approach to perform panendoscopy in clinic; screen for metachronous or synchronous tumors; screen for Barrett's esophagus or gastroesophageal junctional carcinoma; detect and evaluate strictures (anastomotic or esophageal); screen for eosinophilic esophagitis; evaluate gastroesophageal and extraesophageal reflux; review hiatal herniae; identify extrinsic esophageal compression; detect and evaluate gastric features, including lower esophageal competence, gastritis, and gastric polyps; assist in feeding tube placement or biopsies for *Helicobacter pylori*; biopsy anywhere else in the laryngopharynx or esophagus; provide therapeutic injections, e.g., botulinum toxin, anticarcinogenic, or antiviral medications; perform laser therapies or ablations; guide and perform balloon dilation or secondary tracheoesophageal fistula punctures; and perform any number of laryngeal procedures with these maneuvrable endoscopes.

Otolaryngologists are well placed to drive this momentum. We are already facile with endoscope use and care; we understand the anatomy of the upper aerodigestive tract and can branch across what have previously been nominal anatomic boundaries, e.g., the cricopharyngeus or bronchus. In fact, collaboration between specialities is one of the greatest advantages of these tools, as all can see the utility and information that can be obtained by prudent use of these devices. In many situations, treatment of troublesome symptoms that repeatedly present across multiple specialities can be streamlined by a one-stop clinic approach. Channeled endoscopes TNE used in these settings play a central role in facilitating this process, e.g., a MDT cough clinic. Our service takes this approach providing a cough MDT with an otolaryngologist, respiratory physician, and speech language therapist for joint consultation with spirometry, lung assessment, cough reflex testing, in-office bronchoesophagoscopy, and/or biopsies undertaken at the first 45-min assessment.

This chapter will cover the technology and brief technique of TNE examination and provide illustrative cases.

TECHNOLOGY

Expansion of our ability to investigate and manage swallowing problems has been largely due to the rise of fiberoptic technology. Now with the advent of narrow-caliber endoscopes with distal chip camera technology, we have advanced the ability of endoscopists to reach internal luminal spaces through natural orifices with markedly better definition, clarity, and recording ability. Instead of traditional access per oral, with the associated gag response and risk of bite damage to the endoscopes, it is now possible to utilize the transnasal route with channeled endoscopes measuring 60–120 cm long, equipped with a working channel >2 mm, and excellent video capabilities (Fig. 9.1).

Transnasal use of ultrathin endoscopes was first reported in 2001 and again further in 2004.[1] The first large series of transnasal esophagoscopies was reported by Postma et al. in 2005, where more than 700 cases were evaluated demonstrating successful completion of the exam in 97% of the subjects.[2] Obstructive nasal anatomy or vasovagal faint response precluded

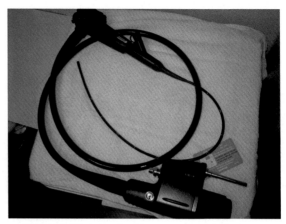

FIG. 9.1 Photograph of transnasal esophagoscope.

completion in 3% of subjects. Most common findings were esophagitis (17%), hiatal hernia (8%), Barrett's metaplasia (BM) (5%), and carcinomata (4%).[2] Accuracy of TNE has been evaluated against standard gastroscopy with equivalent results.[3–6] Similar findings were published by Howell et al., and in our own series of 570 transnasal esophagoscopies, where the completion rate was also 97% (Allen and Johnson, unpublished).

TNE has been assessed for patient tolerance too. Polat et al. evaluated patient perception of TNE, before and after the procedure, in 314 patients.[7] Whilst patients anticipated a painful procedure, their reported postprocedure discomfort scores were low.[7] The noncompletion rate was 4% with minimal complications. In a different comparison study between TNE performed by endosheath and standard per oral gastroscopy for detection of BM, there was equivalent detection of BM but slightly lower biopsy positivity using a transnasal approach.[8] However, 60% of patients preferred TNE, with only 25% preferring standard sedated endoscopy.[8] Sabirin et al. performed a systematic review of TNE and found it to be effective for screening of dysphagia, globus, reflux, and metachronous tumors.[9] A number of papers have identified several procedures suitable for performance by TNE with potential cost-saving and reduced complications.[10–17] Before a new technique is adopted, practitioners need to understand the utility and safety of the technique. Previous manuscripts have evaluated TNE against formal gastroscopy,[3,4] in terms of accuracy, tolerance, and cost.[3–5,8,9] Sensitivity and specificity have been reported as 0.98 and 1.00 when compared to standard endoscopy.[8] Unsedated TNE has also been utilized in children.[18] Friedlander et al. successfully performed 21/22

TNE examinations with biopsies unsedated in the office in children aged 8—17 years.[18]

Current endoscopes vary in caliber (3.5—5.5 mm), contain a working channel (usually around 2—2.8 mm diameter) which also allows for insufflation of air via the processing unit pump. This provides visualization within the esophagus by separating the luminal surfaces and expanding the intraluminal space. Mucosal contour can then be evaluated, as can fixed (noncompliant) or compliant restrictions or compressions. Through the working channel, biopsies may be obtained. If the system contains recording capability, then the patient may review the examination and visualize the findings with the physician. This can be hugely helpful in achieving compliance with treatment recommendations and giving reassurance in worried individuals.

When performing TNE, as with any endoscopic visualization, it is worth considering environmental factors in achieving the best view. These include low ambient light and a good-quality nonreflective screen. If affordable, use of front-to-back high-definition systems produce better images. Warming up the endoscope for 30 s prior to insertion can be useful, and defogging using heat, saliva, or antifog agent gives greater definition. The most important factor though is a relaxed and compliant patient!

TECHNIQUE

Explanation to the patient of the procedure and possible discomfort and the length of time that the procedure will likely take are very useful in achieving successful completion of the endoscopy. Preprocedure advice about breathing, along with coaching during the procedure, can also reassure the patient and focus them on breathing when the endoscope passes the upper esophageal sphincter (most gag-inducing part). Consent is obtained, and then the patient is seated comfortably in straight-back position with the head in neutral. The use of appropriate anesthetic is also crucial. We have found that swallowed lidocaine gel (2% lidocaine gel, Orion Healthcare, Auckland, New Zealand) is extremely helpful in management of gag. An assistant is required if biopsies are to be taken, as they will need to manipulate the biopsy forceps through the working channel whilst the clinician is driving the endoscope. The assistant may also act as a coach for the patient, encouraging them to use a stable breathing pattern of in through the nose and slowly out through the mouth. This tends to help control reflexive gag responses and keep the patient on board when the endoscope traverses the upper esophageal sphincter.

Technique of Flexible Transnasal Esophagoscopy

In brief, TNE is performed with the subject seated. The nose is prepared with two puffs of cophenylcaine spray (5% lidocaine and 0.5% phenylephrine, ENT Technologies, Australia) in each nostril. The subject may also be given a teaspoon (5 mL) of lidocaine gel (2% lidocaine, Orion Healthcare, NZ) to swallow prior to endoscopy. The endoscope is lubricated with aqueous gel and/or 2% lidocaine gel then advanced through the most patent nasal cavity, usually via the middle meatus. Findings are observed throughout, including nasal abnormalities, post nasal space secretions or masses, hypopharyngeal secretions (in either valleculae or piriform apices), tongue base symmetry, piriform fossae patency, mass lesions at any site, laryngeal anatomy, e.g., false vocal fold prominence, true vocal fold mobility and symmetry, mass lesions of the glottis including vocal process granulomata, and findings of laryngeal irritation (as per the reflux finding score[19]). The endoscope is then advanced through the upper esophageal sphincter in conjunction with the patient performing a hard swallow. Rapid but careful advancement of the endoscope to the gastroesophageal junction (GEJ) is performed, to limit gag sensation, with insufflation to provide circumferential views of the mucosa, GEJ, squamocolumnar junction (Fig. 9.2), and then to enter the stomach. This is evaluated in a stepwise fashion including a retroflexed view to assess the cardia region and rule out junctional malignancy. If biopsies are required, these are performed through the 2-mm working channel of the endoscope. Once gastric and GEJ examination is

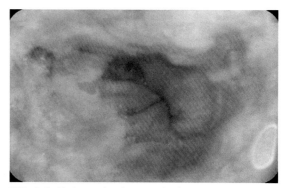

FIG. 9.2 Endoscopic photograph of the squamocolumnar junction demonstrating distinct color change from pale pink esophageal mucosa to salmon pink gastric mucosa at the Z-line. Irregular excursions of gastric mucosa can be seen at 9 o'clock.

complete, the endoscope is slowly retracted and the lumen is inspected throughout its length back to the pharynx. The view on retracting the scope is often better than the initial entry views for two reasons—the patient has usually settled down, and the endoscope tends to drift to the middle as it is retracted, and with a small amount of insufflation, good circumferential views are achieved. Be sure to look for heterotopic gastric mucosal patches in the proximal esophagus as the endoscope nears the upper sphincter. Review of the recorded procedure assists in discussion with the patient and allows the clinician to pause and review frame by frame, particularly in areas which are often passed quickly during performance of the endoscopy. Patients are usually well, following removal of the endoscope. They experience little pain and are able to drive and go home. In addition there is no restriction in diet or vocal use is placed following routine TNE.

CASE EXAMPLES
Case 1

A 56-year-old woman presents with 9 months of cough. It is nonproductive, harsh, and exaggerated, often causing a retch response. It is worse following food and positional change, and may wake her from sleep. Treatment with corticosteroid inhaler, antibiotic, proton-pump inhibitor, and antihistamines have been unhelpful. There is mild intermittent dysphonia following cough and frequent daytime throat clearing. She is a nonsmoker.

TNE performed in the office demonstrates a crowded laryngopharynx with interarytenoid edema, bilateral vocal fold edema, patchy laryngeal mucus, and bulky ventricular folds (Fig. 9.3). Esophageal mucosa was normal; however, there was a borderline hiatal hernia with a Shatzki's ring at the GEJ (Fig. 9.4). The stomach was normal except for a grade-2 flap valve on retroflexed view. Treatment advice was given as a combination of behavioral cough suppression techniques, use of alginate, reflux lifestyle modifications, and plan to perform swallowing study to rule out esophageal dysmotility.

Advantage of TNE
Having immediate feedback about her esophageal changes enabled directed treatment for these to be administered in combination with cough control advice, avoiding unnecessary acid suppression. It also

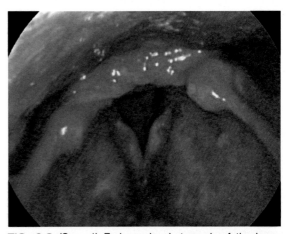

FIG. 9.3 (Case 1) Endoscopic photograph of the larynx demonstrating changes consistent with laryngopharyngeal reflux (laryngeal irritation), including a crowded laryngopharynx with interarytenoid edema, bilateral vocal fold edema, patchy laryngeal mucus, and bulky ventricular folds. These changes may also be seen in other disorders.

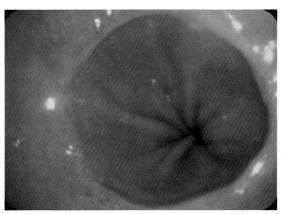

FIG. 9.4 (Case 1) Endoscopic photograph of the gastroesophageal junction illustrating a Shatzki's ring and borderline hiatal hernia with the squamocolumnar junction at the Shatzki ring.

rules out an esophageal adenocarcinoma, which has been associated with cough symptom presentations.[20]

Case 2
A 75-year-old man was treated for metastatic skin carcinoma to the parotid, with parotidectomy, neck

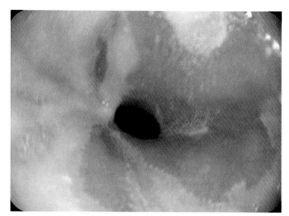

FIG. 9.5 (Case 2) Endoscopic photograph of distal esophagus with florid Barrett's metaplasia and a constricting peptic stricture.

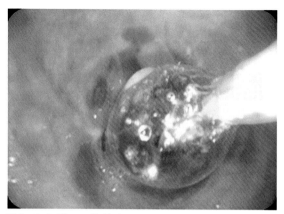

FIG. 9.6 (Case 2) Endoscopic photograph of the same peptic stricture with a controlled radial expansion balloon dilator in place.

dissection, and postoperative radiotherapy. One year later, he presented with solid food dysphagia (SFD) and 3 kg weight loss. Obvious volume deficit was present in the neck at the surgical site and postradiotherapy skin changes noted. Mild-to-moderate trismus was present. TNE demonstrated xeropharyngia, mobile but thinned vocal folds, florid long-segment BM, a peptic stricture, and large paraesophageal hernia (Fig. 9.5).

Management
Management is by biopsy of Barrett's epithelium to check for dysplasia (negative), balloon dilatation of peptic stricture (in-office, Fig. 9.6), and dietary strategies to manage SFD, plus acid suppression medication and alginate suspension.

Advantage of TNE
Avoids issues with trismus, as the flexible esophagoscope can negotiate the laryngopharynx easily; identifies source of SFD; and enables biopsies, then immediate treatment with a balloon dilator in the office, without the need for general anesthesia and without delay. TNE can also be used for long-term surveillance of the Barrett's esophagus.

Case 3
A 40-year-old man with episodes of solid food impaction and globus sensation associated with mild dyspepsia presents to clinic. He has no other medical conditions and is a nonsmoker. TNE demonstrates

trachealization of the esophageal mucosa (Fig. 9.7), and biopsy results demonstrate >50 eosinophils per high power field. This confirms a diagnosis of eosinophilic esophagitis. He is referred for food allergy testing, started on swallowed fluticasone inhaler, and screened for gluten intolerance.

Advantages of TNE
Immediate indication of disease process and biopsies taken to confirm diagnosis. No general anesthesia or sedation is needed. Upright positioning during TNE replicates normal eating position.

Case 4
A 41-year-old male in a high-stress occupation presents with dyspepsia, heartburn, regurgitation, and occasional epigastric discomfort and central chest pain. He also complains of nocturnal waking and globus sensation relieved by eating food. TNE demonstrates Grade A esophagitis (LA Grading) with Barrett's esophagus (biopsy proven) and gastritis (Figs. 9.8 and 9.9). Gastric biopsies are positive for *H. pylori*. Pharmacotherapy is given and interval surveillance endoscopy booked as per American Academy of Gastroenterologist guidelines.

Advantages of TNE
Immediate identification of esophageal and gastric pathology and thus the ability to treat with specific triple therapy regimen and plan appropriate review.

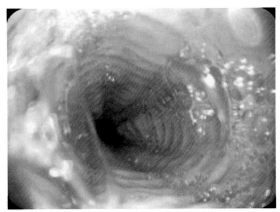

FIG. 9.7 (Case 3) Endoscopic photograph of the mid-esophagus demonstrating trachealization (or ringed appearance) of esophagus typically seen in eosinophilic esophagitis.

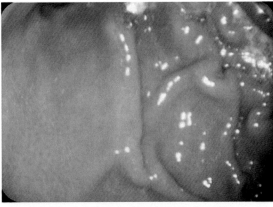

FIG. 9.9 (Case 4) Endoscopic photograph of the stomach with red speckled appearance consistent with gastritis (biopsy proven to be *Helicobacter pylori* positive).

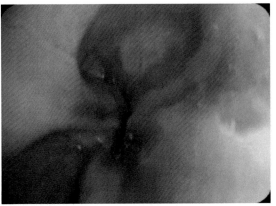

FIG. 9.8 (Case 4) Endoscopic photograph of the gastroesophageal junction (GEJ) with LA grade A esophagitis at 9 o'clock and Barrett's metaplasia around the rest of the circumference of the GEJ.

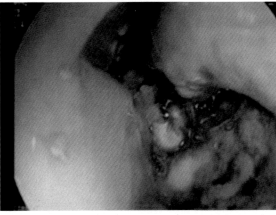

FIG. 9.10 (Case 5) Endoscopic photograph of the junction of the proximal and middle thirds of the esophagus manifesting a circumferential, irregular, ulcerated mass that was biopsy proven to be squamous cell carcinoma.

Case 5

A 60-year-old man presents with cough, regurgitation, slight weight loss (3 kg), and a nasal polyp. Biopsy of the nasal mass reveals inverting papilloma. CT scan of sinuses, neck, and chest is performed. An irregular region of contrast enhancement is identified within the esophagus. TNE demonstrates an eccentric, irregular, friable mass within the mid-esophagus, and biopsies are taken (Fig. 9.10). These are positive for squamous cell carcinoma. Further staging is undertaken and discussion at a tumor board is scheduled for definitive management planning.

Advantages of TNE

Immediate screening for metachronous tumor was undertaken, avoiding delays in diagnosis and allowing full consideration of treatment options. No general anesthesia required.

Case 6

A 45-year-old woman on long-term corticosteroid inhaler for asthma presents with solid food sticking and early satiety. Voice is intermittently dysphonic, and she is a nonsmoker. TNE demonstrates pharyngo-laryngeal and esophageal candidiasis (Fig. 9.11). Treatment is oral fluconazole for 14 days.

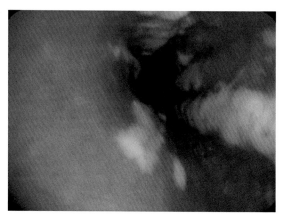

FIG. 9.11 (Case 6) Endoscopic photograph of the distal esophagus with linear tracings and white plaques of esophageal candidiasis.

Advantages of TNE

Visualization of candida affecting the larynx and esophagus, explaining symptoms, and directing therapy with antifungal medicines. Rapid diagnosis and avoidance of unnecessary tests or empiric trials of medication. Allows consideration of inhaler technique, need for a spacer device, or careful dietary probiotic therapy.

CONCLUSION

As the cost of healthcare rises and the population ages, there is a need to be able to assess and treat individuals in the most cost-effective and expedient manner. This has encouraged development of office-based techniques, which are time-saving, generally safer, and reduce overall costs to the health system. Office-based unsedated esophageal evaluation (TNE) can be performed in minutes with use of topical nasal anesthetic only, obviating the need for additional staff time, operating room support and recovery costs, and reducing overall economic burden. Otolaryngologists are required to assess the pharynx and larynx and to provide management of conditions in the head and neck. It is a natural extension for otolaryngologists to examine the esophagus in the same manner, particularly given that many esophageal pathologies contribute to pharyngeal symptoms. TNE provides views of the nasal cavity, nasopharynx, hypopharynx, larynx, esophagus, and stomach. In recent years, TNE has been adopted by otolaryngologists in some centers, but it has not become widespread. The American Bronchoesophagological Association published a position statement in 2008, in support of TNE for diagnosis.[21]

Capital expense and learning curve appear to have reduced uptake of this technique. Otolaryngologists may feel inexperienced in diagnosing esophageal pathology. However, there is much to commend TNE, particularly in light of the current health resource climate. We should encourage and embrace this tool and its use to the benefit of our patients.

REFERENCES

1. Belafsky PC, Postma GN, Daniel E, Koufman JA. Transnasal esophagoscopy. *Otolaryngol Head Neck Surg.* 2001; 125:588–589.
2. Postma GN, Cohen JT, Belafsky PC, et al. Transnasal esophagoscopy: revisited (over 700 consecutive cases). *Laryngoscope.* 2005;115:321–323.
3. Saeian K, Staff DM, Vailopoulos S, et al. Unsedated transnasal endoscopy accurately detects Barrett's metaplasia and dysplasia. *Gastrointest Endosc.* 2002;56:472–478.
4. Shariff MK, Bird-Lieberman EL, O'Donovan M, et al. Randomized crossover study comparing efficacy of transnasal endoscopy with that of standard endoscopy to detect Barrett's esophagus. *Gastrointest Endosc.* 2012;75: 954–961.
5. Peery AF, Hoppo T, Garman KS, et al. Feasibility, safety, acceptability, and yield of office-based screening transnasal esophagoscopy (with video). *Gastrointest Endosc.* 2012;75:945–953.
6. Howell RJ, Pate MB, Ishman SL, et al. Prospective multi-institutional transnasal esophagoscopy: predictors of a change in management. *Laryngoscope.* 2016;126: 2667–2671.
7. Polat B, Karahatay S, Birkent H, Gerek M. The practicability of transnasal esophagoscopy and the evaluation of patient's perception: a prospective study. *Clin Exp Otorhinolaryngol.* 2016;366–369.
8. Shariff MK, Barghese S, O'Donovan M, et al. Pilot randomized crossover study comparing the efficacy of transnasal disposable endosheath with standard endoscopy to detect Barrett's esophagus. *Endoscopy.* 2016;48:110–116.
9. Sabirin J, Abd Rahman M, Rajan P. Changing trends in oesophageal endoscopy: a systematic review of transnasal oesophagoscopy. *ISRN Otolaryngol.* 2013. https://doi.org/10.1155/2013/586973.
10. Huang YC, Lee YC, Tseng PH, et al. Regular screening of esophageal cancer for 248 newly diagnosed hypopharyngeal squamous cell carcinoma by unsedated transnasal esophagogastroduodenoscopy. *Oral Oncol.* 2016;55:55–60.
11. Sanyaolu LN, Jemah A, Stew B, Ingrams DR. The role of transnasal oesophagoscopy in the management of globus pharyngeus and non-progressive dysphagia. *Ann R Coll Surg Engl.* 2016;98:49–52.
12. Shih CW, Hao CY, Wang YJ, Hao SP. A new trend in the management of esophageal foreign body: transnasal esophagoscopy. *Otolaryngol Head Neck Surg.* 2015;153: 189–192.

13. Rees CJ. In-office transnasal Esophagoscopy-guided botulinum toxin injection of the lower esophageal sphincter. *Curr Opin Otolaryngol Head Neck Surg.* 2007;15:409−411.

14. Rees CJ. In-office unsedated transnasal balloon dilation of the esophagus and trachea. *Curr Opin Otolaryngol Head Neck Surg.* 2007;15:401−404.

15. Doctor VS. In-office unsedated tracheoesophageal puncture. *Curr Opin Otolaryngol Head Neck Surg.* 2007;15:405−408.

16. Roof SA, Amin MR. Transnasal esophagoscopy in modern head and neck surgery. *Curr Opin Otolaryngol Head Neck Surg.* 2015;23:171−175.

17. Athanasiadis T, Allen JE. Chronic cough: an otorhinolaryngology perspective. *Curr Opin Head Neck Surg.* 2013;21:517−522.

18. Friedlander JA, DeBoer EM, Soden JS, et al. Unsedated transnasal oesophagoscopy for monitoring therapy in pediatric eosinophilic esophagitis. *Gastrointest Endosc.* 2016;83:299−306.

19. Belafsky PC, Postma GN, Koufman JA. The validity and reliability of the reflux finding score (RFS). *Laryngoscope.* 2001;111:1313−1317.

20. Reavis KM, Morris CD, Gopal DV, Hunter JG, Jobe BA. Laryngopharyngeal reflux symptoms better predict the presence of esophageal adenocarcinoma than typical gastroesophageal reflux symptoms. *Ann Surg.* 2004;239:849−856.

21. Amin MR, Postma GN, Setzen M, Koufman JA. Transnasal esophagoscopy: a position statement from the American Bronchoesophagological Association (ABEA). *Otolaryngol Head Neck Surg.* 2008;138:411−414.

CHAPTER 10

Modified Barium Swallow Study

ANDREW ERMAN, MA, CCC-SLP • DINESH K. CHHETRI, MD

INTRODUCTION

The modified barium swallow study (MBSS) is currently the gold standard assessment used to evaluate oropharyngeal swallow disorders. It is a fluoroscopic swallowing exam, typically performed by speech language pathologist (SLP), to image the head and neck structures while the patient swallows liquid and food of various consistencies. On the macrolevel, the test elucidates swallow safety (i.e., lower airway protection) and swallow efficiency (i.e., time to clear a bolus through the oral cavity and pharynx, and how much residue remains after the swallow). On the microlevel, the MBSS reveals how individual swallow structures function, in regard to the range of motion and timing, and how this relates to postswallow residue and aspiration.

The MBSS can be modified on the spot to answer the clinical questions relevant to a particular patient. Some of these questions are understood before the study starts. Other questions become apparent as the study progresses (e.g., why is material not clearing the upper esophageal sphincter [UES] very well?). At its best, the MBSS is a fluid test that is modified based on moment-to-moment findings. The test is performed to answer a variety of clinical questions, such as the following:

- Is the patient safe for oral intake? If so, what consistencies and bolus sizes of food and liquid will be swallowed with the least aspiration risk?
- If the patient aspirates, why does this occur? What mechanisms lead to aspiration?
- Why does oral cavity and/or pharyngeal residue remain?
- Are anatomical abnormalities present that impede swallow function (e.g., an obstructive epiglottis or cricopharyngeal (CP) bar?
- Are there behavioral techniques that improve lower airway protection and/or swallow efficiency?
- Is the patient a candidate for swallow therapy?
- Did the behavioral and/or surgical intervention work to improve swallow function

The advantages of MBSS in comparison to flexible endoscopic evaluation of swallowing (FEES, see Chapter 8) are (1) the entire swallowing anatomy and function from the oral cavity to the cervical esophagus can be visualized, (2) there is better delineation of the base of the tongue versus pharyngeal constrictor muscle contraction in the pharyngeal phase, (3) pharyngoceles are generally only seen on MBSS, (4) there is no "white out" period during the pharyngeal swallow phase, thus the entire phase (before, during, and after the swallow) is assessed, (5) the function of the UES can be directly visualized, and (6) cervical esophageal phase and other anatomic anomalies in this area, such as a esophageal diverticulum, upper esophageal stenosis, or dysfunction of the esophageal transition zone can be assessed. MBSS is complementary to FEES in the assessment of epiglottic dysfunction, pharyngeal residue, penetration and aspiration, and assessment of the efficacy of behavioral modifications during swallowing. MBSS may provide some insight on the etiology of pharyngeal residue that may be difficult to glean from FEES. For example, pyriform sinus residue is typically due to decreased opening of the esophageal inlet or reduced pharyngeal driving force (which is a product of the tongue base and pharyngeal constrictor contraction). However, it may also result from vallecular residue that passively drains to the pyriform sinuses as pharyngeal structures return to a resting position, but this event may not be clearly visualized on FEES.

The disadvantages of MBSS are the need to transport the patient to a radiology suite and, more importantly, the use of fluoroscopy (continuous X-ray radiation beam) to image the swallowing anatomy and function. Although MBSS simulates normal oropharyngeal swallowing, the naturalistic quality of a meal is absent, because the patient's pace of eating and drinking is controlled to coordinate swallowing with turning on of the fluoroscopic unit. Competing environmental stimuli that may distract the patient during a meal (e.g., TV, conversation) are not present. Additionally, the sample of swallowing events is limited to reduce radiation exposure. This can be an issue because a patient may demonstrate variable swallow function between swallows, using the same consistency and bolus size. Microaspiration events may not be observed. It is not possible to accurately *quantify* the amount of pharyngeal residue present after the swallow since the recorded image is two-dimensional (2D) but the swallowing space is three-dimensional (3D). Software is under development by research groups to measure and quantitate residue, but currently, such tools are too inefficient for routine clinical use. Despite the disadvantages, the MBSS currently is the most comprehensive assessment tool in management of oropharyngeal dysphagia.

TECHNOLOGY

The MBSS is a fluoroscopic assessment procedure and can be performed using an upended fluoroscopy table or a C-arm unit (Figs. 10.1 and 10.2). Currently, the standard is to digitally record studies at 30 frames per second. A normal oropharyngeal swallow takes around 1.5–2 s. Recording at less than 30 frames may not capture some swallow events. For example,

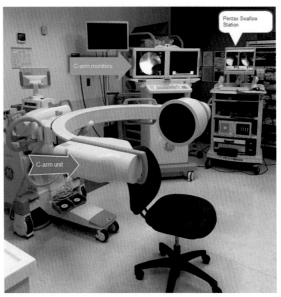

FIG. 10.2 C-arm radiology unit for the modified barium swallow study. The C-arm unit can accommodate a wheelchair that might be too wide to fit within an upended fluoroscopy table.

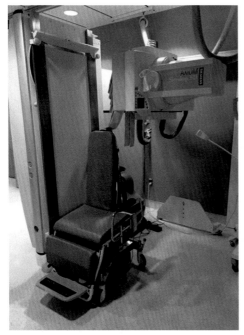

FIG. 10.1 Upended fluoroscopy table with a chair designed specifically for the modified barium swallow study.

aspiration may be seen on fluoroscopy, but the video may not capture the aspiration event. The recording system should have the option to play back frame-by-frame so that the clinician can analyze discrete swallow events (e.g., pharyngeal constrictor contraction or when and why a patient is aspirating). Systems have been developed specifically for MBSSs and fulfill these purposes. Some hospitals have decided to record studies on Picture Archiving and Communication System (PACS), a widespread technology used to store, retrieve, and review radiologic imaging. The PACS has the advantage of allowing the MBSS to be viewed from any terminal connected to the intranet. PACS disadvantages, depending on the system, include limited storage space (and thus, only portions of the study may be recorded or the frames per second stored may be reduced) and there may be limited play back control. Some dedicated systems can include a server, to which studies are saved, allowing viewing from multiple workstations.

Chairs designed specifically for the MBSS exist. These chairs often resemble cardiac chairs but have narrow backs to fit between the upended fluoroscopy table and image intensifier. These chairs also allow the seat to be elevated, back to be reclined, and legs to be elevated, depending on the patient's need.

What the Patient Swallows During Modified Barium Swallow Study

Since the MBSS simulates normal swallowing, food and liquid are given that attempt to mimic consistencies the patient swallows outside the radiology suite. A contrast material (usually barium) must be used to view the bolus movement from the oral cavity, through the oropharynx, and into the upper esophagus. Liquid barium products developed for routine gastrointestinal studies are generally not appropriate for the MBSS, as they are designed to coat endoluminal structures. This coating would obscure the view of swallow structures for subsequent swallows, making it difficult to assess how residue collects or how aspirate can be cleared. Varibar barium sulfate products were developed to address this problem. Varibar products include thin liquid, nectar, honey, and pudding and are designed to minimize coating of the lumen, though residue will remain, depending on the swallow pathology. Additionally, barium tablets (circular in shape) exist, but they are large (half-inch diameter) and do not simulate the shape of a normal pill—they are designed to assess for esophageal stricture. In our institution, we use 16 or 20 French gel caps filled with barium powder, and the patients swallow the gel caps with water or pudding without contrast added.

Modified Barium Swallow Study Candidacy

When using an upended fluoroscopy table, patients must have sufficient trunk support to maintain an adequate upright sitting position. A C-arm fluoroscopy unit is useful for patients on a gurney (with the back raised) or wheelchair. Patients must have adequate cognitive function to participate in the MBSS (i.e., sufficiently alert, able to follow simple instructions or at the very least, be able to initiate an oropharyngeal swallow when material is placed in the patient's mouth). The MBSS should be avoided with pregnant women.

TECHNIQUE

Personnel

A SLP typically runs the MBSS. Occupational therapists may occasionally perform an MBSS. A radiology technologist or a radiologist operates the fluoroscopy equipment.

Chart Review and Patient Interview

The medical record is reviewed for information relating to the etiology of the patient's dysphagia, as well as comorbidities that may impact swallow function. Gastroenterology, pulmonology, head and neck surgery, radiation oncology, medical oncology, internal medicine, neurology, and dietary notes are of particular interest. The patient interview can be critical to understand the individual's goals relative to her/his swallowing, and to further clarify the clinical questions that the MBSS will hopefully answer. It is important to comprehend the patient's perception of his or her swallowing problem, where the problem is felt to occur, when it began, how often it occurs and with what consistencies of food and/or liquid, and what foods or liquids the patient is consequently avoiding. Patients may develop their own useful compensations for their swallow problem. Therefore, it is helpful to ask the patient how they have responded to their dysphagia.

Patient Positioning

An optimal fluoroscopic view includes the entire oral cavity, pharynx and larynx, upper trachea, UES, and cervical esophagus. The *lateral view* gives the best picture of swallow structures important for bolus transit and lower airway protection. The *oblique view* is used when the patient's anatomy interferes with obtaining a good lateral view (e.g., because of a short neck, large shoulders, etc.) of the UES and cervical esophagus. The *anteroposterior (AP) view* is employed to observe laterality of anatomical abnormalities, as well as to explicate if bolus flow and/or residue are symmetric. The AP and lateral views are required to imagine the patient's swallow in three dimensions.

Feeding

Since the MBSS is designed to simulate normal oropharyngeal swallowing, it is best for the patient to be fed in a manner similar to that which occurs in a patient's natural environment. In other words, if a patient feeds himself, he should feed himself during an MBSS. If a caregiver feeds the patient, the caregiver should feed during the MBSS.

Oral Peripheral Examination

We recommend visualizing a patient's oral cavity to shed light on the etiology of oral dysphagia. The findings and hypotheses are corroborated during the MBSS. The oral cavity is examined for structure normalcy and range of motion. Lip, tongue, and velar symmetry are assessed, both at rest and with movement. The patient's ability to achieve an adequate labial seal and to protrude his/her tongue at midline is evaluated. If lingual protrusion is not midline, lingual weakness may be present and tongue will deviate toward the side of the weakness—more residue may accrue to the weak side as well. The presence of adequate dentition for cutting and grinding is evaluated. Bear in mind that some patients masticate without teeth. Additionally, oral mucosa is examined for signs of xerostomia, since oropharyngeal dryness can impede organization and transit of food boluses and result in residue; xerostomia is also associated with increased risk of dental caries. The teeth are observed for any obvious signs of poor condition, since dental decay is associated with aspiration pneumonia, in that the patient may aspirate oral pathogens. The oral cavity is assessed for excess secretions, food residue, and/or lesions. Residue between the lateral dentition and cheeks may suggest buccal weakness. Maximal oral opening is measured between the incisors if trismus is noted. Trismus can impact oral feeding, dental care, and/or the ability to perform endoscopic procedures. Finally, speech and voice deficits are screened, as they may be associated with dysphagia.

Assessment of Swallowing

The MBSS is initially read in real time. The study begins by establishing the optimal lateral view before the patient swallows, and reviewing the anatomy for structural anomalies. This includes looking for a thickened and short epiglottis (seen in radiated patients) and widened or narrowed pharyngeal space (as may occur with muscle atrophy). Any laryngeal or tracheal areas of increased contrast that may indicate calcification should be noted. Otherwise, these areas may be mistaken during the study for penetration or aspiration. Given that there is a great deal of activity of various structures within a 1- to 2-s period, the initial reading may be more of a gestalt impression of the swallow than a specific understanding of how the various swallow structures contribute to the patient's dysphagia. Depending on the complexity of the study, it may be necessary to temporarily halt the study to review the recordings collected thus far, to understand the patient's disorder and how to address the corresponding clinical questions that may arise. Following study completion, the recorded MBSS should be reviewed for further analysis and interpretation.

INTERPRETATION OF MODIFIED BARIUM SWALLOW STUDY

Following are the events and structures examined, and questions considered, from the review of the MBSS recording:

- Labial seal: does contrast leak out of the mouth at any point of the swallow?
- Mastication: does chewing appear to be organized and performed in a rotary fashion? Is mastication thorough?
- Oral cavity bolus formation: does the patient form a cohesive bolus?

- Bolus cohesion during oral transit: is the patient able to propel the bolus from the oral cavity to the pharynx in a single lingual motion? Or is there uncoordinated oral structure movement during oral transit?
- Residue in the oral cavity: does excess oral cavity residue remain? If so, where and how much, and with what consistency of food or liquid?
- Is bolus cohesion maintained during oral transit? If not, it may not be possible to measure when the pharyngeal swallow should trigger.
- Does the pharyngeal swallow trigger in a timely manner (i.e., as the head of the bolus passes the mandibular ramus for young and middle-aged adults or reaches the valleculae for the elderly)?
- If the pharyngeal trigger is not timely, how far does the bolus reach before triggering occurs? How long is the bolus at rest in the pharynx before the pharyngeal swallow triggers?
- If bolus cohesion is *not* maintained during oral transit, how far does the head of the bolus reach, and for how long before the pharyngeal swallow occurs?
- Is tongue base retraction evident? Does retraction appear reduced (Fig. 10.3)?
- Do the pharyngeal constrictors demonstrate a traveling wave (from superior to inferior)? Is there space between the tongue base and pharyngeal constrictors at the height of the swallow (Figs. 10.4–10.6)?

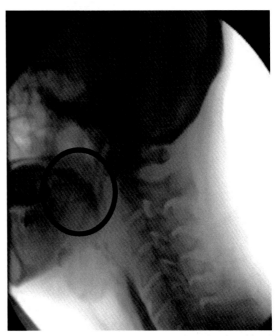

FIG. 10.3 Reduced tongue base contraction resulting in oropharyngeal residue (*circle*).

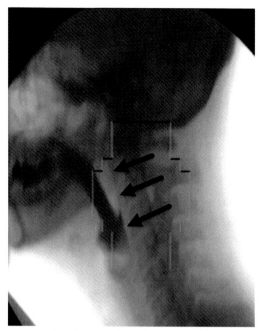

FIG. 10.4 Oropharyngeal swallow onset. No pharyngeal constrictor contraction has occurred yet (*arrows*).

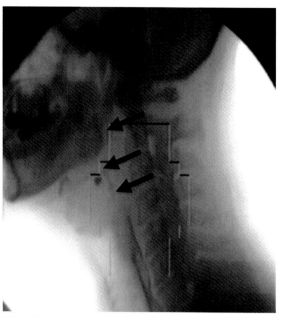

FIG. 10.6 Oropharyngeal swallow. Pharyngeal constrictor contraction complete—no air space is left (*arrows*).

- Epiglottis: does it fully deflect (Fig. 10.7)? If not, does it appear to obstruct the bolus? What is impeding epiglottic deflection? Is deflection (or lack thereof) consistent? Is there associated nasal regurgitation?
- Hyolaryngeal elevation: does the hyolaryngeal complex elevate and move forward? Is the vestibule closed during the swallow?
- Penetration/aspiration: does it occur? If so, with what consistencies, at what point of the swallow (before, during, or after), in what amount, and, importantly, why? Is aspiration consistent? Is the penetrated or aspirated material reflexively expelled during the swallow process or volitionally (at the examiner's request) with a cough or throat clear (Figs. 10.8 and 10.9)?
- Nasal regurgitation: does this occur? If so, why? In what estimated amount? With what consistencies? With what bolus sizes? How far into the nasal cavity does this material reach?
- Pharyngeal residue: is there residue after the swallow? If so, where, and how much is estimated for each consistency and bolus size? What causes this residue? Does the patient swallow to clear the residue (suggesting at least somewhat intact sensation)? Does the patient acknowledge sensing the residue when queried? Does the residue move from one area to another after the swallow

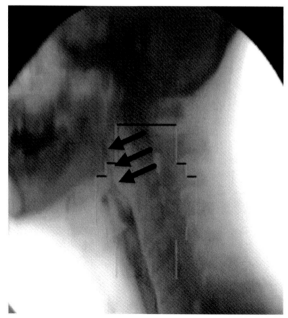

FIG. 10.5 Oropharyngeal swallow. Pharyngeal constrictor contraction begins (*arrows*) and has progressed to the hyoid level.

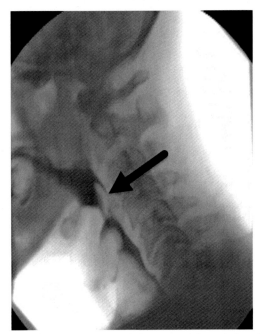

FIG. 10.7 Epiglottis (*arrow*) does not deflect during the swallow.

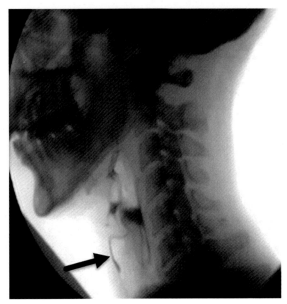

FIG. 10.9 Aspiration. The thin layer of barium (*arrow*) is seen on the anterior wall of the trachea.

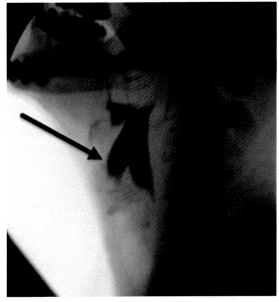

FIG. 10.8 Penetration. In this image of mid-oropharyngeal swallow phase, a large column of barium is seen entering the laryngeal vestibule.

(e.g., from valleculae to the pyriform sinuses or pyriform sinuses to the larynx) because of gravity?
- Does the patient report pain with swallowing? If so, where and how severe and with what consistency?
- UES opening: is UES opening adequate? A good-sized bolus is required to determine UES opening since the UES may not open wide for a small bolus. Is there any obstacle in the UES region obstructing bolus flow? Is UES opening limited, without any observable anatomical deviation? It is important to determine if poor clearance through the UES occurs because of (1) anatomical deviations, such as a Zenker's diverticulum, versus (2) reduced UES opening that may be associated with poor driving force and/or poor hyolaryngeal elevation (Figs. 10.10 and 10.11).
- Esophagus: this may be screened to determine if contrast remains. At our institution, if we suspect an esophageal component to the patient's swallow complaint, we screen the esophagus by turning on fluoroscopy 1 min after the last swallow of food to view the esophagus for residue. If contrast is noted, an esophageal work-up is recommended. During an MBSS, one may also observe if material does not clear the cervical esophagus or re-enters that area from lower in the esophagus.

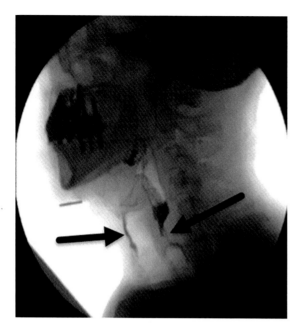

FIG. 10.10 Upper esophageal sphincter dysfunction (*right arrow*) causing aspiration (*left arrow*).

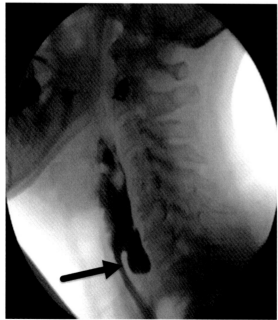

FIG. 10.11 Zenker's diverticulum. The typical cricopharyngeal bar is seen (*arrow*) in front of the pouch.

Anatomical Findings That Appear to Impact Swallowing

The anatomical findings that appear to impact swallowing are as follows:

- Osteophytes: do they narrow the pharynx and appear to impede epiglottic deflection? Does their shape and location divert bolus flow into the larynx or impede the bolus from entering the UES (see Chapter 17)?
- Cervical spine lordosis: does this narrow the pharynx in a manner that impedes epiglottic deflection?
- Pharyngocele: these can be unilateral or bilateral, are usually located at the level of the valleculae, typically fill with liquid more than food, and empty after the swallow. If present, how do they behave with each consistency? Are they bilateral? What happens to the residue after the swallow? Where are they located?
- CP bar: is this present with all consistencies? Does the hypopharynx appear dilated during the swallow (possibly due to increased pressure moving the bolus past the bar)? Does the bar obstruct bolus flow and result in material above the CP? If so, does the material re-enter the hypopharynx? Does swallowing with head turned right or left reduce the postswallow residue?
- Esophageal diverticula: is there a diverticulum in the UES region? Is there a CP bar and is the area of collection above or below the bar? The lateral or oblique view is needed to determine the relationship of the pouch to the CP muscle, while the AP view provides information regarding the relation of the pouch to midline. A Zenker's diverticulum occurs above the CP bar and posterior or posterolateral to the esophagus, whereas Killian–Jamieson diverticulum occurs below the CP muscle and protrudes laterally (best seen on AP view). Also, assess if contrast within the area of collection stays there or moves up or down in the esophagus. Does aspiration result from this area of collection? In patients complaining of pill dysphagia, barium pills can be used to assess if it lodges within the diverticulum (Figs. 10.12 and 10.13).
- Stricture: upper esophageal stenosis and webs often present as a thin band of tissue in the cervical esophageal region. Does this tissue restrict bolus flow past the UES? How much residue remains above the tissue band? Is the hypopharynx dilated during the swallow (Fig. 10.14)?

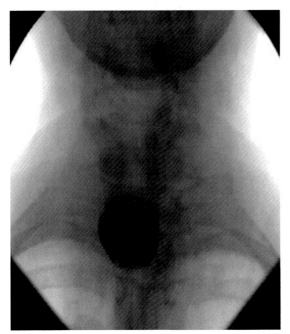

FIG. 10.12 Anteroposterior view of the Zenker's diverticulum from Fig. 10.11. Barium is retained in the pouch after the swallow. The pouch is posterior to the esophagus.

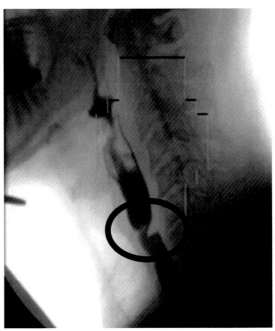

FIG. 10.14 Esophageal stenosis after chemoradiation therapy for oropharyngeal cancer. Note the narrow upper esophageal sphincter region (*circle*) and contrast superior to the stricture.

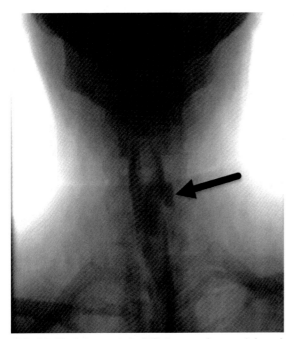

FIG. 10.13 Anteroposterior (AP) view reveals a pouch (*arrow*) lateral to the esophagus consistent with a Killian–Jamieson diverticulum.

COMPENSATORY STRATEGIES

Compensatory strategies are behavioral maneuvers that aim to reduce aspiration and/or improve swallow efficiency. Efficacy of these strategies can be determined during an MBSS. The maneuvers can be grouped into three categories: (1) head postures, (2) lower airway protective maneuvers, and (3) using liquid to facilitate transit of food boluses. Our practice is to only use these maneuvers during an instrumental assessment (as opposed to a clinical evaluation) since they can also cause more residue and aspiration.

Head Postures

Head turns (right or left) presumably cause the contralateral side of the pharynx to do more work—useful if there is unilateral pharyngeal weakness. *Chin down* positions the tongue base closer to the posterior pharyngeal wall and may result in better pharyngeal driving force and hence less residue; this posture can also widen the vallecular space by changing the epiglottis position, which may be useful in protecting a patient from aspiration before and during the swallow (in the case of delayed lower airway closure at the level of the larynx). Head turn (right or left) with chin down combines the effects of both maneuvers. *Chin up* can be useful for patients with poor ability to perform oral transit (and therefore require the assistance of gravity) or with labial incompetence.

Lower Airway Protective Maneuvers

In a *supraglottic swallow*, the patient volitionally holds his/her breath prior to and during the swallow. The patient can also be asked to hold her/his breath between swallows, if multiple swallows per bolus are required. A supraglottic swallow can be followed by a throat clear or cough to expel material that has penetrated the larynx. In a *super supraglottic swallow*, the patient holds the breath same as the supraglottic swallow except that the patient bears down to perform a Valsalva. The super-supraglottic swallow is performed if a patient does not achieve adequate laryngeal closure using the supraglottic swallow. The Valsalva maneuver has been reported to cause arrhythmias in patients with a history of stroke or coronary artery disease, and caution should be exercised.[1]

Using Liquid to Facilitate Food Bolus Clearance

Taking a sip of liquid after swallowing food to clear oral and/or pharyngeal residue is called a *liquid wash*. The *liquid assist* technique requires a pt to swallow food together with liquid, Both techniques facilitate better clearance of the food bolus through the oral cavity and/or pharynx, which may be otherwise impeded by xerostomia and/or reduced oral and/or pharyngeal driving force.

OBJECTIVE MEASURES

Some swallow events may be objectively measured by time or distance. Reasons to measure include quantifying evaluation findings, improving inter- and intrarater reliability, and quantifying if swallow function improves. *Timing of swallow events* such as oral and pharyngeal transit time in normal swallowing have been reported.[2,3] Time required to clear a bolus thru the oral cavity and pharynx may be measured—this is especially useful for patients who have to swallow multiple times per bolus. Likewise, one may measure the number of swallows required to clear a bolus thru the oral cavity and/or pharynx. Timing and magnitude of hyolaryngeal elevation have also been reported but are generally not used clinically. Since MBSS is recorded in two dimensions while swallowing is in three dimensions, it is challenging to quantify the pharyngeal residue. Measuring *pharyngeal constriction ratio* (PCR) has been advocated as a surrogate for pharyngeal strength.[4] PCR is the ratio of the pharyngeal area when food or liquid bolus is held in the oral cavity, divided by

pharyngeal area at the point of maximal pharyngeal squeeze during deglutition. However, calculating this measure is time consuming and therefore, PCR is not in wide clinical use. Software is under development to quantify area and the distance structures move, but is not currently in regular clinical use.

The *penetration/aspiration scale* numerically grades discrete penetration/aspiration events and has been frequently used to report swallowing outcomes.[5] The *MBSS Impairment Profile* includes an online training program and reliability testing.[6] This program provides descriptive language and scores for 17 discrete swallow events from lip closure to esophageal clearance of the bolus. Benefits of these scales include standardizing descriptive language and assessment criteria between and within clinicians. These scales are not truly objective, since they are based on the perception of swallow events by the clinician.

SUBJECTIVE IMPRESSIONS

Most observations made during an MBSS are subjective. This includes structure movement required to propel a bolus through the oral cavity and pharynx, structures involved in opening the UES and protecting the lower airway, the amount of residue present after the swallow, and the amount of material penetrated or aspirated. Factors contributing to the subjectivity of the MBSS are the difficulty in making distance measurements, observing 3D events in 2D, and variability between swallows and bolus size. Subjectivity for repeat studies may be minimized somewhat by displaying two studies side by side for comparison, as some systems allow.

The MBSS cannot measure strength—manometry is a better modality for that function. Strength (or lack thereof) may be inferred by swallow structure range of motion and the amount of residue present after a swallow. The MBSS does not directly measure sensation, but we may infer reduced or preserved sensation given how a patient responds to residue and/or aspiration. We observe that patients with poor sensation for residue and aspiration often do not follow recommendations that improve swallow efficiency and lower airway protection, even with counseling and viewing the MBSS video. We hypothesize that behavioral change is less likely to occur if the patient does not experience physiologic feedback that the proposed strategy is beneficial.

THE MODIFIED BARIUM SWALLOW STUDY REPORT

Otolaryngologists are now increasingly involved in the treatment of swallowing disorders. Therefore, the

MBSS report should convey information to the otolaryngologist that subsequently allows for optimal treatment planning. The MBSS report should describe the clinical question the referring provider seeks an answer to, history related to why the patient may have dysphagia, conditions that may impact the patient's swallow function, and the patient's subjective and objective report of his/her swallowing. The MBSS report should describe what was given, and in what amount. Oral structure observations that may contribute to the patient's dysphagia should be provided (e.g., unilaterally smaller tongue size that suggests atrophy, insufficient dentition for adequate mastication). Abnormal swallow events should be described as observed, with no interpretation. The history and results should be synthesized into an impressions section that describes the following: (1) what the patient aspirates and why; (2) the perceived aspiration risk with various consistencies; (3) description of swallow efficiency and why the patient has an inefficient swallow; (4) if any behavioral maneuvers improve lower airway protection and/or swallow efficiency; and (5) impressions of the patient's sensory function for residue and/or aspiration. Recommendations should follow, listing recommended food and liquid consistencies and behavioral recommendations (e.g., head postures, swallow therapy, oral care, etc.), as well as referrals to other professionals. A recommendation for or against swallow therapy candidacy should also be made.

CONCLUSIONS

The MBSS is the gold standard assessment that allows a physician to understand oropharyngeal swallow function. The test is complementary to FEES. Each test contributes different information. We have found that a collaborative review of FEES and MBSS videos by the otolaryngologist and the speech pathologist to be extremely helpful in understanding a patient's swallowing disorder. Ensuing discussion of each patient's case has resulted in thoughtful and informed treatment planning. Additionally, working together on a continuing basis has deepened our analysis. The oropharyngeal swallow is a collection of well-described behaviors. Nevertheless, aspects of an individual's swallowing function can remain mysterious and open to hypothesis formation. This makes swallowing assessment challenging and stimulating.

REFERENCES

1. Chaudhuri G, Hildner CD, Brady S, Hutchins B, Aliga N, Abadilla E. Cardiovascular effects of the supraglottic and super-supraglottic swallowing maneuvers in stroke patients with dysphagia. *Dysphagia*. 2002 Winter;17(1):19−23.
2. Kendall KA, McKenzie S, Leonard RJ, Gonçalves MI, Walker A. Timing of events in normal swallowing: a videofluoroscopic study. *Dysphagia*. 2000 Spring;15(2):74−83.
3. Leonard R, Kendall K, McKenzie S. UES opening and cricopharyngeal bar in nondysphagic elderly and nonelderly adults. *Dysphagia*. 2004 Summer;19(3):182−191.
4. Leonard R, Belafsky PC, Rees CJ. Relationship between fluoroscopic and manometric measures of pharyngeal constriction: the pharyngeal constriction ratio. *Ann Otol Rhinol Laryngol*. 2006;115(12):897−901.
5. Nam HS, Oh BM, Han TR. Temporal characteristics of hyolaryngeal structural movements in normal swallowing. *Laryngoscope*. 2015;125(9):2129−2133.
6. Rosenbek JC, Robbins JA, Roecker EB, Coyle JL, Wood JL. A penetration-aspiration scale. *Dysphagia*. 1996 Spring;11(2): 93−98.

FURTHER READING

1. Martin-Harris B, Brodsky MB, Michel Y, et al. MBS measurement tool for swallow impairment — MBSImP: establishing a standard. *Dysphagia*. 2008;23:392−405.

CHAPTER 11

The Barium Esophagram

STEVEN S. RAMAN, MD • KARUNA DEWAN, MD • DINESH K. CHHETRI, MD

INTRODUCTION

Fluoroscopic assessment of the oropharynx, hypopharynx, and upper esophagus is commonly performed to assess swallow function and for the workup of the various causes of dysphagia. This chapter will review fluoroscopic findings of the common causes of dysphagia relevant to the otolaryngologist. Most patients referred for fluoroscopic evaluation of oropharyngeal dysphagia have nonspecific symptoms which include difficulty initiating swallowing, globus sensation, regurgitation, hoarseness, coughing, and/or choking while eating.[1] As these symptoms are generally nonspecific, fluoroscopic evaluation of the anatomy can assess for structural and/or functional etiologies of the patient's presenting symptoms.

TECHNOLOGY

Barium esophagram is an older technology that remains relevant today. There is no better esophageal test for the critical analysis of esophageal motility, relative replication of physiologic function, good anatomic definition, and ability to correlate potential symptoms with findings on imaging. With the use of thin barium, this study is used to visualize the anatomic structural aspects of the esophagus. It can be performed as either a single- and/or double-contrast study. Most are performed with both techniques, starting with single contrast. A cine esophagram refers to video recording of the esophagram rather than using only still images.

TECHNIQUE

If possible, patients should avoid smoking for 12 h and eating for 4 h prior to the examination.[1,2] If there is clinical concern for foreign body, plain film, or spot fluoroscopic views should be performed prior to barium evaluation. Standard anteroposterior (AP) and lateral (or at least oblique) views should be obtained at each stage of evaluation. On AP views, the mandible should be superimposed over the occipital bone to avoid obscuring the pharynx.[3] Lateral or oblique views should extend to the inferior portion of the nasopharynx superiorly and should include part of the upper esophagus inferiorly.[4] Both AP and lateral views should be well collimated laterally to minimize veiling glare.[5]

With the patient in standing position, lateral fluoroscopic views are initially obtained after administering a thin suspension of commercially available liquid barium solution (Varibar, barium sulfate, 40% w/v). Nonionic, water-soluble contrast is the initial contrast of choice in postoperative patients or in cases of suspected perforation. Videofluoroscopic lateral views are obtained initially to assess swallowing function and to evaluate for aspiration; if aspiration is significant, the evaluation should be aborted. With thin barium coating the pharyngeal mucosa, modified Valsalva and phonation AP and lateral views are obtained.[3] Additional barium is given as needed to ensure adequate mucosal coating throughout the protocol. Oblique or other additional views are obtained as needed to thoroughly evaluate any structural abnormalities that are encountered.

NORMAL ANATOMY AND SWALLOW FUNCTION

Understanding the normal oropharyngeal/upper esophageal anatomy is crucial for proper delineation of any structural or functional pathology that may be encountered. The pharynx consists of constrictor muscles that originate superiorly from the cranium and hyoid bone with anterior origins from the thyroid cartilage of the adjacent larynx. These muscles extend posteriorly to form a complex tubular structure around the laryngeal inlet that inserts and interdigitates with its contralateral counterpart at the posterior median raphe.[6] The cricopharyngeus (CP) muscle attaches to the lateral aspects of the cricoid cartilage and forms the upper esophageal sphincter (UES); this structure also defines the boundary between the hypopharynx

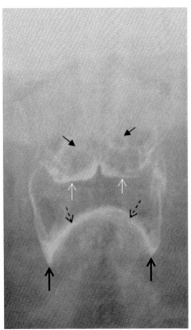

FIG. 11.1 The pharyngoepiglottic folds (*small black arrows*) define the separation of oropharynx and hypopharynx. The valleculae (*white arrows*) are paired pouches that are separated in the midline by the median glossoepiglottic fold. Just below the level of the laryngeal inlet, the paired piriform sinuses are appreciated (*heavy black arrows*). Apposition of the posterior cricoid cartilage against the posterior hypopharynx results in the postcricoid line (*dashed arrows*).

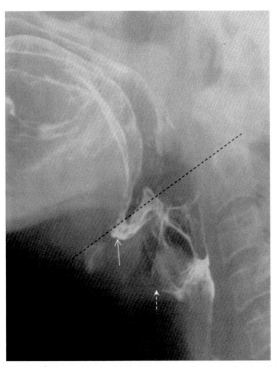

FIG. 11.2 The *black dotted line* runs through the hyoid bone and the free edge of the epiglottis, demarcating the anatomic division between oro- and hypopharynx. The valleculae are superimposed on one another in lateral view, seen in profile as a pouch contiguous with the posterior tongue (*white arrow*). Similarly, the piriform sinuses are also superimposed on lateral view and extend anterolaterally just below the aryepiglottic folds (*dashed white arrow*).

and upper esophagus.[6] Anatomically, the oropharynx and hypopharynx are separated by the pharyngoepiglottic fold which can be seen on AP views after contrast has been given (Fig. 11.1). As this fold is not well seen on lateral views, the hyoid bone and free edge of the epiglottis are commonly used to demarcate the border between the oropharynx and hypopharynx (Fig. 11.2).[3] The remainder of the lateral pharyngeal/upper esophageal anatomy will be discussed in the context of swallowing function in the following sections.

Oral Preparatory Stage: During the initial oral preparatory stage of swallowing, the patient sips the thin barium contrast material and is instructed to hold it orally. On lateral fluoroscopic view, the radiopaque liquid is seen held in place adjacent to the hard palate and upper anterior alveolar ridge by coaptation of the posterior tongue and soft palate (Fig. 11.3). During this stage, some premature leakage of contrast into the pharynx can be seen, particularly in older patients (Fig. 11.3).[6]

Oral Propulsive Stage: The oral propulsive stage is initiated after patients are instructed to begin the swallowing process. Thin barium is propelled from the anterior oral cavity posteriorly by coordinated elevation of the anterior tongue and depression of the posterior tongue. The tongue then progressively increases its area of contact with the palate in an anterior to posterior direction, thereby propelling the contrast bolus posteriorly toward the oropharynx.[6] The contrast bolus courses down along the posterior tongue, over the lingual tonsils and through the fauces into the paired vallecula of the oropharynx (Fig. 11.4). The valleculae can be seen on both AP and lateral fluoroscopic views (Figs. 11.1 and 11.2). The valleculae are just inferior to the free edge of the epiglottis and are separated in the midline by the median glossoepiglottic fold which is best seen on AP view (Fig. 11.1). On lateral view, the valleculae are seen in profile extending anteroinferiorly from the epiglottis at the approximate level of the

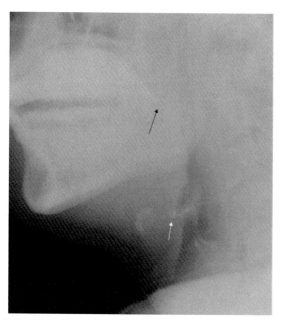

FIG. 11.3 Coaptation of the posterior tongue and soft palate (*black arrow*) keeps ingested barium in the oral cavity during the oral preparatory stage of swallowing. A small amount of premature pharyngeal leakage is also demonstrated (*white arrow*).

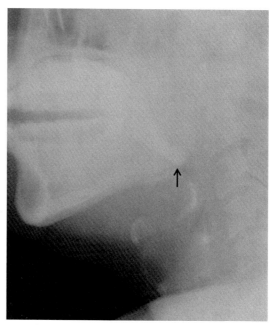

FIG. 11.4 As the oral propulsive stage commences, anterior to posterior coordinated contraction of the tongue pushes the contrast bolus from the oral cavity to the oropharynx (*black arrow*). The passage of swallowed material to the valleculae helps to trigger the pharyngeal stage of swallowing.

hyoid bone.[3] The accumulation of ingested contrast in the valleculae assists in triggering the pharyngeal stage of swallowing. Thin barium can normally move rapidly to the hypopharynx by way of the paired piriform sinuses that can be seen lateral to and just below the level of the laryngeal inlet on AP view (Fig. 11.1). These structures will be superimposed on lateral view and extend anteroinferior from the aryepiglottic folds (Fig. 11.2). On AP view, the arch-shaped postcricoid line appears to connect the paired piriform sinuses. This line results from apposition of the mucosal surfaces of the hypopharynx and cricoid cartilage (Fig. 11.1).

Pharyngeal Stage: The pharyngeal stage of swallowing continues to propel the thin barium toward the esophagus while simultaneously closing off communication with the nasopharyngeal and laryngeal airways. This stage is initiated when the soft palate rises and contacts the lateral and posterior pharyngeal walls, thus preventing reflux of thin barium into the nasopharynx (Fig. 11.5). The contrast bolus is propelled fully into the pharynx by the posterior tongue followed by contraction of the pharyngeal constrictors and downward propulsion of the ingested material toward the hypopharynx. This movement results in superior to

inferior contraction of the pharynx as well as anterior/superior movement of the hyoid bone, which brings the laryngeal inlet closer to the epiglottis. The epiglottis tilts posteriorly during swallowing, closing off the larynx to prevent laryngeal aspiration of thin barium (Fig. 11.5). Anterior movement of the hyoid/larynx also contributes to opening of the UES. Relaxation of the cricopharyngeus and mass effect of the ingested bolus also promotes its passage through the UES.[6]

Esophageal Stage: After passing into the esophagus, the ingested bolus is propelled inferiorly by peristalsis from the UES to the gastroesophageal (GE) junction (Fig. 11.6).[6]

COMMON FINDINGS

Mucus or other debris: Depending on the quality of the preprocedure preparation as well as patient variability in quantity and quality of secretions, accumulation of mucus or swallowed material can mimic a mass on fluoroscopic evaluation, particularly if it leads to coaptation of the pharyngeal walls (Fig. 11.7).[3] If this is suspected, obtaining phonation, Valsalva maneuver,

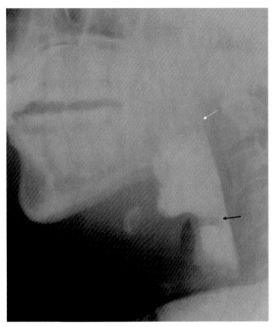

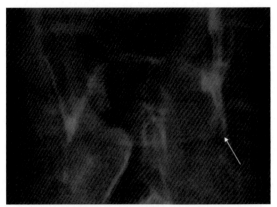

FIG. 11.7 Coaptation of the mucosal surfaces of the left piriform sinus (*white arrow*) results in asymmetry in comparison with the right piriform sinus. Provocative maneuvers and additional swallowing resolved the coaptation, resulting in a more symmetric appearance of the piriform sinuses.

FIG. 11.5 During the pharyngeal stage of swallowing, apposition of the soft palate with the posterolateral pharynx prevents nasopharyngeal reflux (*white arrow*). Anterior/ superior movement of the hyoid bone couples with posterior tilt of the epiglottis (*black arrow*) to prevent laryngeal penetration/aspiration.

and additional views after asking the patient to swallow can help to move the accumulated material. If the finding maintains a similar shape despite provocative maneuvers or if the patient cannot satisfactorily perform provocative maneuvers, further workup for a pharyngeal mass may be indicated.

Lateral protrusion of the lateral wall of the hypopharynx: This variant is best seen on AP views as lateral protrusion of the hypopharynx just above the thyroid cartilage. This can be seen in elderly patients as well as younger patients involved in activities that increase pharyngeal pressure, such as playing a wind instrument.[3,7] This finding, usually a normal variant, may be clinically significant if there is retained ingested material noted within the protrusion, as these patients are at increased risk of aspiration.[3,8]

Lymphoid tissue: Lymphoid tissue in the lingual tonsils results in subtle mucosal irregularity seen fluoroscopically on both AP and lateral views at the base of the tongue with extension into the valleculae. Mild asymmetry of the lingual tonsils is a normal variant (Fig. 11.8).[3]

STRUCTURAL CAUSES OF OROPHARYNGEAL DYSPHAGIA

Foreign bodies: Radiopaque oropharyngeal foreign bodies are best seen on plain film radiographs or spot fluoroscopic views prior to administration of contrast material. In adults, ingested bones are the most common culprit, generally impacting near the cricopharyngeus muscle.[1] The causative objects in

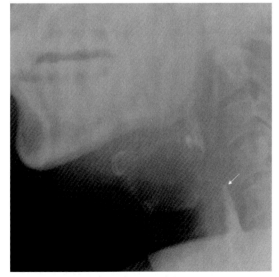

FIG. 11.6 Anterior movement of the larynx coupled with mass effect of the swallowed material opens the cricopharyngeal muscle/upper esophageal sphincter (*white arrow*) thus initiating the esophageal phase of swallowing.

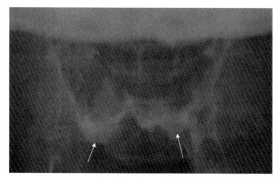

FIG. 11.8 Lymphoid tissue results in mildly asymmetric irregular appearance of the vallecular mucosa (*white arrows*), a normal variant.

children are more varied, including small toys, coins, button batteries, and jewelry. The use of water-soluble contrast material (Gastrografin, Bracco Diagnostics) on initial evaluation is advisable if there is concern for perforation, particularly if the foreign body has been impacted for more than 24 h.[1] If no perforation is noted with water-soluble contrast, thin barium may be subsequently used for any additional evaluation. Filling defects noted after contrast administration will be seen in the setting of a radiolucent foreign body (Fig. 11.9). Foreign bodies are generally amenable to endoscopic removal.[3]

Perforation: Perforation of the pharynx is generally iatrogenic in etiology, secondary to endoscopy, naso/orogastric tube placement, or traumatic intubation. Less likely etiologies include penetrating trauma, emesis, foreign bodies, and spontaneous perforation.[3] Generally, pharyngeal perforation is diagnosed endoscopically. On fluoroscopy, water-soluble contrast material (Gastrografin, Bracco Diagnostics) should be used initially for any suspected perforation. In patients with perforation, contrast material will be seen as irregular linear or stellate collections extending beyond the expected mural pharyngeal contour, seeping into the surrounding tissues from the site of perforation.[3]

INFECTIOUS/INFLAMMATORY CAUSES OF DYSPHAGIA

Infectious and inflammatory etiologies of dysphagia have very similar appearance on fluoroscopic evaluation, generally presenting with a component of pharyngeal thickening. Some infectious etiologies are more highly suspected depending on the pattern of pharyngeal thickening, as discussed in more detail below.

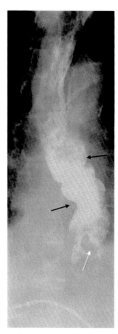

FIG. 11.9 A radiolucent filling defect (*white arrow*) in the distal esophagus prevents passage of contrast to the stomach in a patient who presented with sensation of food caught in their neck. Tertiary waves attempting to pass the impacted food bolus can be seen in the distal dilated esophagus (*black arrows*).

Pharyngitis/Retropharyngeal Abscess: Both bacterial and viral pharyngitis can result in diffuse thickening of the pharynx that can be difficult to detect on fluoroscopy.[3] As such, patients are rarely referred for fluoroscopic evaluation in uncomplicated causes of pharyngitis. Retropharyngeal abscess is the most feared complication of pharyngitis and is a diagnosis that can be readily suspected on fluoroscopy. Lateral views will demonstrate significant thickening of the prevertebral soft tissues and sometimes foci of gas can be seen within the area of thickening.[3]

Epiglottitis: Epiglottitis should be suspected when there is focal thickening of the epiglottis and/or aryepiglottic folds, best seen on lateral fluoroscopic view. Some have described the epiglottis assuming the shape of a thumb when it is inflamed. Prior to implementation of its vaccination, *Haemophilus influenza* B was the most common cause of epiglottitis, and it was most commonly seen in children. Now, Streptococcal species (*S. pneumonia* and *S. pyogenes*) are the more common causes with increasing prevalence in the adult population.[3]

Granulomatous Disease: Granulomatous diseases present with diffuse thickening of the epiglottis and aryepiglottic folds. Tuberculosis and sarcoidosis are the main etiologies, resulting in caseating and noncaseating granulomas, respectively. Of these two etiologies, tuberculosis is the most likely one to present with ulceration.[3]

Amyloidosis: In this disorder, focal or diffuse enlargement of the pharyngeal structures results from extracellular deposition of protein. Patients may have other systemic manifestations of amyloidosis, or it may appear localized to the pharynx.[3]

CHEMORADIATION

The combination of chemotherapy and external beam radiation (chemoradiation) used for treatment of head and neck cancers contributes to diffusely thickened pharyngeal mucosa, an appearance that peaks at 6–8 weeks post treatment and is most pronounced in the radiation treatment port (Fig. 11.10). This initial thickening usually resolves 6 months after completion of treatment.[3] Thickening seen after 6 months must be worked up for tumor recurrence, though chronic strictures secondary to radiation can have a similar appearance on fluoroscopy (Fig. 11.11). Thickening is particularly worrisome for tumor recurrence when associated ulceration is noted.

CAUSTIC INGESTION

In the acute phase after caustic ingestion, mucosal injury is generally assessed endoscopically if not already treated as a surgical emergency. Ingestion-related scarring can have a varied appearance, fluoroscopic evaluation often demonstrates long segment stricture or more complex, multifocal narrowing (Fig. 11.12). These injuries can affect the oro/hypopharynx, cervical esophagus as well as the larynx, particularly if aspiration occurs.

NEOPLASMS

Benign: Benign pharyngeal neoplastic lesions characteristically appear as well-circumscribed, sessile filling defects arising abruptly from the mucosal surface. Lipoma, fibrovascular polyp, and papilloma can appear as pedunculated filling defects, though these entities are uncommon.[9] The differential can be narrowed based on the anatomic location of the benign-appearing filling defect, as delineated in Table 11.1. Generally, these lesions will require further imaging workup with computed tomography (CT) or MRI.

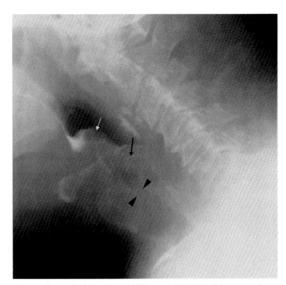

FIG. 11.10 Thickening of the epiglottis (*white arrow*) and aryepiglottic folds (*black arrow*) is noted in this patient with left-sided supraglottic squamous cell carcinoma after chemoradiation therapy. Mass and associated mucosal thickening is contributing to focal narrowing of the laryngeal inlet (*black arrowheads*).

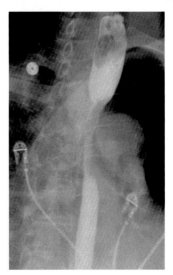

FIG. 11.11 Endoscope was unable to pass beyond a chronic long segment stricture in the mid esophagus of a patient presenting with odynophagia who had received prior radiation therapy.

Squamous cell carcinoma: Squamous cell carcinoma is responsible for 90% of pharyngeal malignancy, with multiple primary lesions seen in the oropharynx, larynx, upper gastrointestinal tract or lung in more

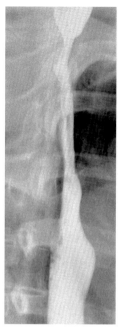

FIG. 11.12 A long segment esophageal stricture is the cause of pill dysphagia in this patient who had ingested Drano weeks previously.

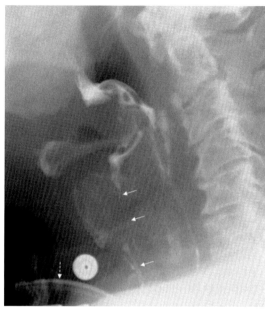

FIG. 11.13 Near complete occlusion of the laryngeal inlet with increased epiglottic and aryepiglottic thickening is secondary to squamous cell carcinoma. A small trickle of contrast results in silent aspiration during swallow evaluation (*white arrows*). Note the presence of a tracheostomy tube, partially visualized (*white dashed arrow*).

TABLE 11.1
Benign Pharyngeal Tumors[9]
Base of the tongue
Retention cyst
Ectopic thyroid
Thyroglossal duct cyst
Granular cell tumor
Benign salivary gland tumors
Aryepiglottic folds
Retention cyst
Saccular cyst
Lipoma
Neurofibroma
Oncocytoma
Granular cell tumors
Laryngeal cartilage
Chondroma
Osteochondroma

than 20% of cases.[3,9] Risk factors include prolonged tobacco use and human papillomavirus exposure. On fluoroscopic evaluation, malignant tumors can present as irregularly shaped focal mucosal asymmetry that can extend from the pharyngeal wall into the lumen. Infiltrative masses can be subtler and may present with irregular pooling of contrast compatible with associated ulceration. Dysmotility brought on by the presence of infiltrative mass may also be appreciated on videofluoroscopic evaluation.[3] The palatine tonsils are most commonly involved, though persistent fluoroscopic irregularity or focal dysmotility of any visualized pharyngeal or laryngeal mucosal surface should prompt further workup (Fig. 11.13).

Lymphoma: Almost all pharyngeal lymphomas are of the non-Hodgkin's variant, comprising ~10% of pharyngeal malignancy.[9] This lesion will present as a bulky mass arising from anywhere along Waldeyer's ring, most commonly involving the palatine tonsils, followed by the adenoids and lingual tonsils as less commonly involved locations. Multiple foci of involvement are common. Patients with HIV and other immune-mediated diseases are at higher risk for lymphoma. This lesion cannot be differentiated from squamous cell carcinoma based on fluoroscopy alone and further workup is warranted.[9]

Kaposi sarcoma: Kaposi sarcoma is an AIDS-defining lesion that involves the pharynx in up to 56% of cases. Nodular, plaque-like, or polypoid pharyngeal filling defects can be seen on fluoroscopy, often resulting in asymmetry of the valleculae or piriform sinuses.[9,10] Ulceration is an uncommon finding with this entity. CT or MRI workup is essential to determine the extent of disease.[10]

Salivary gland tumors: Most minor salivary gland tumors are malignant and appear as irregular masses arising most commonly from the soft palate.[9] In order of descending frequency, the common salivary gland tumor variants are adenoid cystic carcinoma, solid adenocarcinoma, and mucoepidermoid carcinoma. In addition to the soft palate, these tumors can involve the tongue, submandibular gland, and mandible.[9] MRI is specifically helpful in assessment for perineural spread, particularly along the lingual and hypoglossal nerves.

Melanoma: While mucosal melanoma is rare, the head and neck region are common locations for its presentation. These will most commonly involve the palate, though the gingiva, buccal mucosa, tongue, and mouth floor can also demonstrate involvement.[11] These masses may appear as nodular irregularities and may be pedunculated.

DIVERTICULA

Zenker's: This pulsion pseudodiverticulum is a mucosal/submucosal outpouching that occurs just proximal to the cricopharyngeus muscle at Killian's dehiscence, a hypopharyngeal weak point at the junction of pharyngeal constrictor and cricopharyngeal muscle fibers.[12,13] This lesion is traditionally best seen on lateral fluoroscopic evaluation, though these lesions are frequently evident on AP view as they commonly extend laterally as they enlarge (Fig. 11.14).

Killian–Jamieson: This less common pulsion pseudodiverticulum arises from the anterolateral cervical esophagus below the cricopharyngeus muscle, most conspicuous on AP view and most commonly arising from the left side.[13] Similar to Zenker's diverticula, these arise from a focal anatomic weakness lateral to the longitudinal tendon of the esophagus just inferior to the cricopharyngeus known as the Killian–Jamieson space. Killian–Jamieson diverticula tend to be smaller and less symptomatic than Zenker's.[1]

Epiphrenic: Epiphrenic diverticula are pulsion diverticula that occur most commonly on the right side of the distal third of the esophagus, are most common

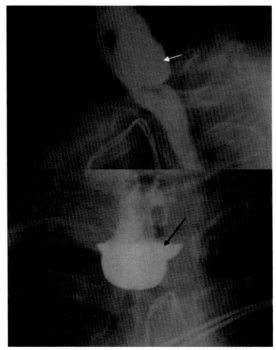

FIG. 11.14 Lateral view (*top*) of a Zenker's diverticulum demonstrates luminal outpouching of the hypopharynx that extends posteriorly (*white arrow*), exerting mild mass effect on the cervical esophagus. Air-fluid level is seen within the luminal outpouching (*black arrow*) on anteroposterior view (bottom).

in the elderly, and are commonly associated with motility disorders (Fig. 11.15).[14] Epiphrenic diverticula can be true, involving all three layers of the esophageal wall, or pseudodiverticula. Larger epiphrenic diverticula are correlated with greater risk of aspiration and esophageal cancer.[15]

ACHALASIA

Achalasia results from poor relaxation of the GE sphincter with associated dysmotility and diffuse dilation of the esophagus.[13] Similar to patients with epiphrenic diverticula, those with severe, long-standing achalasia are at greater risk of aspiration and malignancy in the dilated esophagus. Smooth, beak-like tapering of the distal esophagus is the characteristic finding of this lesion on fluoroscopic evaluation. Patients with irregularity of the tapering mucosa may have pseudoachalasia and should undergo additional workup for a GE mass, as a circumferential lesion at the GE junction can mimic the GE spasm seen in true achalasia (Fig. 11.16).[13]

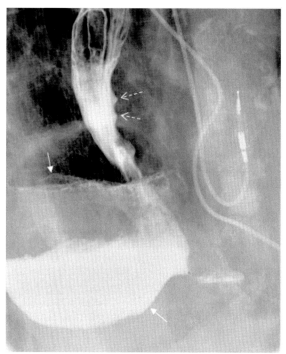

FIG. 11.15 A large epiphrenic diverticulum (*white arrows*) arises from the right side of the esophagus just proximal to the gastroesophageal junction. Evidence of tertiary contractions (*dashed white arrows*) suggests underlying dysmotility in this 90-year-old patient with dysphagia.

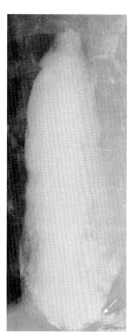

FIG. 11.16 Smooth tapering of the distal esophagus (*white arrow*) denotes gastroesophageal sphincter spasm with proximal dilation of the esophagus, findings characteristic of achalasia. On real-time fluoroscopy, the filling defects in the distal esophagus were determined to be ingested material.

ESOPHAGEAL DYSMOTILITY

If abnormal peristalsis of the esophagus is noted on two or more of five separate videofluoroscopic swallows, esophageal dysmotility must be considered. With the exception of achalasia, which has a known pathophysiology, primary esophageal dysmotility is generally idiopathic and can be associated with aging. Diffuse esophageal spasm is a unique primary cause of esophageal dysmotility and can present with noncardiogenic chest pain that may or may not be related to active swallowing. If esophageal dysmotility occurs in the setting of poorly controlled diabetes, chronic reflux, or scleroderma, dysmotility secondary to these systemic disorders should be considered. Severe cases of esophageal dysmotility may require G-tube support to maintain adequate nutrition and to minimize risk of aspiration (Fig. 11.17).

WEBS/RINGS/STRICTURES

Though these lesions have disparate etiologies and associations, they all can present with focal luminal

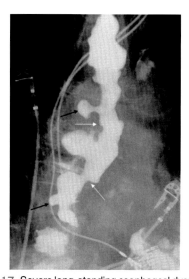

FIG. 11.17 Severe long-standing esophageal dysmotility in an elderly female who required gastric-tube placement to ensure adequate nutrition and to reduce risk of aspiration. Alternating segments of esophageal spasm (white arrows) and saccular outpouching of the esophageal mucosa (black arrows) are seen.

narrowing evident on both AP and lateral views. Esophageal webs consist of 1- to 2-mm thick infoldings of mucosa and lamina propria into the hypopharyngeal and/or cervical esophageal lumina.[9] Webs tend to be eccentric and most commonly involve the anterior hypopharynx/cervical esophagus (Fig. 11.18). When a web appears more circumferential, it can be referred to as a ring, though this appearance is more commonly appreciated in the more distal esophagus. Webs in the valleculae and piriform sinuses are considered normal variants.[9]

Plummer–Vinson syndrome: Plummer–Vinson syndrome consists of the triad of iron deficiency anemia, atrophic glossitis, and cervical esophageal webs. Thorough evaluation of these patients is crucial, as they are at increased risk of developing squamous cell carcinoma.[9]

Secondary to gastroesophageal reflux disease: Chronic GE reflux is also cited as an etiology of web formation in the cervical esophagus, similar to its role in causing more distal webs nearer the GE junction. These patients are also at increased risk of esophageal cancer.[9] Webs secondary to GE reflux disease should not be confused with CP muscle dysfunction.[13] Reflux can also contribute to symptoms of dysphagia by CP spasm. Spasm of this muscle inhibits smooth passage of the ingested bolus from the hypopharynx to the cervical esophagus and places the patient at increased risk of laryngeal penetration/aspiration. This finding is generally seen on lateral fluoroscopic views and is considered significant if the muscle persistently occupies greater than 50% of the expected luminal diameter with proximal dilatation of the hypopharynx. This entity is associated with Zenker's diverticulum as well as other forms of pharyngeal and esophageal dysmotility.

EXTRINSIC IMPRESSIONS

Extrinsic mass: Both benign and malignant thyroid masses can be large enough to produce dysphagia symptoms and can contour and compress upon the pharyngeal wall (Fig. 11.19). Bulky lymphadenopathy from lymphoma or other metastatic lesion may also impart mass effect and a similar appearance on fluoroscopic evaluation.[13]

Cervical osteophytes: Cervical osteophytes, if large enough, can produce mass effect on the esophagus significant enough to produce dysphagia (Fig. 11.18). Symptomatic osteophytes are most likely to occur at the C5–C6 level, as the esophagus is fixed between the spine and cricoid cartilage at this level. Given the high prevalence of anterior cervical osteophytes in the general population, this should be treated as a diagnosis of exclusion, as only 6% of patients with anterior cervical osteophytes endorse dysphagia symptoms. This finding is most conspicuous on lateral views obtained during swallowing.[13]

CONGENITAL ANOMALIES

Branchial arch anomalies: Branchial cysts are the most common branchial arch anomaly and usually arise from the second and third arches. They often present with cutaneous drainage tracts and most commonly present in childhood. Large cysts can compress the pharynx resulting in extrinsic convex mass effect on fluoroscopic evaluation and symptoms of dysphagia or stridor at presentation. Fluoroscopic evaluation is also used to assess for sinus tracts associated with the branchial arch anomaly. Second branchial arch anomalies are most common and are associated with the tonsillar fossae. Third arch anomalies are associated with the piriform sinuses.[3]

Laryngeal clefts: Laryngeal clefts result from incomplete separation of the laryngeal and pharyngeal structures during fetal development. Patients with laryngeal clefts generally appear early in childhood and can commonly present in association with both CHARGE and VACTERL syndromes. Laryngeal clefts can range in

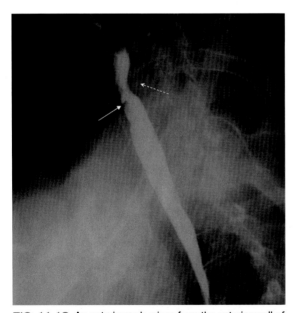

FIG. 11.18 An anterior web arises from the anterior wall of the cervical esophagus, contributing to luminal narrowing (*white arrow*). Large osteophytes also contribute to luminal narrowing just above the esophageal web (*dashed white arrow*).

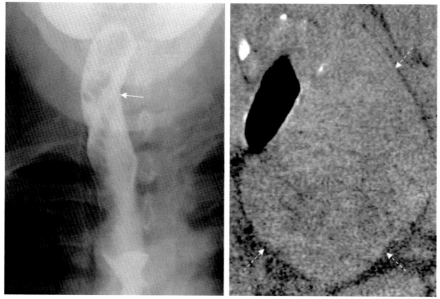

FIG. 11.19 Fluoroscopic anteroposterior view demonstrates rightward displacement of the trachea and cervical esophagus (*white arrow*) secondary to a large left-sided goiter, as demonstrated on coronal CT (*dashed white arrows*).

size from small, interarytenoid lesions to larger clefts that extend into the trachea. Contrast will be seen in both the airway and esophagus at approximately the same time, depending on the size of the lesion.[3]

Tracheoesophageal fistula and Esophageal atresia: These lesions are commonly associated and are generally detected early in life. On fluoroscopic evaluation, a fistulous connection between the trachea and esophagus will usually only be detected in H-type or proximal tracheoesophageal lesions. Esophageal atresia will present as a blind pouch on fluoroscopic study. Though a tracheoesophageal fistula will not be reliably seen in patients with esophageal atresia, the presence of esophageal atresia should prompt further workup for a distal tracheoesophageal fistula. Tracheoesophageal fistula and esophageal atresia are part of the VACTERL syndrome.[3]

POSTSURGICAL/POSTPROCEDURAL

Total Laryngectomy: Fluoroscopic evaluation in patients after total laryngectomy demonstrates a smooth neopharynx that extends as a tube from the oropharynx to the cervical esophagus. The neopharynx may deviate toward the side of lateral neck dissection on AP views, if one was performed. The hyoid bone and laryngeal cartilage are removed and will not be

evident on fluoroscopic evaluation. There is increased prevertebral soft-tissue density at the level of C4–C5 in patients after laryngectomy secondary to retracted thyropharyngeal and cricopharyngeal muscles that have been surgically detached from their usual anterior attachments.[3]

Partial Laryngectomy: Depending on the size and location of the tumor, partial laryngectomy can sometimes be performed. In these cases, some amount of swallowing function can be preserved depending on the postoperative anatomy. The appearance of the larynx can vary widely depending on the type of resection and reconstruction performed.[3,16] Close attention to the operative report is crucial for accurate interpretation of fluoroscopic evaluation after partial laryngectomy. Evaluation for aspiration is particularly important given the risk for postoperative compromise of swallow function.

COMPLICATIONS

Pharyngocutaneous fistula and Pseudodiverticulum: Both of these postoperative complications most commonly occur secondary to breakdown of the anastomosis between the tongue base and the neopharynx. Pharyngocutaneous fistula occurs when this dehiscence results in a sinus tract between the anastomotic breakdown and the skin that can be identified on fluoroscopic evaluation. Fluoroscopic evaluation of pseudodiverticulum is defined by a blind-ending pouch arising from the neopharyngeal-tongue base anastomotic breakdown (Fig. 11.20). Both of these entities are more commonly seen in the setting of radiation/chemoradiation therapy.[3]

Tumor recurrence: Tumor recurrence can have a variety of appearances. Mucosal nodularity is most common, this finding will not change shape with swallowing, a feature that helps differentiate this finding from webs or CP muscle on fluoroscopy. As a nodule enlarges, it may present as an eccentric mass that partially obstructs the neopharyngeal lumen. Strictures with more irregular or angular features should also be worked up for tumor recurrence (3).

PROPULSIVE CAUSES OF OROPHARYNGEAL DYSPHAGIA

While Tables 11.2 and 11.3 list many diverse causes of propulsive oropharyngeal dysphagia, the clinically significant fluoroscopic findings are generally very

TABLE 11.2 Neurogenic Causes of Propulsive Oropharyngeal Dysphagia
Stroke
Neurodegenerative disease
Amyotropic lateral sclerosis
Parkinson's disease
Huntington's disease
Demyelinating disease
Multiple sclerosis
Guillain–Barré
Brainstem lesion
Cerebral palsy
Postpolio syndrome

similar, regardless of specific etiology. Tongue pumping is a notable exception, as it is a pathognomonic fluoroscopic finding of Parkinson's disease. Best seen on lateral view during swallow evaluation, the tongue can be observed moving back and forth repeatedly in an anterior/posterior direction.[4]

Penetration of the laryngeal vestibules is a general finding of propulsive oropharyngeal dysphagia. Contrast material is observed passing into the supraglottic space from the oral cavity, sometimes with apparent delay in initiation of the pharyngeal phase of swallowing. While supraglottic penetration can be seen in asymptomatic individuals, the presence of material in the supraglottic space should promptly initiate the pharyngeal swallow. Material that lingers in the supraglottic space is at risk for aspiration. Patients with premature oral spillage of ingested bolus and delayed initiation of pharyngeal swallow are at

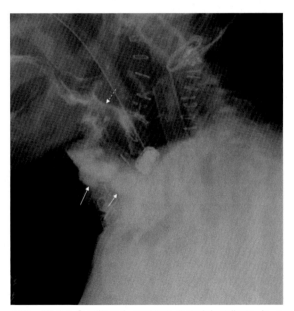

FIG. 11.20 Swallowed contrast material collects in a pseudodiverticulum in the anterior neck soft tissues (*white arrows*) in this patient who has undergone chemoradiation and total laryngectomy for laryngeal squamous cell carcinoma. This leak originates from a breakdown of the anastomosis between the base of the tongue and nasopharynx (*dashed white arrow*). A pharyngocutaneous fistula was confirmed upon clinical evaluation.

TABLE 11.3 Myogenic Causes of Propulsive Oropharyngeal Dysphagia
Myasthenia gravis
Polymyositis
Mixed connective tissue disorders
Oculopharyngeal muscular dystrophy
Paraneoplastic syndrome
Myotonic dystrophy
Sarcoidosis

increased risk of laryngeal vestibule penetration and secondary aspiration.

When contrast material extends beyond the true vocal cords on fluoroscopic evaluation, aspiration has occurred (Fig. 11.13). Immediate cough reflex is expected as a normal response to aspiration. During speech therapy swallow evaluation, scales are used to qualitatively grade severity of aspiration. Food consistency recommendations are made based on which textures place the patient at risk for aspiration.[4]

Poor food bolus propulsion can also result in retained contrast material in the valleculae, piriform sinuses, or other spaces of the pharynx. This can be seen as a result of weak pharyngeal constrictors, dysfunction of the CP muscle, and/or inefficient function of the upper esophagus. Pharyngeal residue places patients at risk for secondary aspiration.

SUMMARY

The barium esophagram, though an old test, remains important to the understanding of pharyngoesophageal physiology and the diagnosis of swallowing disorders. It is valuable in providing additional and confirmatory information in evaluating dysphagia, globus sensation and chronic cough. Its advantage lies in the demonstration of esophageal anatomy, easily correlated with patient symptoms.

REFERENCES

1. Brant William E, Helms Clyde A. *Fundamentals of Diagnostic Radiology*. Wolters Kluwer Health. Lippincott Williams & Wilkins; 2012.
2. Kasper Dennis L, et al. Dysphagia. In: *Harrison's Principles of Internal Medicine*. McGraw-Hill Education; 2015.
3. Tao TY, Menias CO, Herman TE, McAlister WH, Balfe DM. Easier to swallow: pictorial review of structural findings of the pharynx at barium pharyngography. *RadioGraphics*. 2013;33(7):e189–208.
4. Jaffer Nasir M, et al. Fluoroscopic evaluation of oropharyngeal dysphagia: anatomic, technical, and common etiologic factors. *Am J Roentgenol*. 2015;204(1):49–58.
5. Wang Jihong, Blackburn Timothy J. The AAPM/RSNA physics tutorial for residents: X-Ray image intensifiers for fluoroscopy. *RadioGraphics*. 2000;20(5):1471–1477.
6. Matsuo K, Palmer JB. Anatomy and physiology of feeding and swallowing: normal and abnormal. *Phys Med Rehabil Clin N Am*. 2008;19(4):691–707.
7. Costa, Melciades Barbosa Milton, et al. Lateral laryngopharyngeal diverticula: a videofluoroscopic study of laryngopharyngeal wall in wind instrumentalists. *Arq De Gastroenterol*. 2012;49(2):99–106.
8. Lindbichler F, Raith J, et al. Aspiration resulting from lateral hypopharyngeal pouches. *Am J Roentgenol*. 1998;170(1):129–132.
9. Ekberg Olle. *Radiology of the Pharynx and the Esophagus*. Springer; 2004.
10. Restrepo Carlos S, et al. Imaging manifestations of Kaposi sarcoma. *RadioGraphics*. 2006;26(4):1169–1185.
11. Jena A, Alamuri A, et al. A rare case of oropharyngeal melanoma: case report and brief review of literature. *Indian J Oral Sci*. 2016;7(1):63–66.
12. Kanne Jeffrey P, et al. Eponyms in radiology of the digestive tract: historical perspectives and imaging appearances. *RadioGraphics*. 2006;26(1):129–142.
13. Carucci LR, Turner MA. Dysphagia revisited: common and unusual causes. *RadioGraphics*. 2015;35(1):105–122.
14. Rubesin SE, Levine MS. Killian-Jamieson Diverticula: radiographic findings in 16 patients. *Am J Roentgenol*. 2001;177(1):85–89.
15. Abdollahimohammad A, Masinaeinezhad N, Firouzkouhi M. Epiphrenic esophageal diverticula. *J Res Med Sci*. 2014;19:795–797.
16. Ferreiro-Arguelles Concepcion, et al. CT findings after laryngectomy. *RadioGraphics*. 2008;28(3):869–882.

CHAPTER 12

Evaluation of Esophageal Motor Function With High-Resolution Manometry

JEFFREY L. CONKLIN, MD, FACG

INTRODUCTION

The reliable assessment of esophageal function with manometry became possible in the 1970s when Wyle (Jerry) Dodds, a radiologist, and Ron Arndorfer, an engineer, developed the first high-fidelity manometry system.[1,2] Variations of their methods remained the state-of-the-art until the 1990s when Ray Clouse and his colleagues invented high resolution manometry (HRM). With the miniaturization of solid-state pressure sensors, they were able to decrease the spacing between pressure sensing sites along the manometry catheter from 3−5 cm to 1 cm. This decreased the quantity of pressure data lost due to widely spaced sensors. They also lengthened the sensing segment of the catheter. Current HRM catheters consist of up to 36 pressure sensors positioned 1 cm apart. This configuration makes it possible to simultaneously observe motor function of the upper esophageal sphincter (UES), esophagus, and lower esophageal sphincter (LES) with each swallow. This allows us a much more comprehensive spatial and temporal depiction of esophageal motor function than was previously possible. Dr Clouse and his collaborators developed of a new way to think about the display of manometry pressures. They assigned colors to pressures, with high pressures represented by warmer colors (reds and yellows) and low pressures by cool colors (blues and greens), and presented the data as a color topographical map of esophageal pressure, which has been called the Clouse plot or esophageal pressure topography (EPT) (Fig. 12.1).[3,4] This type of representation is analogous to weather radar images that assign color to rain intensity or topographical maps of terrain. After getting comfortable with the EPT, many esophageal motility disorders are recognizable as distinct patterns. HRM has changed how we categorize and define esophageal motor disorders.

WHAT PROCESSES DOES ESOPHAGEAL MANOMETRY REVEAL?

The tongue, pharynx, esophagus, and its sphincters convey what is eaten from the mouth to the stomach, protect against reflux of injurious gastric contents into the esophagus and airways, and clear the esophagus, should reflux happen. HRM allows clinicians to observe normal and abnormal swallowing function.

The esophagus is a roughly 20-cm long muscular tube that is closed at its upper and lower ends by sphincters. The UES partitions the pharynx from the esophagus and is seen manometrically as a zone of high pressure at the cephalad extent of the esophagus. The structure and function of the UES will be described elsewhere.

The muscular components of the esophagus consist of inner circular and outer longitudinal muscle layers named according to the axial orientation of their muscle cells. Striated muscle, which makes up the top 5% of the esophagus, has a somatic innervation. Peristalsis in this part of the esophagus is produced by patterned activation of brainstem neurons that sequentially innervate the striated esophageal muscle.[5] The muscle of the middle 35%−40% is a mixture of striated and smooth muscles, which is called the transition zone (TZ). The bottom 50%−60% of the esophagus consists of smooth muscle. A flat plexus of neurons called the myenteric plexus is sandwiched between the muscle layers. It receives neural inputs from the central nervous system (CNS), and is the terminal motor innervation of the smooth muscle esophagus.[6] Peristalsis in the smooth muscle esophagus is controlled by complicated interactions of the CNS, myenteric plexus, and smooth muscle.[7,8] Esophageal peristalsis is a ring of circular muscle contraction, which starts when pharyngeal peristalsis arrives at the UES and moves down the

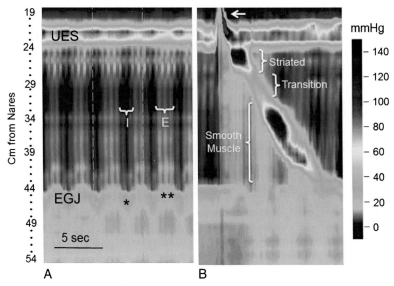

FIG. 12.1 **High-Resolution Color Topographical Pressure Plot of Normal Esophageal Anatomy and Function at Rest (A) and Following a Swallow (B).**   These recordings were made using a catheter with 36 pressure sensors positioned at 1-cm intervals along the catheter. This gives a sensing segment of 35 cm, which is long enough to span from the pharynx to the stomach. It allows recording of the entire esophageal motor response to each swallow. In these color topographical plots, pressure is depicted as colors, with higher pressures being warmer colors and lower pressures being cooler colors. The relationship between color and pressure is seen in the color bar on the right. On the y-axis is distance of pressure sensors from the nares, and time is on the x-axis. *The esophageal pressure topography at rest (A).* The band of warmer color at the top of the figure indicates tonic contraction of the resting upper esophageal sphincter (*UES*). The band of higher pressure around 46 cm from the nares is the esophagogastric junction (*EGJ*). Pressures recorded from the EGJ are a composite of tonic lower esophageal sphincter (LES) contraction (**) and cyclical crural diaphragm contraction with inspiration (*). Pressure in the chest decreases during inspiration (I) and increases during expiration (E). The opposite is true in the abdominal cavity. The point at which pressure across the EGJ during inspiration becomes negative relative to intraabdominal pressure is called the respiratory or pressure inversion point (PIP). The PIP indicates the location of the crural diaphragm. In this figure, positioning of EGJ and crural diaphragm is at the same location, which is normal. *Normal esophageal motor events initiated by swallowing (B).* Opening of the UES and LES are depicted as changes of color to hues that represent lower pressures. A short-lived rise in pressure above the UES represents peristalsis generated by the tongue and pharyngeal constrictors (*arrow*). A diagonal band of color running from the UES to the LES represents a peristaltic pressure wave. Variations in peristaltic pressure are normal along the length of the esophagus. The vigorous contraction just below the UES is generated in the striated muscle esophagus. Below this, there is a pressure trough that is called the transition zone, because it is the region over which the esophageal musculature transitions from striated to smooth muscle. The rise in peristaltic pressure below the pressure trough is the result of contraction in the smooth muscle esophagus. When peristalsis reaches the EGJ, the LES contracts.

esophagus to the esophagogastric junction (EGJ). It is observed by manometry as a wave of increased pressure that propagates down the esophagus (Fig. 12.1B). The amplitude of peristalsis normally declines in the TZ and increases in the smooth muscle segment. With swallowing, the esophagus shortens about 2.0 cm, as a result of longitudinal muscle contraction. Esophageal shortening and restoration of the original length at the end of peristalsis are seen with HRM.

The LES is composed of specialized muscle structures at the EGJ, which generate tone at rest.[9] The LES is identified by manometry as a 2- to 4-cm-wide zone of higher pressure at the EGJ (Fig. 12.1A). Elevated resting pressure at the EGJ is a composite of muscular activity from the LES, and the diaphragmatic crura, which normally border the LES. The component of the resting pressure contributed by the LES depends on the tonic contraction of the sphincter muscles, which is governed by cellular properties intrinsic to the sphincter muscle and activity of its excitatory and inhibitory innervations.[7,9,10] Pressure contributed by the diaphragmatic crura is seen as a cyclical rise and fall of pressure produced by crural contraction and relaxation during respiration[11,12] (Fig. 12.1A).

Just after a swallow is initiated, the tonically contracted LES relaxes and the EGJ opens (Fig. 12.1B). This occurs because swallowing activates vagal efferent neurons in the dorsal motor nucleus of the vagus, which terminate on myenteric neurons of the LES.[13,14] These neurons penetrate the smooth muscle layer and generate nitric oxide, which activates cellular processes in the LES muscle that result in its relaxation.[15,16] EGJ opening is recorded manometrically as a 5- to 10-s drop in pressure at the EGJ (Fig. 12.1B). The sphincter remains relaxed until the peristaltic contraction arrives. At this time, the LES contracts vigorously and then settles back to its resting pressure.

INDICATIONS FOR ESOPHAGEAL MANOMETRY

The primary indication for esophageal manometry is the evaluation of dysphagia when entities like esophagitis, eosinophilic esophagitis, esophageal ulcers or strictures, and esophageal cancers are not present. Manometry is also used to evaluate atypical or noncardiac chest pain, but only after cardiac disease, the esophageal disorders listed above, musculoskeletal pain syndromes and anxiety disorders are excluded.

Esophageal manometry is the best way to identify the upper border of the LES for accurate pH probe placement.[20] It is recommended before fundoplication: the surgical approach might be modified or the surgery abandoned when peristalsis in the smooth muscle esophagus is weak or absent. It is frequently used before bariatric surgery, especially when the patient has esophageal symptoms. HRM is used to evaluate chest pain or dysphagia following surgical antireflux and bariatric procedures. Its use is invaluable when evaluating patients with dysphagia after Heller myotomy.

HOW IS ESOPHAGEAL MOTOR FUNCTION ANALYZED?

Esophageal manometry elucidates resting characteristics of the esophageal sphincters, and esophageal motor functions initiated by swallowing. The analysis is carried according to the Chicago Classification, which uses a hierarchical approach to identify disorders of the EGJ, major disorders of peristalsis, and minor

disorders of peristalsis.[17] A number of computer tools are used to define these disorders.

The first step in the classification process is to evaluate EGJ anatomy and function. The resting characteristics of the esophageal sphincters are observed during a 30-s period when no swallowing is allowed (Fig. 12.1A). The UES and LES are recognized in the EPT as horizontal bands of color near the top and bottom of the recording. Variations in pressure generated by respiration are observed as cyclical changes in color. EPT allows a detailed analysis of the anatomical and functional properties of the EGJ. At the normal EGJ, both the resting LES and diaphragmatic crura contribute to the pressure profile. Contraction of the diaphragmatic crura is seen as cyclical variations in pressure. The isolated, resting LES pressure is observed between crural contractions (Fig. 12.1A). During inspiration, pressure goes down in the chest and up in the abdomen. The opposite is true with expiration (Fig. 12.1A). The location along the vertical axis of the EGJ at which the more negative intrathoracic pressure produced by inspiration inverts to a more positive intragastric pressure is called the pressure inversion point (PIP). The PIP essentially defines where the diaphragm partitions the chest from the abdomen. Spatial separation of the PIP from pressure produced by a resting LES identifies a hiatal hernia (Fig. 12.2).[18] By convention, resting LES pressure is the respiratory minimum LES pressure; that is, the mean of the lowest EGJ pressures during expirations in the 30-s period when no swallowing occurred. This excludes pressures generated by diaphragmatic contraction and is thought to more accurately reflect true resting LES pressure. Although resting LES pressure is not used in the Chicago Classification, a hypertensive LES might indicate dysfunction of inhibitory motor neurons supplying the LES, and herald a spastic motor dysfunction. A hypotensive LES might be associated with a number of disorders predisposing to gastroesophageal reflux disease.

Next, sphincteric motor responses to water swallowing are evaluated (Fig. 12.1B). Normally, the UES and EGJ open shortly after swallowing. This is depicted in the EPT as changes in color to tones representing lower pressures. At the UES, the pressure/color approximates that in the proximal esophagus, and at the EGJ, the pressure/color approximates that in the stomach (Fig. 12.1B). A tool called the *integrated relaxation or residual pressure* (IRP) was developed to assess sufficiency of EGJ opening (Fig. 12.3).[19] To calculate the IRP, a computer algorithm first detects the upper and lower margins of the EGJ and then identifies a 10-s time window that begins at the start of swallow-induced UES

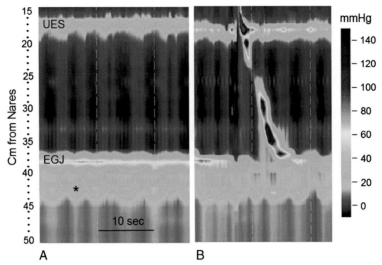

FIG. 12.2 *Hiatal hernia* at rest **(A)** and with esophageal peristalsis **(B)**. There is a spatial separation of the diaphragm (*) from the esophagogastric junction (*EGJ*), indicating a hiatal hernia. The size of the hernia varies from patient to patient. *UES,* upper esophageal sphincter.

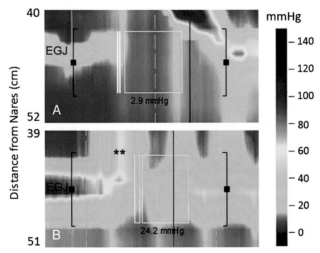

FIG. 12.3 **Evaluation of Esophagogastric Junction (*EGJ*) Function During Swallowing.** Panels **(A)** and **(B)** are focused on swallow-induced events at the EGJ. The top panel **(A)** is an esophageal pressure topography of normal EGJ function following a wet swallow. As you can see, pressure at the EGJ normally drops ahead of the advancing peristaltic pressure wave. It is not a direct measure of lower esophageal sphincter (LES) relaxation but of pressure in the swallowed bolus as it opens and traverses the EGJ. EGJ function during swallowing is determined by a measurement called the 4-s integrated relaxation (residual) pressure (IRP). It is determined within a "deglutitive relaxation window," a window that straddles the EGJ and stretches for 10 s after opening of the UES (*black brackets*). This is the spatial and temporal domain within which EGJ function is evaluated. A tool called the eSleeve (Sierra Scientific Instruments) is used to set the spatial extent of the window, which is 6 cm in length by default. The eSleeve determines the highest pressure within the deglutitive relaxation window at each point in time. The 4-s IRP algorithm takes these pressures and averages the lowest of them over four continuous or discontinuous seconds (*white boxes*). This discontinuous measurement avoids inclusion of elevated pressures produced by contraction of the crural diaphragm or cardiovascular structures in the calculation of IRP. The lower panel **(B)** is an example of an abnormal IRP seen in achalasia. In this case, pressure at the EGJ results from failed LES relaxation and pressurization of the swallowed bolus above the LES (**).

relaxation. A tool called the eSleeve, that measures pressure simultaneously over a 6-cm length, is positioned to straddle the LES. It calculates maximum pressure along the 6-cm segment at each time point within the 10-s time window. The algorithm averages the lowest of these pressures over four continuous or discontinuous seconds. This is called the 4-s IRP. Using four discontinuous seconds to determining nadir pressure eliminates pressures produced by contraction of the crural diaphragm during inspiration from calculation of the IRP. In the Chicago Classification, the normal IRP is <15 mmHg (Fig. 12.3A).[17,19] Any mechanical or functional process that impedes flow across the EGJ might elevate the IRP. Some of these abnormalities include achalasia, eosinophilic esophagitis, neoplasms, or strictures at the EGJ, and surgical complications related to Nissen fundoplication or laparoscopic band (Fig. 12.3B).

Normal esophageal peristalsis is observed in the EPT as contraction running diagonally from the UES to EGJ (Fig. 12.1B).[4] The first thing we would like to know about esophageal function is whether or not peristalsis is present and, if so, is it complete. To determine completeness of peristalsis, a 20-mmHg isobaric contour line is applied to the EPT. It appears as a black line over all parts of the EPT where the pressure is 20 mmHg and identifies if pressure drops below 20 mmHg during the peristaltic pressure wave (Fig. 12.4A). A threshold value of 20 mmHg above

which intact esophageal peristalsis is defined was chosen because this is the peristaltic pressure required for normal bolus transit when the EGJ is functioning normally. Peristaltic integrity is evaluated by looking for gaps in the 20-mmHg contour along the length of the esophagus (Fig. 12.4A). Gaps of >5 cm are thought to represent loss of peristaltic integrity and are likely to result in poor bolus transit.

Another tool developed to evaluate propagation of esophageal pressure waves is called distal latency (DL) (Fig. 12.5A). DL identifies the time from the start of swallow-induced UES opening to arrival of esophageal contraction at EGJ. Arrival of peristalsis at the EGJ is defined in the EPT by the contractile deceleration point (CDP).[20] The CDP is the point during a peristaltic pressure wave at which peristalsis in the distal esophagus appears to slow appreciably (Fig. 12.5A). Functionally, the CDP is the time at which esophageal peristalsis terminates, and the LES contracts and begins to descend to its resting position. Descent of the LES is defined radiographically as emptying of the phrenic ampulla.

The DL is presumed to measure adequacy of inhibitory neuromuscular function in the smooth muscle esophagus.[20,21] A short DL indicates early arrival of esophageal contraction in the distal esophagus. According to the Chicago Classification, esophageal spasm is defined as a DL <4.5 s and normal opening of the EGJ (Fig. 12.5B).[17,21,22]

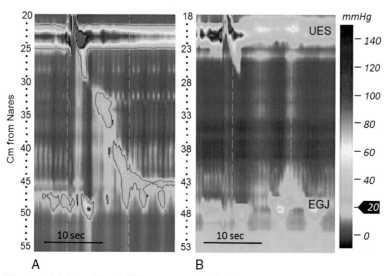

FIG. 12.4 **Weak Peristalsis.**   Panel **(A)** is an example of ineffective esophageal motility. It is defined in the Chicago Classification as a distal contractile integral (DCI) between 450 and 100 mmHg/cm s. Panel **(B)** is an example of absent peristalsis. It is defined by a DCI of <100 mmHg/cm s. The *black line* is the 20 mmHg isobaric pressure line. *UES,* upper esophageal sphincter.

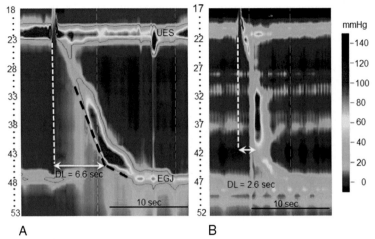

FIG. 12.5 **Distal Latency.** Panel **(A)** demonstrates normal function of the esophagus and its sphincters. The thin *black line* is a 30-mmHg isobaric contour line. It identifies all loci in the esophageal pressure topography where the pressure is 30 mmHg. The thick *dashed black line* indicates the velocity of peristalsis. Notice that there is a point at which the slope of the line changes, indicating apparent slowing of peristalsis in the distal smooth muscle esophagus. This point is called the *contractile deceleration point* (CDP). Functionally, the CDP is the time at which esophageal peristalsis terminates, and the lower esophageal sphincter descends to its resting position. The distal latency (*DL*) is the time from opening of the upper esophageal sphincter (*UES*) during swallowing (*dashed white line*) to the CDP. A normal DL is >4.5 s. A DL of <4.5 s defines esophageal spasm **(Panel B)**. *EGJ*, esophagogastric junction.

The distal contractile integral (DCI) is a tool used to measure the vigor of peristaltic contraction in the smooth muscle esophagus (Fig. 12.6). It is the integral of time, pressure, and distance of the peristaltic contraction along the smooth muscle esophagus.[23] To calculate DCI, the computer makes a box that encompasses all swallow-induced motor activity in the smooth muscle esophagus, that is, from the TZ to the CDP (Fig. 12.6). It then applies a 20-mmHg isobaric pressure line to the EPT. The DCI is calculated by summing pressures >20 mmHg from all of the time/length foci within the box. Said another way, it is basically an aggregate of the contraction amplitude of the smooth muscle esophagus, the length over which that contraction propagates, and duration of contraction. The easiest way to think about the DCI is to visualize the color topographical plot of pressure as altitude. When you do this, you can think of the topographical plot of peristalsis as a mountain range. The DCI is analogous to the volume of the mountain range. It is reported as mmHg/cm s. A peristaltic pressure wave with DCI of >8000 mmHg/cm s defines a hypercontractile peristalsis, also called jackhammer esophagus (Fig. 12.7), between 8000 and 450 as normal peristalsis (Fig. 12.6), between 450 and 100 as ineffective peristalsis (Fig. 12.4A), and <100 as failed peristalsis (Fig. 12.4B).[17,23]

Another important characteristic of the EPT is a pattern of pressurization (Fig. 12.8). Pressurization is seen as isobaric pressure (consistent pressure, i.e., the same color) simultaneously along a segment of the esophagus.[17,24,25] It is indicative of bolus entrapment, which is usually seen between the peristaltic esophageal contraction and a mechanical or functional obstruction. The obstruction is in most cases at the EGJ (Fig. 12.8). Pathological processes that cause pressurization include esophageal strictures or neoplasms, Nissen fundoplications and lap bands, and sometimes a variant of achalasia. An isobaric pressure that spans from the EGJ to the UES is called panesophageal pressurization. It is one of the common features of achalasia, which defines achalasia type II (Fig. 12.9B).[17,24,26]

After all of the swallows are analyzed with the tools described above, the data are applied to the Chicago Classification to make a diagnosis. The Chicago Classification is seen in Table 12.1. The classification scheme divides esophageal motor abnormalities into major disorders of the EGJ or esophagus that are not seen in normal subjects and minor disorders that might impair bolus clearance.

Achalasia is clinically and pathophysiologically the best understood of esophageal motor disorders. For many years, it has been defined manometrically as failure of LES relaxation and the absence of peristalsis in

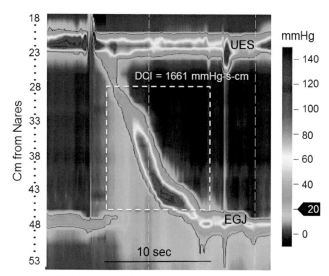

FIG. 12.6 *The distal contractile integral (DCI)* is a measure of how robust peristalsis is in the smooth muscle esophagus. It is determined by first making a box that encompasses all swallow-induced motor activity from the transition zone to the contractile deceleration point (*white dashed line*). Next, the 20-mmHg isobaric contour line is determined (*black line*). The DCI is calculated by summing pressures from all of the time/length foci within the field constrained by the box and 20-mmHg isobaric contour line. *EGJ*, esophagogastric junction; *UES*, upper esophageal sphincter.

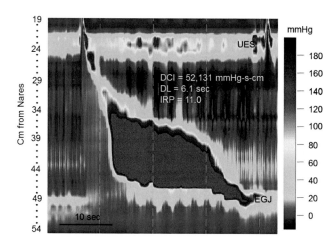

FIG. 12.7 The *jackhammer esophagus* is characterized by a distal contractile integral (*DCI*) of >8000 mmHg/cm s, with normal distal latency (*DL* > 4.5 s) and normal integrated residual or relaxation pressure (*IRP* < 15 mmHg). *EGJ*, esophagogastric junction; *UES*, upper esophageal sphincter.

the smooth muscle esophagus. With HRM, we now recognize three types of achalasia.[26] All are characterized by failure of LES relaxation, and each has a different esophageal motor pattern (Fig. 12.9). Type I achalasia has no appreciable motor activity in the smooth muscle esophagus (Fig. 12.9A), type II is defined by panesophageal pressurization (Fig. 12.9B), and type III exhibits premature contractions

(Fig. 12.9C).[26] Knowing the type of achalasia guides therapy. Type I is the most difficult to treat but is best treated with Heller myotomy, Type II responds well to all therapies, and Type III is best treated with peroral endoscopic myotomy (POEM).[26,27]

EGJ outflow obstruction is defined by failed or incomplete opening of the EGJ, some peristalsis in the smooth muscle esophagus and pressurization of the swallowed

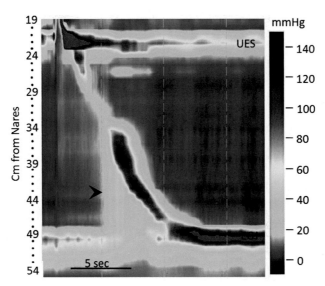

FIG. 12.8 *Esophagogastric junction (EGJ) outflow obstruction* is characterized by failed or incomplete opening of the EGJ (integrated relaxation or residual pressure >15), some peristalsis in the smooth muscle esophagus and pressurization of the swallowed bolus between an unyielding EGJ and peristaltic contraction (*arrowhead*). Peristalsis can be normal, weak or hypercontractile. *UES*, upper esophageal sphincter.

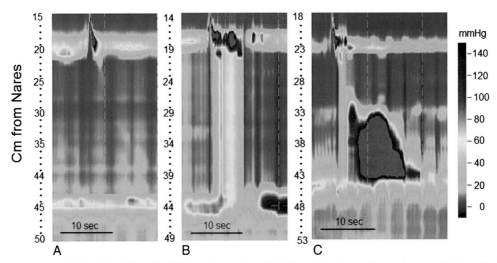

FIG. 12.9 *Achalasia* is defined by failure of normal peristalsis and inadequate esophagogastric junction opening (integrated relaxation or residual pressure >15). The disorder is further subclassified based on the morphology of esophageal pressure patterns. Type I is characterized by little if any discernible pressure activity in the esophagus **(A)**, type II by panesophageal pressurization **(B)**, and type III by premature esophageal contraction (short distal latency) **(C)**.

bolus between the unyielding EGJ and peristaltic contraction (Fig. 12.8).[24,25] This motility pattern is seen with obstructing lesions like strictures, neoplasms, tight fundoplications or tight lap bands and in some cases of eosinophilic esophagitis. Finding EGJ outflow obstruction should trigger an evaluation with upper gastrointestinal endoscopy and perhaps endoscopic ultrasound. When no mechanical obstruction is found, this motor pattern might indicate a variant of achalasia, which often responds to achalasia treatment.

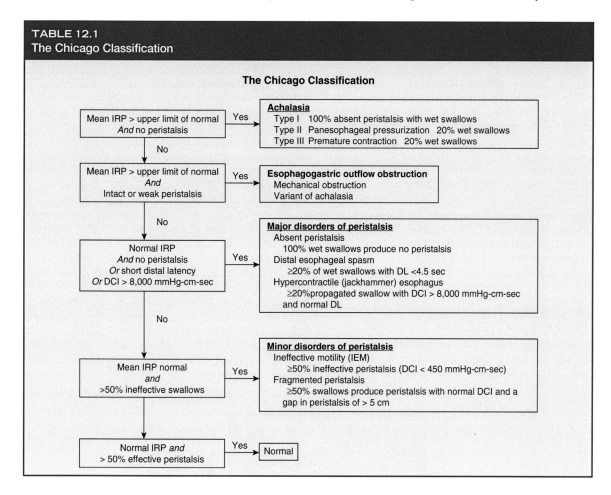

TABLE 12.1
The Chicago Classification

The classification of major disorders of esophageal peristalsis is a diverse group of esophageal motor abnormalities that are not seen in asymptomatic individuals. They include absent peristalsis, distal esophageal spasm, and jackhammer esophagus.

Absent peristalsis (Fig. 12.4B) is characterized by a normal opening of the EGJ and no peristalsis in the smooth muscle esophagus. This pattern is seen with collagen vascular disease, particularly scleroderma, amyloidosis, and occasionally diabetes or hypothyroidism.

Distal esophageal spasm (Fig. 12.5B) is an uncommon motility disorder that is characterized by a short DL (<4.5 s) and normal opening of the EGJ (Fig. 12.8A). This esophageal motor abnormality is associated with dysphagia, chest pain, and regurgitation. It is sometimes a harbinger of achalasia and can be treated with peppermint oil, type 5 phosphodiesterase inhibitors, nitrates, BoTox injection, or now by POEM.

Jackhammer esophagus (Fig. 12.7) is a relatively rare EPT pattern that is defined by wet swallows producing a peristaltic contraction in the smooth muscle with a DCI >8000 mmHg/cm s, normal DL, and normal opening of the EGJ. These contractions are usually prolonged and can be multiphasic. The symptoms and treatment of jackhammer esophagus are the same as for spasm. It is typically associated with dysphagia and/or noncardiac chest pain, which might be amenable to medications that modulate visceral pain and/or relax smooth muscle. Jackhammer esophagus is occasionally associated with the pattern of EGJ outflow obstruction. This suggests that the esophagus is working very hard against an obstruction at the EGJ. This finding should spark a search for an obstruction lesion at the EGJ. This combination of EPT patterns has also been suggested as another form of achalasia.

The other major category of motor abnormalities in the Chicago Classification is called *minor disorders of peristalsis*. One of these abnormalities is called ineffective esophageal motility, which is characterized by weak peristalsis (DCI between 450 and 100 mmHg/cm s) (Fig. 12.4A). The other abnormality is fragmented peristalsis which is defined as a larger than 5-cm gap in peristaltic contractions which have a normal DCI (between 8000 and 450 mmHg/cm s) (Fig. 12.10). These motor abnormalities are associated with poor bolus transit, which can be seen with impedance measurement or radiographically as the bolus being left behind in the esophagus after the peristaltic contraction. When this occurs in the proximal esophagus at the level of the TZ, it is called proximal bolus escape.[28] Failed bolus clearance might be sensed as dysphagia or even regurgitation.

WHAT DOESN'T THE CHICAGO CLASSIFICATION TELL US?

The Chicago Classification does not address all abnormalities of the swallowing apparatus.[29] These abnormalities include disorders of the pharynx, UES, or striated muscle esophagus; postsurgical problems; supragastric belching; and the rumination syndrome.

HRM facilitates evaluation of UES function. A hypertensive UES is the most common UES abnormality. It is usually an artifact from irritation caused by the catheter. It is often accompanied by prolonged, hypertensive peristaltic contractions of the striated muscle esophagus. These elevated pressures tend to disappear over time, as the patient accommodates to the catheter. Occasionally, the UES is hypotensive. This is usually seen as the study progresses, probably because the patient accommodates to the catheter. All of this suggests that UES evaluation might be the most reliable at the end of study. A hypotensive UES is observed in patients with neuromuscular diseases that affect the striated muscle[18,30,31] but might be a part of the aging process.[32] UES pressure usually varies during the respiratory cycle, increasing during inspiration. The UES opens spontaneously in several situations: to vent the esophagus when bolus transit is compromised, as with achalasia, and during transient LES relaxation (tLESR), rumination events, or supragastric belches.[18]

It is possible to evaluate pharyngeal motor function with HRM (Fig. 12.11A). The catheter is positioned so that some sensors are in the nasopharynx and some in

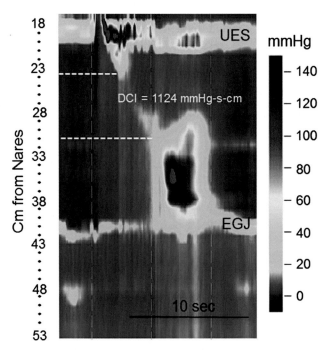

FIG. 12.10 *Fragmented peristalsis* is defined by a normal distal contractile integral (*DCI*), between 450 and 8000 mmHg/cm s, and a gap in the peristaltic pressure wave of >5 cm. This pattern is associated with poor bolus transit. *EGJ*, esophagogastric junction; *UES*, upper esophageal sphincter.

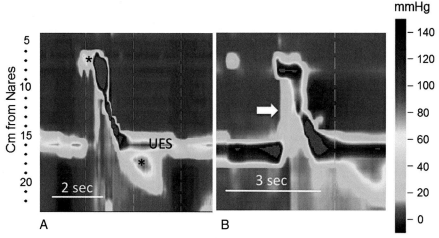

FIG. 12.11   Panel **(A)** is a topographical plot of normal pharyngeal motor function produced by a 5-cc water swallow. The *asterisk* indicates velopalatine closure. Above this is the nasopharynx. Between it and the upper esophageal sphincter (*UES*) is the mesopharynx. Pharyngeal peristalsis is seen as the pressure wave propagating from the end of velopalatine closure to the UES. Normally, during swallow-induced opening of the UES pharyngeal bolus, pressure approximates that in esophageal bolus. In panel **(B)**, there is an elevated pharyngeal bolus pressure (*arrow*). Pharyngeal pressurization raises the possibility of pharyngeal outlet obstruction by a cricopharyngeal bar. *DCI,* distal contractile integral; *DL,* distal latency; *IRP,* integrated relaxation or residual pressure.

the proximal esophagus. In this position, velopalatine closure, peristalsis resulting from tongue and pharyngeal constrictor contraction, and UES opening are easily observed (Fig. 12.11A). Hypotensive or absent peristalsis in the pharynx and/or striated muscle esophagus is seen with neuromuscular diseases that affect striated muscle, e.g., myositis and myasthenia gravis, and Parkinson disease.[18,29–31] Radiation injury can also produce profound weakness of the pharynx, UES, and striated muscle esophagus.[18] A pattern of pressurization in the pharynx indicates obstruction to flow across the UES (Fig. 12.11B). This pattern is typical of a symptomatic cricopharyngeal bar.

tLESR, rumination, and supragastric belch can be differentiated with high-resolution esophageal manometry. A description of these abnormalities and their genesis is beyond the scope of this review but can be found elsewhere.[33–35]

HRM can also be used to evaluate patients with esophageal symptoms after operations like Nissen fundoplication, Heller myotomy for achalasia, and bariatric surgery.[36]

CONCLUSIONS

HRM provides us with a complete spatial and temporal view of esophageal motor function for the first time.

Almost all disorders of esophageal motor function produce different EPT patterns that are easily distinguished from one another. There are now efforts to apply this technology to pharyngeal motor function. They have not reached the sophistication of the Chicago Classification.

REFERENCES

1. Steff JJ, Dodds WJ, Hogan WJ, Linehan JH, Stewart ET. Intraluminal esophageal manometry: an analysis of variables affecting recording fidelity of peristaltic pressures. *Gastroenterology.* 1974;67:221–230.
2. Arndorfer RC, Steff JJ, Dodds WJ, Linehan JH, Hogan WJ. Improved infusion system for intraluminal esophageal manometry. *Gastroenterology.* 1977;73:23–27.
3. Clouse RE, Staiano A. Topography of the esophageal peristaltic pressure wave. *Am J Physiol.* 1991;261:G677–G684.
4. Clouse RE, Staiano A, Alrakawi A, Harolan A. Application of topographical methods to clinical esophageal manometry. *Am J Gastroenterol.* 2000;95:2720–2730.
5. Roman C. Nervous control of esophageal peristalsis. *J de Physiol.* 1966;58:79–108.
6. Christensen J, Robison BA. Anatomy of the myenteric plexus of the opossum esophagus. *Gastroenterology.* 1982; 83:1033–1042.
7. Conklin JL, Christensen J. Motor functions of the esophagus. In: Johnson LR, Christensen J, Alpers D, Jacobsen ED, Walsh J, eds. *Physiology of the Gastrointestinal Tract.* 3rd ed. 1994:33–40 [Chapter 4].

8. Doty RW. Neural organization of deglutition. In: Code CF, ed. *Handbook of Physiology, Section 6. Alimentary Canal.* Vol. 4. 1968:1861–1902.

9. Goyal RK, Rattan S. Genesis of basal sphincter pressure: effect of tetrodotoxin on lower esophageal sphincter pressure in opossum in vivo. *Gastroenterology.* 1976;71:62–77.

10. Holloway RH, Blank EL, Takashashi I, Dodds WJ, Dent J, Sarna SK. Electrical control activity of the lower esophageal sphincter in unanesthetized opossums. *Am J Physiol.* 1987; 252:G511–G521.

11. Mittal RK, Rochester DF, McCallum RW. Sphincteric action of the diaphragm during a relaxed lower esophageal sphincter in humans. *Am J Physiol.* 1989;256:G139–G144.

12. Boyle JT, Altschuler SM, Nixon TE, Tuchman DN, Pack AI, Cohen S. Role of the diaphragm in the genesis of lower esophageal sphincter pressure in the cat. *Gastroenterology.* 1985;88:723–730.

13. Rossiter CD, Norman WP, Jain M, Hornby PJ, Benjamin S, Gillis RA. Control of the lower esophageal sphincter pressure by two sites in the dorsal motor nucleus of the vagus. *Am J Physiol.* 1990;256:G899–G906.

14. Paterson WG, Anderson MA, Anand N. Pharmacological characterization of lower esophageal sphincter relaxation induced by swallowing, vagal efferent nerve stimulation, and esophageal distension. *Can J Physiol Pharmacol.* 1992; 70:1011–1015.

15. Murray J, Du C, Ledlow A, Bates JN, Conklin JL. Nitric oxide: mediator of nonadrenergic noncholinergic responses of opossum esophageal muscle. *Am J Physiol.* 1991;261: G401–G406.

16. Tøttrup A, Svane D, Forman A. Nitric oxide mediating NANC inhibition in opossum lower esophageal sphincter. *Am J Physiol.* 1991;260:G385–G389.

17. Kahrilas PJ, Bredenoord M, Gyawali S, Roman S, Smout AJPM, Pandolfino JE. The international working group on high resolution esophageal manometry. The Chicago classification of esophageal motility disorders, v3.0. *Neurogastroenterol Motil.* 2015;27:160–174.

18. Conklin JL, Pimentel M, Soffer E. *A Color Atlas of High-Resolution Manometry.* New York: Springer; 2009.

19. Ghosh SK, Pandolfino JE, Rice J, Clarke JO, Kwiatek M, Kahrilas PJ. Impaired deglutitive EGJ relaxation in clinical esophageal manometry: a quantitative analysis of 400 patients and 75 controls. *Am J Physiol Gastrointest Liver Physiol.* 2007;293:G878–G885.

20. Pandolfino JE, Leslie E, Luger D, Mitchell B, Kwiatek MA, Kahrilas PJ. The contractile deceleration point: an important physiological landmark on oesophageal pressure topography. *Neurogastrenterol Motil.* 2010;22:395–400.

21. Pandolfino JE, Roman S, Lin Z, Kahrilas PJ. Distal contraction latency: a measure of propagation velocity optimized for esophageal pressure topography studies. *Am J Gastroenterol.* 2011;106:443–451.

22. Pandolfino JE, Roman S, Carlson D, et al. Distal esophageal spasm in high-resolution esophageal pressure topography: defining clinical phenotypes. *Gastroenterology.* 2011;141:469–475.

23. Pandolfino JE, Ghosh SK, Rice J, Clarke JO, Kwiatek MA, Kahrilas PJ. Classifying esophageal motility by pressure topography characteristics: a study of 400 patients and 75 controls. *Am J Gastroenterol.* 2008;103:27–37.

24. Scherer JR, Kwiatek MA, Soper NJ, Pandolfino JE, Kahrilas PJ. Functional esophagogastric junction obstruction with intact peristalsis: a heterogeneous syndrome sometimes akin to achalasia. *J Gastrointest Surg.* 2009;13: 2219–2225.

25. Gyawali CP, Kushnir VM. High-resolution manometric characteristics help differentiate types of distal esophageal obstruction in patients with peristalsis. *Neurogastroenterol Motil.* 2011;23:502–e197.

26. Pandolfino JE, Kwiatek MA, Nealis T, Bulsiewicz W, Post J, Kahrilas PJ. Achalasia: a new clinically relevant classification by high-resolution manometry. *Gastroenterology.* 2008;135:1526–1533.

27. Salvador R, Costantini M, Zaninotto G, et al. The preoperative manometric pattern predicts the outcome of surgical treatment for esophageal achalasia. *J Gastrointest Surg.* 2010;14:1635–1645.

28. Ghosh SK, Janiak P, Fox M, Schwizer W, Hebbard GS, Brasseur JG. Physiology of the oesophageal transition zone in the presence of chronic bolus retention: studies using concurrent high-resolution manometry and digital fluoroscopy. *Neurogastroenterol Motil.* 2008;20:750–759.

29. Wan UT, Yazaki E, Sifrim D. High-resolution manometry: esophageal disorders not addressed by the Chicago classification. *J Neurogastroenterol Motil.* 2012;18:365–372.

30. Ebert EC. Review article: the gastrointestinal complications of myositis. *Aliment Pharmacol Ther.* 2010;31:359–365.

31. Huang MH, King KL, Chien KY. Esophageal manometric studies in patients with myasthenia gravis. *J Thorac Cardiovasc Surg.* 1988;95:281–285.

32. Fulp SR, Dalton CB, Castell JA, Castell DO. Aging-related alterations in human upper esophageal sphincter function. *Am J Gastroenterol.* 1990;85:1569–1572.

33. Pandolfino JE, Zhang QG, Ghosh SK, Han A, Boniquit C, Kahrilas PJ. Transient lower esophageal sphincter relaxations and reflux: mechanistic analysis using concurrent fluoroscopy and high-resolution manometry. *Gastroenterology.* 2006;131:1725–1733.

34. Tucker E, Knowles K, Wright J, Fox MR. Rumination variations: aetiology and classification of abnormal behavioural responses to digestive symptoms based on high-resolution manometry studies. *Aliment Pharmacol Ther.* 2013;37:263–274.

35. Kessing BF, Bredenoord AJ, Smout AJ. Mechanisms of gastric and supragastric belching: a study using concurrent high-resolution manometry and impedance monitoring. *Neurogastroenterol Motil.* 2012;24:e573–e579.

36. Burch M, Conklin JL. Post-surgical dysphagia: post-Nissen fundoplication, C-spine surgery, thyroid surgery, gastric banding, gastric bypass. In: Shaker R, Belafsky P, Postma G, Easterling C, eds. *Principles of Deglutition: A Multidisciplinary Text for Swallowing and its Disorders.* New York: Springer; 2012:631–644.

CHAPTER 13

Developing the Optimal Treatment Strategy for Dysphagia

DINESH K. CHHETRI, MD

INTRODUCTION

Contemporary management of oropharyngeal dysphagia is a multidisciplinary effort. The otolaryngologist and the speech language pathologist (SLP) must play central roles in evaluation and co-management of dysphagia. Other specialties such as gastroenterology and general surgery also play significant roles, especially for esophageal dysphagia. The optimal treatment can be developed and offered to the patient only after a thorough assessment of swallowing dysfunction via targeted history, physical exam, instrumental exams of swallowing, and consideration of relevant comorbid medical conditions and cognitive functioning of the patient. Treatment decisions may be primary surgery, primary swallow therapy, or both. Sometimes, observation and routine surveillance is an acceptable treatment approach. A collaborative multidisciplinary approach for the assessment and treatment of dysphagia will lead to better medical decisions and superior swallowing outcomes.

DEVELOPING THE OPTIMAL TREATMENT PLAN TOGETHER

The optimal dysphagia treatment is developed if the otolaryngologist and SLP with dedicated clinical focus on dysphagia work closely together. Ideally, both should convene a face-to-face meeting and review the core triad of instrumental swallow assessments for dysphagia: flexible endoscopic evaluation of swallowing (FEES), modified barium swallow study (MBSS), and transnasal esophagoscopy (TNE). At the minimum, there should be open channels of communication between the two to co-manage the patient. At our institution, we convene weekly meetings to go over all swallow studies. This collaborative effort has many benefits. For the otolaryngologist, it is

very useful to review the MBSS personally with the SLP to correlate and corroborate the anatomic and swallowing dysfunction seen on FEES, especially for surgical planning. An indepth discussion of swallowing evaluations, and the pros and cons of the different treatment options is discussed. The face-to-face discussion also benefits the SLP, as it brings out in discussion the physician's assessment and plans as well as what MBSS images, interpretations, and reporting is needed to facilitate those treatment decisions. The SLP can also view the endoscopic images to more fully understand the patient's anatomy and swallow function and provide input about how a surgical intervention may impact swallow function or swallow therapy. The approach also improves the coordination of care. For example, a decision can be made for a staged treatment approach, with surgery followed by swallow therapy or vice versa. Most importantly, the patient benefits from better treatment decisions and swallowing outcomes that result when cases are discussed and the patient's dysphagia complaints and swallow dysfunction are clarified prior to treatment. This collaboration also allows the swallow team to speak with a single voice, which may improve the patient's understanding of the problem and plans for managing dysphagia.

The dysphagia history is first discussed during the case reviews. A key question to consider is how the medical history may be expected to relate to the patient's swallowing problems. For example, is there a history of chronic neurologic disease, chemoradiation therapy, head and neck surgery, or other acute exacerbating factors such as recent stroke? What is the patient's age? This may be an important consideration since some elderly individuals have multiple medical conditions and reduced functional reserve. Generally, older patients in their 80s and 90s poorly tolerate acute worsening of swallow function and its complications. How long has the patient had a swallowing problem? The time since the onset of dysphagia is particularly important in dysphagia from chemoradiation therapy for head and neck cancer. We also consider the patient's description of the swallowing problems as well as medical conditions that may have a bearing on treatment considerations, such as dementia. Next, the swallow studies are reviewed. FEES provides anatomic details of swallowing apparatus and severity of pharyngeal residue as well as penetration/aspiration. MBSS allows a closer review of all phases of swallowing. The pharyngeal phase of swallowing is quick and lasts about a second, thus reviewing the study in real time often misses the relevant swallow events. Thus, frame-by-frame analysis of the pharyngeal phase of the swallow is performed to fully discern the anatomic and physiologic details of swallow dysfunction. Commercially available video software capable of pausing/advancing/rewinding each frame is needed for this task. After the MBSS review, other tests that may have been obtained—TNE, esophagram, high-resolution esophageal manometry—are discussed. We find it particularly useful to document the severity and details of the following findings in making treatment decisions: presence or absence of (1) pharyngeal weakness, (2) epiglottic dysfunction, (3) penetration, (4) aspiration, (5) upper esophageal sphincter (UES) dysfunction, (6) findings of an esophageal screen on MBSS, if performed, and (7) overall impression of the swallow dysfunction and the contributing factors.

A consensus treatment plan is then developed. First, an overall impression of the key factors that explains the swallow dysfunction should be made. For example, a patient with long-standing dysphagia from radiation therapy or neurodegenerative disease may have had an acute worsening of swallowing after a recent surgical procedure even if the surgery was not in the head and neck region. In such cases, one could anticipate that the swallow dysfunction may be improved at least to baseline before the latest exacerbation in swallowing. The overall treatment plan is documented, including recommendations for (1) currently safe diet, (2) surgical intervention(s), and/or (3) swallow therapy. If both surgery and swallow therapy are recommended, the timing of either should be decided, as well as the swallow therapy technique(s) that may be most effective. For example, if surgery could worsen penetration/aspiration, then it makes sense to train the patient in the supraglottic or super-supraglottic swallow technique to protect the airway prior to surgery. On the other hand, if significant obstructions to swallowing are present, then those obstructions should be removed prior to swallow therapy (assuming that treating the obstruction will not increase the risk of aspiration—each patient

must be viewed as a unique case). Finally, potential barriers to improving swallow function should be considered and documented. Such considerations include the length of time from chemoradiation therapy, whether the pharynx is insensate, the cognitive status of the patient, insurance/financial considerations, the current living arrangements of the patient (e.g., home vs. skilled nursing facility), etc. Finally, the patient is contacted and the plan presented, along with estimated risks and likelihood of improvement.

DECISION MAKING FOR SURGICAL INTERVENTION

Significant obstructions to bolus flow generally require surgical intervention. These include (1) pharyngeal stenosis, (2) epiglottic dysfunction, (3) cricopharyngeal dysfunction, (4) Zenker's diverticulum, (5) esophageal stenosis, and (6) esophageal achalasia (especially type II). A patient with a history of chemoradiation therapy for pharyngeal cancer may develop pharyngeal stenosis, epiglottic dysfunction, and esophageal stenosis (see Chapters 15 and 16). Such obstructions are best treated prior to swallow therapy (Fig. 13.1). Obstructive cricopharyngeus (CP) muscle is generally quite obvious on radiologic swallow tests, and residue also remains above the obstructive CP bar after the swallow. When obstruction is not quite obvious then an anteroposterior view on an MBSS, showing positive "cobra sign," is useful in deciding for surgery (see Chapter 19). During dysphagia rounds, cricopharyngeal bars are carefully assessed since some bars are nonobstructive or only result in small amounts of stasis—surgery is typically not recommended in these situations. The definitive treatment for Zenker's diverticulum is surgical, and these entities are quite obvious on swallow exams as well (see Chapter 20). Esophageal strictures should be treated surgically (see Chapters 9, 10, 15, and 22).

Other cases require further discussion, careful planning, and discussion with patients regarding the risks and benefits of interventions. Epiglottic dysfunction may be treated surgically; however, cases should be selected carefully. Ideal candidates have epiglottis that does not deflect and obstructs the food bolus, have good base of tongue strength and laryngeal sensation, and have pharyngeal crowding that is in part due to the epiglottis (see Chapter 16). Aspiration before the swallow or penetration to the vocal folds is a negative predictor for success with epiglottic surgery (Fig. 13.2). A Killian–Jamieson (KJ) diverticulum typically does not require treatment because the pouch is below the UES and therefore easily empties toward the esophagus. On occasion, it is truly symptomatic

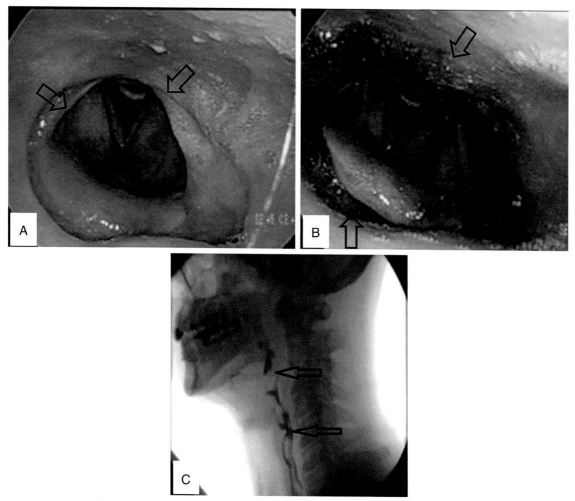

FIG. 13.1 Swallow evaluation in a 78-year-old male patient with a history of chemoradiation therapy for left base of tongue squamous cell carcinoma. (A) Flexible laryngoscopy reveals pharyngeal stenosis at the level of the mid-suprahyoid epiglottis (*arrows*). (B) Flexible endoscopic evaluation of swallowing shows vallecular (*bottom arrow*) and posterior pharyngeal residue (*top arrow*). (C) Modified barium swallow study corroborates epiglottic dysfunction (*top arrow*) and also reveals a "stricture sign" consistent with esophageal stenosis (*bottom arrow*).

because of its size or because it does not empty with certain materials such as pills. In such cases, open surgical resection of KJ diverticulum is warranted (Fig. 13.3). Cervical osteophytes also require careful consideration. The location of the osteophyte determines the mechanisms of dysphagia. Osteophytes at the level of the hypopharynx can narrow the UES area and require external approach for removal, whereas osteophytes at the level of the epiglottis may cause epiglottic dysfunction and may be treated with epiglottic trimming (see Chapter 17). Osteophytes

are often present in older patients who also have concurrent pharyngeal weakness, thus osteophyte resection may lead to further pharyngeal weakness for a variable length of time, and patients should be appropriately counseled. Dysphagia related to radiation therapy for head and neck carcinoma also require careful evaluation of the various contributions to dysphagia; these include obstructions from scars and stenosis, pharyngeal muscle weakness, UES dysfunction, and sensory loss. Each of these dysfunctions should be addressed.

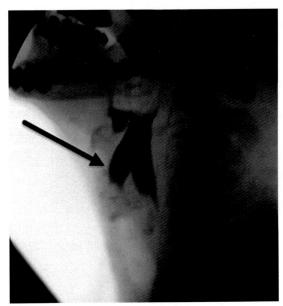

FIG. 13.2 Modified barium swallow study image illustrating significant laryngeal penetration (*arrow*). Epiglottic surgery has the potential to worsen swallowing.

A systematic approach to dysphagia management generally ensures all relevant issues have been covered before treatment is recommended. Dysphagia etiology and duration is an important consideration. Dysphagia after stroke generally improves with time, whereas dysphagia after chemoradiation therapy generally worsens with time. New onset dysphagia is generally more treatable than long-term dysphagia. The likelihood of improving dysphagia without intervention should be considered and discussed with the patient. Is there obstructive anatomy? If so, what is it and what is the functional impact? Will surgery improve or harm swallow function? Sometimes, it is necessary to place a gastric tube concurrently with the dysphagia surgery if oropharyngeal surgery is expected to temporarily worsen swallowing in those with severe dysphagia and aspiration risk. Other swallow deficits that negatively impact the effectiveness of surgery should be considered. Barriers to surgical treatment (e.g., severe trismus, poor physical reserve, severity of swallow deficit, requirement for G-tube during recovery, etc.) should be considered and discussed. If there is no obstructive anatomy, then discussion moves to other possible methodologies to improve swallow function.

After systematic analysis, the determination may be made to not offer any surgical treatment or swallow therapy. For example, a patient with mild weakness of pharyngeal constrictors with trace residue but good base of tongue contraction and no penetration/aspiration may be observed because it is challenging to target pharyngeal constrictors for therapy. If dysphagia symptoms do not match the oropharyngeal swallow findings on FEES or MBSS, then symptoms may be referred from esophageal dysfunction. In those cases, further evaluation with esophageal phase swallow assessments such as TNE, barium esophagram, and high-resolution esophageal manometry may be ordered. Occasionally, dysphagia evaluation from the lips to esophagus reveals no objective dysfunction or very mild dysfunction. In such situations, reassurance and observation is justified.

DECISION MAKING FOR SWALLOW THERAPY

Swallow therapy is a critical component of dysphagia treatment (see Chapter 24). An instrumental assessment of swallowing is required prior to initiation of swallow therapy. This is to assess for the deficits present and what exercises will address the patient's dysphagia, the aspiration risks to using liquid and food for swallow therapy, and the results of compensatory techniques. Either FEES or MBSS can be used for this assessment, but the main advantage of FEES is that since radiation is not used, a prolonged and leisurely time to evaluate the results of compensatory techniques is possible. On the other hand, MBSS is better for assessing why a patient aspirates and the severity of aspiration during the swallow.

After physical obstructions to swallowing are treated surgically, a repeat instrumental assessment may be required to determine optimal swallow therapy technique. The timing of therapy in relation to surgery may vary depending on the initial swallow assessment. For example, in patients with epiglottic dysfunction but significant penetration or aspiration, a super-supraglottic swallow technique can be taught and the surgery performed subsequently once adequate airway protection is demonstrated. On the other hand, a patient with significant pharyngeal stenosis and weakness is better served with pharyngeal surgery for stenosis to remove the obstruction followed by swallow therapy.

Swallow therapy focuses on swallow deficits. Swallow therapy targets some muscles better than others. Tongue muscles and strap muscles are more easily targeted for therapy than pharyngeal constrictor muscles. Compensatory maneuvers (e.g., head turn, chin tuck) are also relatively straightforward to teach compared to swallow techniques (e.g., Mendelsohn maneuver or super-supraglottic swallow). Also, all parties should understand that swallow therapy is more beneficial in patients with mild dysphagia, those with new onset

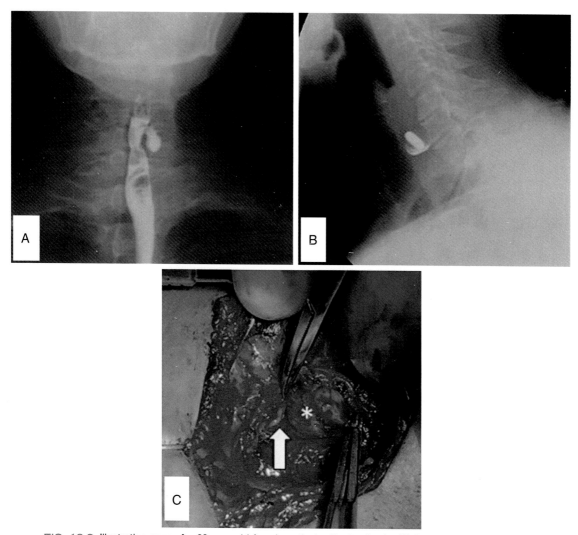

FIG. 13.3 Illustrative case of a 63-year-old female patient with dysphagia. (A) Anteroposterior view of the barium esophagram shows a left lateral diverticulum consistent with a Killian–Jamieson diverticulum. (B) Lateral view shows a barium capsule stuck in the diverticulum. (C) Intraoperative view of the diverticulum (*) shows the proximity of the diverticulum to the recurrent laryngeal nerve (*arrow*).

dysphagia, those with more intact muscular function, those with intact pharyngeal sensation to food bolus, and those who sense aspiration. Other barriers to success with swallow therapy include inadequate cognition, language impairment, poor physical reserve, and poor motivation (see Chapter 24).

THE TERRIBLE TRIAD TO OVERCOME
Safe and adequate swallowing requires the following three major physiologic functions: (1) adequate sensation, (2) adequate driving force, and (3) adequate UES

function. If all three are functioning normally, the swallow should be efficient and safe. Patients may potentially still swallow with rehabilitation if at least one of those functions is normal. A "terrible triad" is present when all three functions are severely compromised. In such cases, the swallow will invariably be abnormal, inefficient, and unsafe for per oral intake. Considering these basic physiologic requirements can help focus the dysphagia clinician to work on rehabilitation of driving force and UES opening. Unfortunately, we do not know how to treat sensory deficits for pharyngeal residue and aspiration.

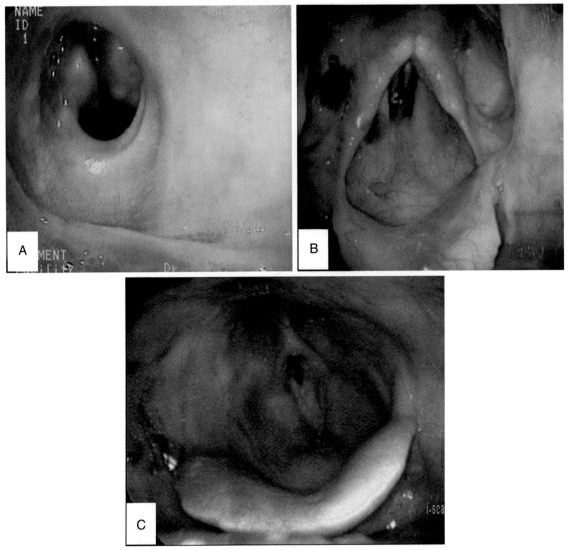

FIG. 13.4 (A–C) Illustrative cases of severe swallowing dysfunction and "Terrible triads" (see text).

Despite all efforts, some patients may not be successfully rehabilitated. Some examples of such patients include (Fig. 13.4): (1) the patient after a supraglottic laryngectomy and partial glossectomy, a free flap reconstruction of the supraglottis and base of tongue, and a pharyngoesophageal stricture. He is asensate, and cough is not triggered until the food bolus is aspirated. He cannot generate adequate pharyngeal driving force and aspirates despite learning a good super-supraglottic swallow maneuver and successful dilation of the stricture (Fig. 13.4A); (2) the patient who comes 30 years after radiation treatment for nasopharyngeal cancer with severe radiation fibrosis and multiple cranial neuropathies involving CN IX, CN X, and CN XI. Swallow is nonfunctional (Fig. 13.4B); (3) the patient with radiation therapy for hypopharyngeal cancer who has pharyngeal scarring, no lateral channels, and narrowing of the hypopharynx (Fig. 13.4C). All of these cases suffer from the terrible triad. In such cases, continued nonoral alimentation (i.e., gastric tube) is recommended. Diversion of the food way from the airway via surgery such as a laryngectomy is a perfectly reasonable approach in these patients but not all agree to undergo this radical operation for their dysphagia. In addition, free-flap reconstruction is frequently needed in these patients, and postoperative swallowing may continue to be dysfunctional. Therefore, such patients should be counseled appropriately.

CONCLUSIONS

Optimal treatment planning for dysphagia is made if the otolaryngologist and the SLP work closely together to assess the anatomic and physiologic basis for dysphagia and develop an individualized dysphagia management plan. Such a working relationship not only makes it enjoyable to become a dysphagia clinician but also improves swallowing outcomes. A multidisciplinary team including otolaryngologists, SLPs, gastroenterologists, and general surgeons should be developed for comprehensive dysphagia treatment. Obstructive etiologies should be treated first to clear the "pipe" (i.e., obstructions), following by treatment of muscular weakness to treat any "pump" failure. Treatment should consider improving the three physiologic requirements for swallowing: adequate sensation, adequate pharyngeal strength, and adequate UES opening.

CHAPTER 14

Neurologic Dysphagia

KENNETH W. ALTMAN, MD, PHD

INTRODUCTION

The concept of "neurologic dysphagia" is both obvious and profound. While it is well established that the phases of swallowing involve oral preparatory, oropharyngeal and esophageal components, the roles of the brain, brainstem, and larynx are often assumed or forgotten.[1] Reflexive swallowing occurs about 500 times a day (2–3 times a minute), driven by unconscious brainstem pacing.[2] Swallowing involves the central neurologic control of 30 muscles through 5 cranial and 3 peripheral nerves.[3] The brainstem is reflexively involved to coordinate cessation of breathing during the swallow.[4] The cortex and primitive brain drive hunger, thirst, and satiety, and have control over awareness of food in the mouth and throat. And afferent nerves are critical to sensation of food in the mouth, pharynx, and larynx with both conscious and reflexive responses.

Central and peripheral neurologic diseases, such as neurodegenerative disease, stroke, and dementia that reflect the spectrum of neurologic contributions to swallowing dysfunction have a profound impact on deglutition. While the etiologies of these diseases are very different, they have a number of commonalities when it comes to the presentation of dysphagia. These include (1) they typically occur in an aging population, (2) there is potential for cognitive impairment (either through direct effects of the disease, comorbidities, or indirect effects of medication), (3) neuromuscular atrophy is often present and progressive, (4) discoordination is also present from deconditioning and central neurologic disease, (5) patients eventually become less active and have a sedentary lifestyle, and (6) they are associated with predominantly oropharyngeal dysphagia and aspiration risk.[5]

Paradoxically, as the diseases progress with age, there is also an increasing nutritional requirement to stave off muscular atrophy. This leads to increased need for oral intake, further taxing the vulnerable deglutition and increasing aspiration risk. This chapter reviews the commonly encountered central and peripheral neurologic diseases presenting with dysphagia, discusses the likelihood of encountering dysphagia, and introduces a management approach that focuses on preserving nutritional requirements and quality of life.

COMMON NEUROLOGIC DYSPHAGIA CONDITIONS

Neurodegenerative Disease

Neurodegenerative diseases are among the most important causes of dysphagia among patients seen by neurologists. Muscular dystrophy, myasthenia gravis (MG), multiple sclerosis (MS), amyotrophic lateral sclerosis (ALS), and Parkinson's disease (PD) are the most commonly encountered, although there are variants with each that may affect different aspects to the swallow. Nevertheless, they all share the consequences of malnutrition, aspiration risk, and ultimately the potential for respiratory failure as a terminal event.

Advancing disease in combination with the aging process frequently leads to an aspiration event that requires hospitalization. When the treatment team recognizes aspiration, they are faced with the dilemma of supplying the patient's nutritional needs, often recommending nil per os (NPO) status along with placement of an enteral feeding tube. The lengthy hospitalization leads to confusion, delayed cognition, inconsistency with medication, and physical deconditioning. Coupled with social stigmata and isolation, they are also prone to depression, sedentary lifestyle, and further increased aspiration. Despite these discouraging events, some new perspectives on these diseases relative to dysphagia are beginning to emerge.

The correlation of functional decline in neurodegenerative diseases with increased dysphagia and aspiration risk is intuitive, but only partly supported by existing literature in a comprehensive review.[6] In a prospective cross-sectional study, over 700 patients with MS were evaluated for dysphagia on self-reported questionnaires, and worsening dysphagia was correlated with

TABLE 14.1 Sentinel Indicators of Decline With Dysphagia and Increased Aspiration Risk			
Demographic	**History**	**Physical Exam**	**Swallowing Evaluation**
Advanced age	Falls	Impaired cognition	Decreased oral bolus manipulation
Medical comorbidities	Wheelchair-bound	Confusion	Delayed initiation of tongue thrust
Poor nutritional status	Recent hospitalization	Drooling	Decreased laryngeal elevation
Depression/anxiety	Recent surgery	Wet voice	Decreased laryngeal sensation
Nursing home resident	Respiratory symptoms	Weak voice	Pooled secretions in the vallecular
	Fatigue and weakness	Cough	and pyriforms
		Dysarthria	Gross or microaspiration

Adapted from Altman KW, Richards A, Goldberg L, Frucht S, McCabe DJ. Dysphagia in stroke, neurodegenerative disease, and advanced dementia. *Otolaryngol Clin N Am*. 2013;46(6):1137–1149.

neurologist-observed functional status.[7] While this study needs to be extended to other neurodegenerative populations, it lends support for screening and early intervention to delay an eventual aspiration event.

Sentinel indicators of decline are clues to dysphagia and aspiration. In addition to functional performance scales for specific neurologic diseases, there are demographic generalizations, patient history, physical exam findings, and swallowing evaluation outcomes that may portend functional decline with swallowing (as listed in Table 14.1). Recognizing both functional status, as well as these sentinel indicators of decline, allows for early intervention in delaying the aspiration event, additional nutritional support to stave off muscular atrophy, and may prolong *quality* of life.

Dysarthria is an indication of oral/oropharyngeal dysphagia. This principle is also intuitive, and now supported by a systematic review showing co-prevalence between dysarthria and dysphagia, although not necessarily proving a causal relationship.[8] Manipulation of the bolus in the oral preparatory phase utilizes the same tongue muscles as articulation when speaking. In addition to adequately preparing the food bolus for swallowing, the posterior tongue thrust plays a vital role in triggering the involuntary sequence of the oropharyngeal swallow. The loss of tongue muscle control and coordination (especially associated with the fasciculation's and atrophy appreciated in ALS) is an extreme example resulting in dysarthria with oral/oropharyngeal dysphagia.

Table 14.2 summarizes these important neurodegenerative diseases with relevance to dysphagia, listing the incidence in the general population, associated prevalence of dysphagia, and the aspect of deglutition affected. PD with dysphagia is likely to be more frequently encountered based on relatively higher

disease incidence coupled with high prevalence of dysphagia, whose onset is earlier in the disease process. A summary of each neuromuscular degenerative disease follows.

Muscular Dystrophy

Muscular dystrophy is a classic example of a peripheral degenerative disease, affecting muscle, which causes dysphagia in the advanced stages of illness. Duchenne muscular dystrophy (DMD) is an x-linked disease affecting 1 in 3600–6000 live male births.[9] Mutations of the dystrophin gene (Xp21.2) result in progressive muscle degeneration and replacement with interstitial fat and fibrosis.[9–11] Diagnosis at presentation is typically around the age of 5 years and precipitated by divergent physical ability compared with peers. Children commonly exhibit progressive muscle weakness resulting in loss of ambulation. In late stages, cardiopulmonary sequelae result in life-threatening complications and, in the absence of intervention, the mean age of death is 19 years.[9]

Dysphagia in DMD is most symptomatic in the late nonambulatory phase of disease. In children with DMD and feeding difficulties, videofluoroscopy showed oral phase difficulties predominated and resulted from masticatory muscle weakness, malocclusion, and macroglossia.[10] The swallow trigger was mildly delayed and weak pharyngeal propulsion resulted in pharyngeal residue. Patients were also desensitized to residue. Choking episodes occurred with more advanced disease, although no patients showed aspiration.

Myasthenia Gravis

MG is a degenerative autoimmune neuromuscular disease with increasing damage to the neuromuscular junction over time.[12] Dysphagia may be prominent in

TABLE 14.2
Neurodegenerative Diseases and Their Effect on Deglutition

Disease	Incidence in General Population	Prevalence of Dysphagia	Aspect of Deglutition Effected	Risk of Aspiration
Muscular dystrophy	17–28:100,000[9]	18%[10]	Oral > pharyngeal[10,11]	Low early stages, high late stages
Myasthenia gravis	1.7–10:1,000,000[13]	40%[14]	Pharyngeal > oral[15]	High 35%[15]
Multiple sclerosis	2–7:100,000[16]	24%–65%[18–20]	Oral/pharyngeal[18–20] Cortical	High
Amyotrophic lateral sclerosis	2:100,000[21,22]	83%[24]	Oral > pharyngeal[22] Cortical	High
Parkinson's disease	13:100,000[25]	82%[28]	Esophageal > oral/pharyngeal[27,28] Cortical	High

Adapted from Altman KW, Richards A, Goldberg L, Frucht S, McCabe DJ. Dysphagia in stroke, neurodegenerative disease, and advanced dementia. *Otolaryngol Clin N Am*. 2013;46(6):1137–1149.

some myasthenia patients, and all myasthenic patients are at risk for dysphagia due to side effects from their medications and intercurrent respiratory illness which may exacerbate their symptoms. It predominantly affects women in the third and fourth decades of life, although men exhibit a bimodal peak in the third and sixth decades of life.[12] Antiacetylcholine receptor antibodies reduce the available number of ACh receptors and result in subthreshold endplate potentials.[12,13] The clinical features involve painless weakness of the striated muscle. Whilst ocular manifestations are the most common, bulbar weakness may be the presenting symptom in up to 6%–15%.[13,14] Patients may also present with dysphonia characterized by vocal weakness and fatigue and may even demonstrate vocal fold paresis with consequent increased aspiration to liquids. The natural history of the disease is progression to maximum severity within 2 years.[13]

The oral preparatory phase is generally affected with poor bolus formation, with extended chewing time, and reduced buccal tension.[15] Oral phase abnormalities included slow transit, piecemeal deglutition, increased residue, and poor seal. The most common findings are in the pharyngeal phase, with delays in initiation, and a reduction in tongue base and epiglottic mobility. Weak constrictor muscles result in pharyngeal residue. Laryngeal penetration was common (35%) and often silent. Electromyography (EMG) studies reveal prolongation of suprahyoid laryngeal elevators in MG, which may compensate in those with subclinical swallow impairment.[14] In this disorder, cricopharyngeal muscle

function is usually normal. Proper diagnosis is critical to management of disease, and fortunately, aggressive medical therapy should result in dramatic improvement of dysphagia.

Multiple Sclerosis

MS is a central immune-mediated demyelinating disorder with a high incidence of dysphagia, particularly when white matter lesions affect the brainstem. There's a female predominance, with an overall incidence of 2–7:100,000 with peak onset at around 30 years.[16] MS is triggered by environmental factors in genetically at-risk patients, and a focal lymphocytic infiltrate results in myelin and axonal damage. The median time to death is approximately 30 years from disease onset.[17]

The incidence of dysphagia varies depending on the severity of the disability from 24% to 65%[18–20] and is most severe in those with brainstem involvement.[18,19] Consequently, aspiration pneumonia is the leading cause of death in MS.[19] Abnormalities include reduced lingual control and tongue base retraction, delayed swallow trigger, reduced laryngeal closure, and pharyngeal contraction and diminished sensation.[19,20] The oral phase is more often affected in those with severe dysphagia.[18] Oro-motor impairment also results in the characteristic dysphonia with "scanning speech," with a complex interplay between dysarthria and cortical compensation. Upper esophageal sphincter dysfunction is also common and most pronounced with disease progression.[19,20] In addition to these aspects of dysphagia, the typical patient with MS has impaired motor control of their limbs and hands with reduced ability to feed themselves.

Amyotrophic Lateral Sclerosis

ALS, otherwise known as Lou Gehrig's disease, uniformly produces dysphagia, and management of speech and swallowing are ideally handled with an interdisciplinary approach in the ALS clinic. Its incidence is approximately 2:100,000, and it affects males greater than females.[21,22] The overwhelming majority of disease onset is at 58–63 years and is mostly idiopathic; however, there are cases of familial disease with Mendelian inheritance.[21,22] Pathophysiology involves degeneration and loss of motor neurons with astrocytic gliosis,[23] and 50% of patients die within 30 months of symptom onset, but the prognosis is better in those with isolated bulbar disease.[22]

These patients often have delayed diagnosis due to the relative rarity in the general population, but the presence of dysarthria with tongue fasciculations warrants proper evaluation. The hallmark clinical feature is the presence of upper and lower motor neuron (LMN) features involving the brainstem and spinal cord. Presentation with limb-onset disease predominates (70%); however, bulbar onset occurs in approximately 25%. On physical exam, the tongue is severely involved showing atrophy, weakness, and characteristic fasciculations, so the oral preparatory and oral phases are most affected. Upper motor neuron dysfunction results in a brisk gag and jaw jerk, while LMN involvement causes tongue fasciculations, wasting and weakness, palatal weakness, and poor cough.[22]

In addition, the swallow trigger reflex is delayed, disordered, and eventually absent, but the oropharyngeal swallow reflex is preserved until the end-stage disease.[24] The cricopharyngeus muscle becomes hyperreflexive and hypertonic, with a resultant loss of coordination during voluntary initiated swallowing, and laryngeal protection is eventually lost with increasing aspiration risk. The natural history of this disease warrants the interdisciplinary clinic, which can also offer palliative care.

Parkinson's Disease

PD is a common progressive disorder with an incidence of approximately 13:100,000[25] and a 1.5% life time risk of development.[26] The median age of onset is 60 years and mean duration of disease is 15 years, with aspiration pneumonia being the most common cause of death.[26] The disease is characterized by bradykinesia, muscular rigidity, mask-like face, shuffling gait with little arm swing, and often a 4–6 Hz resting tremor.

However, atypical Parkinson's and Parkinson's plus syndromes such as progressive supranuclear palsy are increasingly recognized and usually do not include the tremor. The underlying pathophysiology is severe loss of dopaminergic neurons in the pars-compacta nigral cells of the basal ganglia.[26] As the dorsal motor nucleus of vagus and esophageal myenteric plexus degenerate, both pharyngeal and esophageal phase dysphagia become more obvious.

The prototypical Parkinsonian voice is weak, soft, and hypokinetic, suggestive of the muscular weakness and hypokinetic coordination that also contribute to Parkinson's dysphagia. EMG and esophageal scintigraphy studies reveal that there is a high rate of objective dysphagia, even in asymptomatic patients,[27] and overall prevalence rates of dysphagia are 82%.[28] While the oral preparatory and oral phase become affected later in disease accompanied by characteristic drooling, there is far earlier evidence of prolongation of the lower esophageal bolus transport in many patients.[27]

While there are increasing options for the treatment of PD medically and surgically with brainstem electrical stimulation, there are hallmark "on–off" effects of medication that limit seamless management of dysphagia. For example, timing of traditional medication results in a peak of agility followed by a decline in function until the next dose, so it is important to recognize that swallowing is safer during the period of agility rather than when the medication is wearing off. This also applies to the timing of objective swallowing evaluation such as with a modified barium swallow study or flexible endoscopic evaluation of swallowing. Fatigue is also a common problem with PD patients and similarly affects aspiration risk, as well as the emergence of dementia later in the disease process.

Advanced Dementia

While there are changes to the brain parenchyma in everyone with aging often associated with microvascular ischemia, Alzheimer's disease, and other related illnesses causing dementia are progressive, are incurable, and lead to a complete loss of cognitive function and subsequently death. A characteristic feature of the final phase of dementia, which can last from 6 months to 2 years, is loss of interest in eating or dysphagia, again paying tribute to the cognitive, cortical, and central coordination involved with swallowing.

In 2001, there were 24.3 million people in the world with dementia, while in 2040, the number is estimated to increase to over 81 million. The prevalence of dementia is estimated to double every 5 years after the age of 65 years, and at the age of 85 years, the

TABLE 14.3
Advanced Stages of Dementia

Stage	Manifestations	Mean Duration
6a	Ability to perform ADLs becomes compromised (i.e., put clothing on correctly)	2.5 years
6b	Lose the ability to bathe independently	2.5 years
6c	Lose the ability to manage the mechanics of toileting correctly	2.5 years
6d	Urinary incontinence	2.5 years
6e	• Fecal incontinence • Speech overtly breaks down in the ability to articulate. Stuttering, neologisms, and/or an increased paucity of speech are noted. Still able to respond to nonverbal stimuli and communicate pleasure and pain via behavior	2.5 years
7a	• Evident rigidity upon examination of the passive range of motion of major joints, such as the elbow, in majority of AD patients • Require continuous assistance with basic ADLs for survival • Speech is limited to six or fewer intelligible words	1 year
7b	• Approximately 40% of AD patients manifest contractures of the elbow, wrists, and fingers to the extent that they cannot move a major joint more than halfway. • Speech limited to a single intelligible word	1.5 years
7c	• Lose the ability to ambulate independently • Speech is lost	1 year
7d	Lose the ability to sit up independently	1 year
7e	Lose the ability to smile, only grimacing facial movements are observed	1.5 years
7f	Lose the ability to hold up their head independently	

AD, Alzheimer's disease; *ADLs,* activities of daily living.
Adapted from Altman KW, Richards A, Goldberg L, Frucht S, McCabe DJ. Dysphagia in stroke, neurodegenerative disease, and advanced dementia. *Otolaryngol Clin N Am.* 2013;46(6):1137–1149; Martino R, Foley N, Bhogal S, Diamant N, Speechley M, Teasell R. Dysphagia after stroke: incidence, diagnosis, and pulmonary complications. *Stroke.* 2005;36(12):2756–2763; Altman KW, Schaefer SD, Yu G-P, et al. The voice and laryngeal dysfunction in stroke: a report from the neurolaryngology subcommittee of the AAO-HNS. *Otolaryngol Head Neck Surg.* 2007; 136(6):873–881; Smithard DG, O'Neill PA, Park C, et al. Complications and outcome after acute stroke does dysphagia matter? *Stroke.* 1996; 27(7):1200–1204.

prevalence is approximately 50%.[29] Dementia is a leading cause of death in the United States, with mortality affected by aspiration, hydration, and nutritional status. Data in the year 2000 show approximately 4.5 million people in North America with a diagnosis of dementia, and more than half progressed to the moderate-to-severe stages of their disease.[29] An estimated 60% of nursing home residents have dementia with approximately half (480,000) in the last stages of their disease.[30]

The mean survival after dementia diagnosis varies between 1 and 16 years, whereas one-third of these individuals live to advanced stages.[30] Activities of daily living (ADLs) are typically lost in a hierarchical fashion, and the severe phase of dementia is characterized by loss of capacity to provide self-care in basic ADLs such as eating, bathing, and walking independently. Advanced stages of dementia are listed in Table 14.3.[31] In these stages, there are also many behavioral symptoms that compromise the quality of life for both patients and caregivers and are sources of great stress, with institutionalization being the ultimate consequence.

Many patients and their families have limited understanding of the terminal nature of a dementia diagnosis. With these complex characteristics of advanced dementia, there are moral, ethical, religious, and medical dilemmas that arise. These include appreciating the risks, benefits, and alternatives to adjunctive enteral feeding percutaneous endoscopic gastrostomy tubes (PEGs), NPO status, and the role of "comfort care" or "compassionate oral intake." A recent systematic review concluded that there is no objective evidence demonstrating that PEG prolongs life in this population; however, it provides a reliable route for medications and may help maintain nutritional and hydration status.[32]

As with many patients with advanced dysphagia and depending on prognosis and the above-mentioned factors, there is a role for supplemental PEG feeding to maintain baseline nutritional and hydration status, but also allowing compassionate oral intake. Quantifying the level of aspiration risk also allows for patients and their families to decide whether to pursue PEG based on their philosophy. While this approach may not ultimately prolong life, the quality of life is expected to be enhanced by enjoying the consistency and taste of foods, as well as the ritual human interaction at mealtime. Recognizing the indicators of decline provides opportunities to maximize patient status with preferred food consistencies and allows for initiation of compensatory maneuvers during this transition period.

Dysphagia in Stroke

Dysphagia is a common finding in the setting of acute stroke and may occur in up to 78% of patients.[33] It adversely affects the length of hospitalization and also increases the risk of mortality.[34–37] Although about half of patients with dysphagia improve (or die) in the first week,[34] dysphagia is a frequently underrecognized complication of acute stroke. The severity of dysphagia relates to the degree of pharyngeal representation in the unaffected cerebral hemisphere, with the most severe problems in those with an involved dominant hemisphere.[38] Recovery is thought to be related to neuroplasticity in the nonaffected hemisphere.[39] The rate of dysphagia in hemispheric strokes is lower than in those affecting the brainstem,[33] which reflects the cortical neuroplasticity as well as the primitive importance of the brainstem in swallowing reflexes.

Prolonged hospital stay in stroke patients with dysphagia is most evident in those with hemorrhagic disease, with a 55% increase in the duration of stay, although thrombotic strokes are also associated with significant dysphagia.[35] The discharge destination of stroke patients is also dramatically altered, with dysphagia patients having more than double the rate of requiring long-term care.[34] Pneumonia represents a major consequence of dysphagia due to aspiration and is associated with 24%–30% of deaths in acute stroke patients.[37,40] Those with dysphagia have a threefold increase in pneumonia, and aspiration evidenced on videofluoroscopy markedly increases the risk of pneumonia.[33] The effects of dysphagia on stroke patients through their hospitalization are listed in Table 14.4.

Rehabilitation of deglutition following stroke depends on many factors, primarily the geographic

TABLE 14.4
Acute Stroke and the Impact of Dysphagia

	No Dysphagia	Dysphagia
Prevalence	22%–70%	30%–78%
Average hospital length of stay		
≤7 days	85.34%	55.39%
>7 days	14.66%	44.61%
Discharge destination		
Home	59.79%	20.72%
Long-term care	15.7%	33.93%
Incidence of pneumonia	2%–16%	16%–33%
Mortality	6%	37%

Adapted from Altman KW, Richards A, Goldberg L, Frucht S, McCabe DJ. Dysphagia in stroke, neurodegenerative disease, and advanced dementia. *Otolaryngol Clin N Am.* 2013;46(6):1137–1149.

distribution and extent of the stroke. If a patient demonstrates progress with cognition, mobility, and dysphagia in the first week following a stroke, then there is a good prognosis for significant recovery. Therapy is aimed at oral sensation, oromotor manipulation, and compensatory maneuvers to protect from aspiration. It is also important to recognize and monitor aspiration risk with certain food consistencies and maintain adequate nutrition during the rehabilitation period.

In addition to the above findings, vocal paralysis may be associated with vertebral artery brainstem stroke and can result in poor laryngeal protection and ineffective cough.[34] Rehabilitation in this setting starts with examining the larynx with bedside laryngoscopy in order to identify laryngeal immobility. Vocal augmentation with injection or medialization is beneficial to improve the efficacy of a cough, which can help compensate for small amounts of aspiration through pulmonary toilet.

The development of screening protocols for dysphagia is a key step in early identification of the patient at high risk for aspiration and the consequences of dysphagia such as malnutrition. High-risk patient should be considered following stroke, with neurodegenerative disease, later stages of dementia, advanced age, and certain other medical and surgical conditions in order to reduce the complication rates of aspiration.[36] This early identification and intervention approach has been shown to reduce the economic burden of disease.[36]

TREATMENT OPTIONS FOR GLOBAL LARYNGEAL DYSFUNCTION

In patients with acute stroke with persisting dysphagia and those with advanced-stage neurodegenerative disease, the resulting global laryngeal dysfunction can result in major morbidity and mortality. Following early risk stratification, those patients with significant penetration or aspiration should be made NPO and provided with enteral feeding methods. This allows adequate nutrition while oral intake is then cautiously advanced, if appropriate. Although NG or PEG feeding has not been shown to reduce aspiration pneumonia, their role in adequate nutrition and hydration is clear.[41] Early NG feeding reduces mortality, although early PEG insertion has been associated with an increased mortality.[42] PEG should therefore be considered when dysphagia persists but can be initially delayed in the acute stages of illness.

Tracheotomy can improve secretion management and pulmonary toilet, and patients with advanced neurodegenerative disease may already require a tracheostomy for respiratory support. The tracheotomy tube, however, can only limit aspiration and secretions, and thin liquids will still bypass the cuff. Despite the traditional view that tracheotomy causes laryngeal dysfunction, the underlying neurologic dysfunction is more likely the overriding factor.[43] In very select patients who fail to respond to more conservative measures, tracheoesophageal diversion and laryngotracheal separation can be considered. Due to the radical nature of these procedures, however, they are largely reserved for the pediatric population in desperate circumstances.[44] Total laryngectomy has the benefit of eliminating aspiration since there is no conduit connecting the mouth to the trachea. However, it is rarely performed since many patients with global laryngeal dysfunction also have significant cognitive impairment and oromotor and oropharyngeal components to their dysphagia as well.

CONCLUSIONS

Neurodegenerative disease, advanced dementia, and stroke are all characterized by the presence of potentially life-threatening dysphagia. The nature of the baseline diseases both causes dysphagia and makes the patients more prone to the consequences. Early recognition through a systematic approach helps stave off aspiration, maintains nutrition, and seeks to preserve quality of life.

REFERENCES

1. Altman KW. Understanding dysphagia: a rapidly emerging problem. *Otolaryngol Clin N Am.* 2013;46(6):xiii–xvi.
2. Crary MA, Carnaby GD, Sia I, Khanna A, Waters MF. Spontaneous swallowing frequency has potential to identify dysphagia in acute stroke. *Stroke.* 2013;44:3452–3457.
3. Shaw SM, Martino R. The normal swallow: muscular and neurophysiological control. *Otolaryngol Clin N Am.* 2013; 46(6):937–956.
4. Bolser DC, Gestreau C, Morris KF, Davenport PW, Pitts TE. Central neural circuits for coordination of swallowing, breathing, and coughing: predictions from computational modeling and simulation. *Otolaryngol Clin N Am.* 2013; 46(6):957–964.
5. Altman KW, Richards A, Goldberg L, Frucht S, McCabe DJ. Dysphagia in stroke, neurodegenerative disease, and advanced dementia. *Otolaryngol Clin N Am.* 2013;46(6): 1137–1149.
6. Peicher VS, Carter FL, Altman KW. Correlation of dysphagia and functional decline in neurodegenerative diseases – a systematic review. *J Otolaryngol ENT Res.* 2017;7(4): 00214. https://doi.org/10.15406/joentr.2017.07.00214.
7. Altman KW, Mahmoud R, Hutton GJ, Carter FL, Dunham R, Minard CG, "Prevalence of Dysphagia in Multiple Sclerosis and Correlation with Disability".
8. Want BJ, Carter FL, Altman KW. Relationship between dysarthria and oral-oropharyngeal dysphagia: the current evidence. *ENT J.* 2018;97(3):E1–E9.
9. Bushby K, Finkel R, Birnkrant DJ, et al. Diagnosis and management of Duchenne muscular dystrophy, part 1: diagnosis, and pharmacological and psychosocial management. *Lancet Neurol.* 2010;9(1):77–93.
10. Aloysius A, Born P, Kinali M, Davis T, Pane M, Mercuri E. Swallowing difficulties in Duchenne muscular dystrophy: indications for feeding assessment and outcome of video-fluoroscopic swallow studies. *Eur J Paediatr Neurol.* 2008; 12(3):239–245.
11. van den Engel-Hoek L, Erasmus CE, Hendriks JC, et al. Oral muscles are progressively affected in Duchenne muscular dystrophy: implications for dysphagia treatment. *J Neurol.* 2013;260(5):1295–1303.
12. Meyer A, Levy Y. Geoepidemiology of myasthenia gravis. *Autoimmun Rev.* 2010;9(5):A383–A386.
13. Meriggioli MN, Sanders DB. Autoimmune myasthenia gravis: emerging clinical and biological heterogeneity. *Lancet Neurol.* 2009;8(5):475–490.
14. Ertekin C, Yüceyar N, Aydogdu I. Clinical and electrophysiological evaluation of dysphagia in myasthenia gravis. *J Neurol Neurosurg Psychiatry.* 1998;65(6):848–856.
15. Colton-Hudson A, Koopman WJ, Moosa T, Smith D, Bach D, Nicolle M. A prospective assessment of the characteristics of dysphagia in myasthenia gravis. *Dysphagia.* 2002 Spring;17(2):147–151.
16. Koch-Henriksen N, Soelberg Sørensen P. The changing demographic pattern of multiple sclerosis epidemiology. *Lancet Neurol.* 2010;9:520–532.

17. Compston A, Coles A. Multiple sclerosis. *Lancet.* 2008; 372(9648):1502–1517.
18. Calcagno P, Ruoppolo G, Grasso MG, De Vincentiis M, Paolucci S. Dysphagia in multiple sclerosis – prevalence and prognostic factors. *Acta Neurol Scand.* 2002;105:40–43.
19. Prosiegel M, Schelling A, Wagner-Sonntag E. Dysphagia and multiple sclerosis. *Int MS J.* 2004;11(1):22–31.
20. De Pauw A, Dejaeger E, D'hooghe B, Carton H. Dysphagia in multiple sclerosis. *Clin Neurol Neurosurg.* 2002;104(4): 345–351.
21. Mitchell JD, Borasio GD. Amyotrophic lateral sclerosis. *Lancet.* 2007;369(9578):2031–2041.
22. Kiernan MC, Vucic S, Cheah BC, et al. Amyotrophic lateral sclerosis. *Lancet.* 2011;377(9769):942–955.
23. Rowland LP, Shneider NA. Amyotrophic lateral sclerosis. *N Engl J Med.* 2001;344(22):1688–1700.
24. Ertekin C, Aydogdu I, Yüceyar N, Kiylioglu N, Tarlaci S, Uludag B. Pathophysiological mechanisms of oropharyngeal dysphagia in amyotrophic lateral sclerosis. *Brain.* 2000;123(Pt 1):125–140.
25. Van Den Eeden SK, Tanner CM, Bernstein AL, et al. Incidence of Parkinson's disease: variation by age, gender, and race/ethnicity. *Am J Epidemiol.* 2003;157(11):1015–1022.
26. Lees AJ, Hardy J, Revesz T. Parkinson's disease. *Lancet.* 2009;373(9680):2055–2066.
27. Potulska A, Friedman A, Królicki L, Spychala A. Swallowing disorders in Parkinson's disease. *Parkinsonism Relat Disord.* 2003;9(6):349–353.
28. Kalf JG, de Swart BJM, Bloem BR, Munneke. Prevalence of oropharyngeal dysphagia in Parkinson's disease. *Parkinsonism Relat Disord.* 2012;18(4):311–315.
29. Prince M. Epidemiology of dementia. *Psychiatry.* 2007;6: 488–490.
30. Gillick M. When the Nursing home resident with advanced dementia stops eating: what is the medical director to do? *J Am Med Dir Assoc.* 2001;2(5):259–263.
31. Reisberg B. *The Encyclopedia of Visual Medicine Series. An Atlas of Alzheimer's Disease.* Pearl River, NY: Parthenon; 1999.
32. Goldberg L, Altman KW. The role of gastrostomy tube placement in advanced dementia with dysphagia: a critical review. *Clin Interv Aging.* 2014;9:1733–1739.
33. Martino R, Foley N, Bhogal S, Diamant N, Speechley M, Teasell R. Dysphagia after stroke: incidence, diagnosis, and pulmonary complications. *Stroke.* 2005;36(12): 2756–2763.
34. Altman KW, Schaefer SD, Yu G-P, et al. The voice and laryngeal dysfunction in stroke: a report from the neurolaryngology subcommittee of the AAO-HNS. *Otolaryngol Head Neck Surg.* 2007;136(6):873–881.
35. Altman KW, Yu GP, Schaefer SD. Consequences of dysphagia in the hospitalized patient. *Arch Otolaryngol Head Neck Surg.* 2010;136(8):784–789.
36. Altman KW. Dysphagia evaluation and care in the hospital setting: the need for protocolization. *Otolaryngol Head Neck Surg.* 2011;145(6):895–898.
37. Smithard DG, O'Neill PA, Park C, et al. Complications and outcome after acute stroke does dysphagia matter? *Stroke.* 1996;27(7):1200–1204.
38. Hamdy S, Aziz Q, Rothwell JC, et al. Explaining oropharyngeal dysphagia after unilateral hemispheric stroke. *Lancet.* 1997;350(9079):686–692.
39. Hamdy S, Aziz Q, Rothwell JC, et al. Recovery of swallowing after dysphagic stroke relates to functional reorganization in the intact motor cortex. *Gastroenterology.* 1998; 115(5):1104–1112.
40. Katzan IL, Cebul RD, Husak SH, Dawson NV, Baker DW. The effect of pneumonia on mortality among patients hospitalized for acute stroke. *Neurology.* 2003;60(4): 620–625.
41. Singh S, Hamdy S. Dysphagia in stroke patients. *Postgrad Med J.* 2006;82(968):383–391.
42. Dennis MS, Lewis SC, Warlow C. FOOD Trial collaboration Effect of timing and method of enteral tube feeding for dysphagic stroke patients (FOOD): a multicentre randomised controlled trial. *Lancet.* 2005;365(9461): 764–772.
43. Donzelli J, Brady S, Wesling M, Theisen M. Effects of the removal of the tracheotomy tube on swallowing during the fiberoptic endoscopic exam of the swallow (FEES). *Dysphagia.* 2005;20(4):283–289. Fall.
44. Cook SP. Candidate's thesis: laryngotracheal separation in neurologically impaired children: long-term results. *Laryngoscope.* 2009;119(2):390–395.

CHAPTER 15

Chemoradiation-Induced Dysphagia

NAUSHEEN JAMAL, MD • ALEXANDER MICHAEL, BA • RESHA SONI, MD •
DINESH K. CHHETRI, MD

INTRODUCTION

Over the past decade, the prognosis for patients with head and neck cancer (HNC) has been improving, as evidenced by a 12% increase in the overall 5-year survival rate.[1] This improvement in survival is accompanied by an evolving challenge: how can we maximize a patient's quality of life (QOL) after treatment of HNC? These concerns are especially relevant given that laryngeal and pharyngeal cancers alone account for up to 29,000 new cancer diagnoses in the United States per year.[2] Both surgical and nonsurgical treatment options for HNC exert considerable influence on a patient's QOL, and careful consideration of these effects is paramount. The most common complaints in posttreatment patients include dysphagia, dysphonia, dysarthria, trismus, xerostomia, tracheostomy tube dependence, shoulder dysfunction, neuropathy, chronic pain, feeding-tube dependence, lymphedema, and cosmetic deformity.[3-8] The initial choice of cancer treatment is an important factor in QOL-related complaints.[9,10] Dysfunction is more likely to arise after multimodality treatment, high-dose or wide-field radiation, and duration of nil per os (NPO) status.[11,12] In this chapter, we will focus specifically on dysphagia related to chemoradiation therapy (CRT).

Careful assessment of a patient's swallow function is the first step in maximizing QOL and must be done serially through long-term follow-up. A thorough history, physical examination, and an awareness of the timeline and varied presentation of dysphagia in HNC survivors is important in treating this patient population. Furthermore, familiarity with the diagnostic tools for swallow evaluation and the treatment modalities available becomes essential to the treating physician.

PATHOPHYSIOLOGY OF DYSFUNCTION

Radiotherapy (RT) with or without concurrent chemotherapy is a mainstay in organ-preserving treatment of primary laryngeal and pharyngeal cancers. The use of radiation harbors the risk of acute and delayed toxicity, both of which can contribute to dysphagia. The primary mechanism for cell death from ionizing radiation is development of hydroxyl radicals that damages DNA. Apoptosis ensues at the cellular level followed by an acute inflammatory response. Much of the acute toxicity of RT to the head and neck can be explained by this acute inflammation. Dermatitis, mucositis, odynophagia, and dysphagia secondary to pharyngeal swelling are mediated by an acute inflammatory response. Eventually, the acute inflammation gives way to chronic inflammation. The presence of macrophages, differentiation of fibroblasts into postmitotic fibrocytes, and excess production and deposition of extracellular matrix proteins and collagen in the blood vessels are typical histologic findings in this stage. These processes can lead to a substantial fibrosis in the neck, leading to a stiff neck. Blood vessels may develop stenosis, and telangiectasias also form with time on mucosal surfaces.

It was initially believed that tissue dysfunction from ionizing radiation was due to a decrease in cell populations.[13] After the initial damage to cells, there is a silent period in which failed mitosis and compromised function develop slowly. This "target-cell hypothesis" prevailed into the early 20th century but came under scrutiny as newer observations came to light. In particular, the target cell hypothesis did not adequately explain the so-called late side effects of radiation, namely radiation-induced fibrosis.[14] The continued deposition of collagen by fibroblasts, years after the initial radiation exposure, did not mesh well with the idea of a silent period following initial cell death. More recently, the idea of a continuous and active biological response driving radiation toxicity has come to prominence.

Fibrosis is an important contributor to impaired function. The wound healing response is characterized by an early inflammatory phase involving the upregulation of proinflammatory cytokines, including TNFα, IL-1, and IL-6. Deposition of collagen is promoted primarily by TGF-β, an important cytokine associated with fibrosis. The complex interplay of these cytokines is not completely understood, though ionizing radiation is one of several factors that has been shown to induce TGF-β.[15,16] This process is thought to be ongoing and can continue to evolve months to years after active treatment has ceased. In addition to radiation, advanced stage tumors, advanced age, and female gender have been reported as risk factors associated with increased rates of dysphagia.[16–19]

Several studies have detailed the effects of RT on swallowing mechanics. Lazarus et al. reported RT causing a delay in triggering the pharyngeal swallow, reduced posterior motion of the tongue base toward the posterior pharyngeal wall, reduced laryngeal elevation, and reduced laryngeal closure during the swallow.[20] Some patients aspirate during the swallow due to reduced laryngeal closure, while others aspirate after the swallow due to residue that accumulates in the vallecula and posterior pharyngeal wall. Kendall et al. also reported a general decrease in the mobility in pharyngeal structures following single-modality treatment with RT, contributing to dysphagia.[21] Sensory loss due to the late effects of CRT also contributes significantly to long-term swallow dysfunction and aspiration risk.

SYMPTOMS

In general, symptoms of dysphagia can be classified broadly as direct or indirect,[22] and include a constellation of symptoms (see Table 15.1). Symptoms that occur during any phase of swallowing are considered to be direct. Such symptoms include choking or coughing during or immediately after the swallow, throat clearing during meals, drooling, nasal regurgitation, and/or oral regurgitation. Direct symptoms are likely to come to the attention of the patient or the patient's caregiver. Indirect symptoms, as the name implies, do not manifest as symptoms related to phases of swallowing but arise in the setting of dysphagia. These symptoms are more varied and can include weight loss, recurrent fevers, bronchitis, pneumonia, and heartburn.[22] A query of indirect symptoms may be the only indication that a patient is experiencing aspiration

TABLE 15.1
Signs and Symptoms of Dysphagia in the Head and Neck Cancer Population
Aspiration
Coughing
Throat clearing during meals
Prolonged meal times
Avoidance/difficulty with certain consistencies
Oropharyngeal residue
Expectoration
Reduced pleasure with oral intake
Difficulty managing secretions/drooling
Difficulty chewing
Difficulty initiating a swallow
Nasal/pharyngeal regurgitation during eating
Sensation of food sticking in the throat or chest
History of pneumonia
Weight loss
Evidence of malnutrition

events, and therefore indirect symptoms should not be overlooked.

One of the most important symptoms to assess for is aspiration and subsequent pneumonias. The presence or absence of aspiration may not always be obvious; patients with impaired laryngeal sensation or cough reflex may experience silent aspiration. There exists a wide variability in how patients tolerate aspiration events. Some patients may tolerate aspiration of as much as 10% of a food bolus, whereas other individuals will cough or choke on small amounts of saliva.[22] The potential for undetected aspiration means that the clinician must thoroughly evaluate and assess the patient's symptoms. This is of utmost importance, particularly in the elderly patient population and those with dementia, where the risk of aspiration and resultant pneumonias is elevated and merits vigilance. Of equal importance, weight loss can indicate compromised nutritional status, leaving the patient more susceptible to infection.

DIAGNOSIS/EVALUATION

Evaluation of a patient with impaired swallowing begins with a thorough history of the patient's illness. The clinician should take care not to ask overly broad and open-ended questions regarding the patient's swallow function. A general query of the patient's swallowing may be met with a response that "swallowing is fine." However, the use of more direct questions regarding the patient's eating habits may reveal swallow dysfunction. Clinicians should inquire about the avoidance of certain foods or medications, coughing or choking episodes, globus sensation, pain, unexplained fevers, pneumonias or upper respiratory tract infections, throat clearing, weight loss, and other evidence of malnutrition, if meals have taken longer, and if prior placement of a feeding tube was required. Furthermore, social isolation or lifestyle alternations may offer indirect evidence of swallowing dysfunction. Clinicians should make every effort to employ validated, patient-rated symptom questionnaires in order to ensure that all symptoms are brought to their attention (such as the Eating Assessment Tool-10 or the MD Anderson Dysphagia Inventory).[13]

Otolaryngologists should be aware that there is discordance regarding the relationship between patient-reported dysphagia and swallow function. Some patients may present without significant complaints but have considerable aspiration based on objective evaluation. Alternatively, significant subjective complaints may be met with minimal objective findings. In light of this, it is important to systematically interview the patient regarding their symptoms, and supplement the interview with objective testing. In addition to a thorough head and neck physical examination, clinicians should specifically assess for the following: oral hygiene, the absence of dentition, the presence of trismus, dry mucosa, strength and mobility of the tongue, abnormal gag reflex, cough, dysphonia, and dysarthria.

A clinical swallow examination should be performed and is important in assessing the patient's risk of aspiration.[2] Flexible endoscopic evaluation of swallowing (FEES) or FEES with Sensory Testing allows for a comprehensive evaluation of a patient's swallowing from both an anatomical and a functional perspective in the clinic or bedside setting. During such testing, a flexible fiberoptic laryngoscopy is performed, and a variety of food consistencies with a colored dye are then presented to the patient to assess for pooling, laryngeal penetration, frank aspiration, and reflux. Air-pulse stimuli can be delivered to elicit the laryngeal adductor reflex to test supraglottic sensation. FEES is described in detail in Chapter 8. FEES does not allow the clinician to directly observe the oral phase or the upper esophageal sphincter (UES) function. However, it is an excellent and essential tool in correlating anatomical and functional information of the

pharyngeal swallow, and thus is especially useful for the otolaryngologist. A modified barium swallow study (MBS) is a videofluoroscopic swallow procedure for further evaluating dysphagia (see Chapter 10). This differs from an esophagram in that an MBS evaluates the oral and pharyngeal phases of swallowing but not the entire esophagus or esophageal motility. An MBS consists of administering various solid and liquid consistencies coated with barium and is performed in a fluoroscopic suite by a speech-language pathologist. It allows the clinician to assess the function of the UES, develop an impression of the strength of the pharyngeal muscles, and the degree of penetration and aspiration. Epiglottic dysfunction and nasopharyngeal reflux of food is also better seen. However, it does not provide clear anatomical information, unlike FEES. MBS and FEES have shown similar sensitivity with respect to detecting aspiration, although some believe FEES to be more sensitive.[22] While either test is suitable for evaluating for aspiration, the dysphagia clinician may consider using both tests, as they each offer unique and complementary diagnostic information that can aid the clinician. Using both tests offers the clinician a thorough assessment of the patient's anatomical and functional deficits and aids in planning optimal treatment. One may also consider pharyngoesophageal impedance manometry for measurement of pharyngeal contraction, which may be impacted by progressive fibrosis.[23,24]

TREATMENT

Arguably, an important consideration in treating patients who have undergone HNC treatment may be a simple one—pain control. The presence of pain can impair a patient's ability to participate in rehabilitation, which is an important component of recovery. In particular, radiation-induced mucositis can cause pain via both nociceptive and neuropathic pathways,[24–26] which requires that the clinician consider and address both types. Several small retrospective studies have assessed gabapentin's use in treating neuropathic or opioid resistant pain. Gabapentin is associated with a decreased dose of opioid needed to achieve analgesia, is relatively well tolerated, and is without significant drug interactions.[27–30] While gabapentin has a milder side effect profile relative to opioids, further investigation is needed to elucidate its role in treating posttreatment pain in the HNC population.

In reviewing the literature, several large studies have shed light upon the clear role of rehabilitation and behavioral therapy for treatment of dysphagia in HNC patients. A multidisciplinary approach with a team

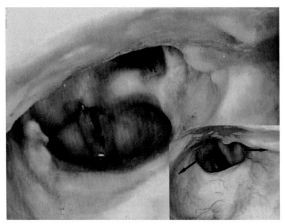

FIG. 15.1 Treatment of supraglottic stenosis visualized on flexible laryngoscopy (inset) with CO_2 laser radial incisions (*arrows*) to enlarge the supraglottis (main figure).

comprising physicians, speech therapists, physical therapists, and occupational therapists allows the patient to benefit from the varied expertise of several professionals, each focusing on different elements of function. Several studies have focused on prophylactic swallow exercises before the initiation of radiation therapy with significant long-term benefit when compared to controls. For example, Peng et al. implemented a swallow preservation protocol comprising swallowing, jaw, and tongue exercises administered to patients prior to or within 2 weeks of beginning CRT. They found that patients enrolled in the protocol had improved swallow function during and shortly following cancer treatment. Other studies have demonstrated the usefulness of exercises for maintaining oral intake during therapy.[30–32,43]

There are occasions where adjunctive surgical procedures may be beneficial. Sites of swallow dysfunction that are typically amenable to surgery include the pharynx, epiglottis, UES, and esophagus. For example, fibrosis and stenosis of the pharynx after CRT can lead to scarring, reduced velopharyngeal closure, reduced medial pharyngeal contraction, or decreased retraction of the tongue base. Surgical treatment consists of surgical laser dilation of scar bands. A carbon dioxide (CO_2) laser is used to create multiple radial incisions within each scar and is followed by balloon dilation to stretch the area of fibrosis and scar[33] (Fig. 15.1).

Fibrosis occurs similarly at the epiglottis. Epiglottal fibrosis may occur following chemoradiotherapy and can manifest as thickening of the epiglottis. FEES may demonstrate the presence of residue in the vallecula and lateral channels, while MBS may reveal the absence of retroflexion with vallecular accumulation of residue (Fig. 15.2A and B). Surgical trimming of the suprahyoid epiglottis may improve swallow function with minimal impact on aspiration risk.[34] This surgery is performed endoscopically through a laryngoscope, with a CO_2 laser used to perform partial resection (Fig. 15.2C).

The UES and cervical esophagus are susceptible to fibrosis, much like the pharynx and the epiglottis. One may visualize pooled secretions or residue in the postcricoid region or the pyriform sinuses. As mentioned previously, MBS is particularly useful in visualizing the UES and may indicate limited passage or obstruction of the food bolus at the level of the UES (Fig. 15.3). When such obstruction is encountered, one may employ transnasal esophagoscopy to further visualize the esophagus, with special attention taken to note a stenotic area or scarring (Fig. 15.4). Inadequate UES opening may be a subtle finding, evidenced by haptic feedback of increased resistance when passing the scope through the UES.[35] Endoscopic cricopharyngeal myotomy is the typical treatment for UES fibrosis. A CO_2 laser is used to incise the fibrotic tissue and is followed by balloon dilation of the area of resection (Fig. 15.5).

In the case of esophageal stenosis, dilation with a balloon catheter or over a guidewire is often required (Fig. 15.6). This procedure should be performed with direct visualization with an ultraslim, flexible esophagoscope when possible.[35–40] In many cases, a single dilation will be insufficient, and subsequent dilations will be required. The surgeon should perform several serial dilations if the patient's stenosis is particularly severe. Serial dilations should be performed until a caliber 15–18 mm is obtained. Complete stenosis may require a simultaneous transoral and transgastric endoscopy (occasionally referred to as transgastric retrograde esophagoscopy with antegrade dilation) to re-establish an esophageal lumen.[36,37] In this procedure, retrograde esophagoscopy allows for safer placement of the guidewire, reducing the risk of false lumen creation or frank perforation.[38] An existing gastrostomy tube may be used in this procedure, allowing more confident passage of a guidewire.[39] This procedure may be performed by an otolaryngologist alone, but depending on the otolaryngologist's comfort and experience with the procedure, they may perform the procedure with a gastroenterologist or general surgeon.

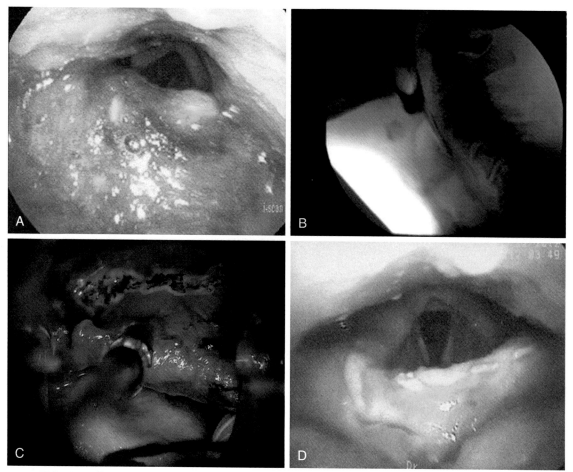

FIG. 15.2 Treatment of epiglottic dysfunction. Vallecular residue is visualized on flexible endoscopic evaluation of swallowing (FEES) **(A)** and modified barium swallow **(B)**. Treated with CO_2 laser partial epiglottidectomy **(C)**. Posttreatment FEES shows minimal residue **(D)**.

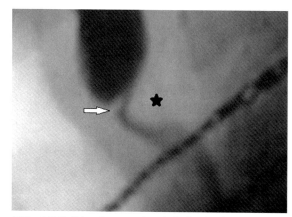

FIG. 15.3 Cricopharyngeal achalasia (*star*) as well as esophageal stenosis (*arrow*) seen in a lateral modified barium swallow view from a chemoradiation therapy patient.

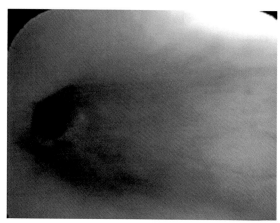

FIG. 15.4 Esophageal stenosis visualized by transnasal esophagoscopy from a chemoradiation therapy patient.

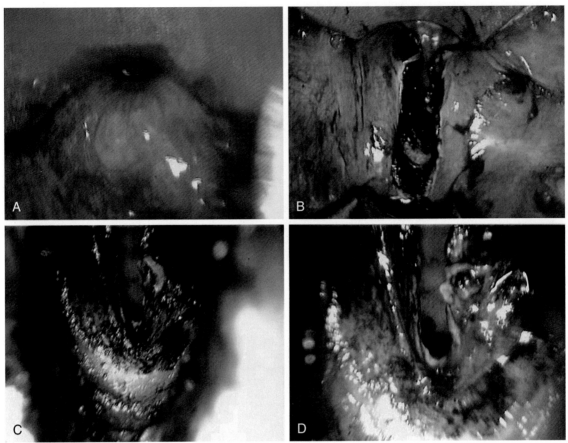

FIG. 15.5 Cricopharyngeal achalasia due to radiation fibrosis **(A)**. CO_2 laser myotomy was performed **(B)**. Closeup views show fibrosis resulting in a rigid fibrotic incision line that requires balloon dilation for maximal effect of myotomy **(C** and **D)**.

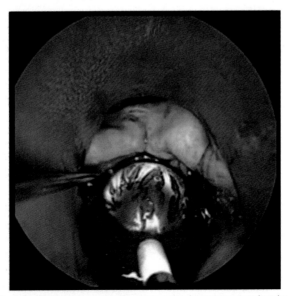

FIG. 15.6 Intraoperative view through the bore of a suspension laryngoscope showing dilation of esophageal stenosis using controlled radial expansion balloon. The wire to the left of the balloon dilator is a guidewire used for initial Savary-Guidewire dilation.

SUMMARY

The management of dysphagia in HNC survivors is a long-term endeavor that requires multidisciplinary collaboration. Dysphagia is the most important consideration in QOL following HNC therapy and requires the coordinated efforts of several specialists.[20,40–42] Therapy must be tailored to the patient's particular functional deficits with the intention of restoring function and preserving the function that remains.[21,43] Most importantly, it is crucial to remember that patients may experience slowly progressive dysfunction years after their initial treatment.[13] HNC survivors are a growing patient population and particular care must be taken to ensure that increased survival is met with improved QOL.

REFERENCES

1. Pulte D, Brenner H. Changes in survival in head and neck cancer in the late 20th century and early 21st century: a period analysis. *Oncologist*. 2010;15(9):994–1001.
2. Rieger JM, Zalmanowitz JG, Wolfaardt JF. Functional outcomes after organ preservation treatment in head and neck cancer: a critical review of the literature. *Int J Oral Maxillofac Surg*. 2006;35(7):581–587.
3. Connor NP, Cohen SB, Kammer RE, et al. Impact of conventional radiotherapy on health-related quality of life and critical functions of the head and neck. *Int J Radiat Oncol Biol Phys*. 2006;65(4):1051–1062.
4. Nguyen NP, Frank C, Moltz CC, et al. Impact of dysphagia on quality of life after treatment of head-and-neck cancer. *Int J Radiat Oncol Biol Phys*. 2005;61(3):772–778.
5. Duke RL, Campbell BH, Indresano AT, et al. *Laryngoscope*. 2005;115(4):678–683.
6. Blanchard D, Bollet M, Dreyer C, et al. Management of somatic pain induced by head and neck cancer treatment: pain following radiation therapy and chemotherapy. *Eur Ann Otorhinolaryngol Head Neck Dis*. 2014;131(4):253–256.
7. Smith BG, Hutcheson KA, Little LG, et al. Lymphedema outcomes in patients with head and neck cancer. *Otolaryngol Head Neck Surg*. 2015;152(2):284–291.
8. Servagi-Vernat S, Ali D, Roubieu C, et al. Dysphagia after radiotherapy: state of the art and prevention. *Eur Ann Otorhinolaryngol Head Neck Dis*. 2015;132(1):25–29.
9. Lee S, Park Y, Byeon H, et al. Comparison of oncologic and functional outcomes after transoral robotic lateral oropharyngectomy versus conventional surgery for T1-T3 tonsillar cancer. *Head Neck*. 2014;6(8):1138–1145.
10. Rosenthal D, Lewin J, Eisbruch A. Prevention and treatment of dysphagia and aspiration after chemoradiation for head and neck cancer. *J Clin Oncol*. 2006;24(17):2636–2643.
11. Caudell JJ, Schaner PE, Meredith RF, et al. Factors associated with long-term dysphagia after definitive radiotherapy for locally advanced head-and-neck cancer. *Int J Radiat Oncol Biol Phys*. 2009;73(2):410–415.
12. Hutcheson KA, Lewin JS, Barringer DA, et al. Late dysphagia after radiotherapy based treatment of head and neck cancer. *Cancer*. 2012;118(23):5793–5799.
13. Lango MN. Multimodal treatment for head and neck cancer. *Surg Clin North Am*. 2009;89(1):43–52.
14. Bentzen SM. Preventing or reducing late side effects of radiation therapy: radiobiology meets molecular pathology. *Nat Rev Cancer*. 2006;6(9):702–713.
15. Ewan KB, et al. Transforming growth factor-β1 mediates cellular response to DNA damage in situ. *Cancer Res*. 2002;62:5627–5631.
16. Ehrhart EJ, et al. Latent transforming growth factor β1 activation in situ: quantitative and functional evidence after low-dose gamma-irradiation. *FASEB J*. 1997;11:991–1002.
17. Shune SE, Karnell LH, Karnell MP, et al. Association between severity of dysphagia and survival in patients with head and neck cancer. *Head Neck*. 2012;34(6):776–784.
18. Jiang N, Zhang LJ, Li LY, et al. Risk factors for late dysphagia after (chemo)radiotherapy for head and neck cancer: a systematic methodological review. *Head Neck*. 2016;38(5):792–800.
19. Pauloski BR, Rademaker AW, Logemann JA, et al. Comparison of swallowing function after intensity-modulated radiation therapy and conventional radiotherapy for head and neck cancer. *Head Neck*. 2015;37(11):1575–1582.
20. Lazarus CL, Logemann JA, Pauloski BR, et al. Swallowing disorders in head and neck cancer patients treated with radiotherapy and adjuvant chemotherapy. *Laryngoscope*. 1996;106:1157–1166.
21. Kendall KA, McKenzie MS, Leonard RJ, Jones C. Structural mobility in deglutition after single modality treatment of head and neck carcinomas with radiotherapy. *Head Neck*. 1998;20:720–725.
22. Langmore SE, Schatz K, Olson N. Endoscopic and videofluoroscopic evaluations of swallowing and aspiration. *Ann Otol Rhinol Laryngol*. 1991;100:678–681.
23. Daniels SK, McAdam CP, Brailey K, et al. Clinical assessment of swallowing and prediction of dysphagia severity. *Am J Speech Lang Pathol*. 1997;6:17–24.
24. Bar Ad V, Weinstein G, Dutta PR, et al. Gabapentin for the treatment of pain syndrome related to radiation induced mucositis in patients with head and neck cancer treated with concurrent chemoradiotherapy. *Cancer*. 2010;116:4206–4213.
25. Portenoy RK. Tolerance to opioid analgesics clinical aspects. *Cancer Surviv*. 1994;21:49–65.
26. Cherry NI, Thaler HT, Friedlander-Klar H, et al. Opioid responsiveness of pain syndromes caused by neuropathic or nociceptive mechanisms: a combined analysis of controlled, single-dose studies. *Neurology*. 1994;44:857–886.
27. Caraceni A, Zecca E, Bonezzi C, et al. Gabapentin for neuropathic cancer pain: a randomized controlled trial from the Gabapentin Cancer Pain Study Group. *J Clin Oncol*. 2004;22:2909–2917.

28. Eckhardt K, et al. Gabapentin enhances the analgesic effect of morphine in healthy volunteers. *Anesth Analg.* 2000;91: 185–191.

29. Gilron I, Bailey JM, Tu D, et al. Morphine, gabapentin, or their combination for neuropathic pain. *N Engl J Med.* 2005;352:1324–1334.

30. Kataoka T, Kiyota N, Funakoshi Y, et al. Randomized trial of standard pain control with or without gabapentin for pain related to radiation-induced mucositis in head and neck cancer. *Auris Nasus Larynx.* 2016;43(6):677–684.

31. Shinn E, Basen-Engquist K, Baum G, et al. Adherence to preventive exercises and self-reported swallowing outcomes in post-radiated head and neck cancer patients. *Head Neck.* 2013;35(12):1707–1712.

32. Lazarus CL. Effects of chemoradiotherapy on voice and swallowing. *Curr Opin Otolaryngol Head Neck Surg.* 2009; 17(3):172–178.

33. Vira D, DeConde A, Chhetri DK. Endoscpoic management of supraglottic laryngopharyngeal stenosis. *Otolaryngol Head Neck Surg.* 2012;146(4):611–613.

34. Jamal N, Erman A, Chhetri DK. Transoral partial epiglottidectomy to treat dysphagia in post-treatment head and neck cancer patients: a preliminary report. *Laryngoscope.* 2014;124(3):665–671.

35. Peng KA, Feinstein AJ, Salinas JB, et al. Utility of the transnasal esophagoscope in the management of chemoradiation-induced esophageal stenosis. *Ann Otol Rhinol Laryngol.* 2015;124(3):221–226.

36. Jamal N, Ebersole B, Erman A, Chhetri D. Maximizing functional outcomes in head and neck cancer survivors: assessment and rehabilitation. *Otolaryngol Clin North Am.* 2017;50(4):837–852.

37. Sullivan CA, Jaklitsch MT, Haddad R, et al. Endoscopic management of hypopharyngeal stenosis after organ sparing therapy for head and neck cancer. *Laryngoscope.* 2004;114(11):1924–1931.

38. Steel NP, Tokayer A, Smith RV. Retrograde endoscopic balloon dilation of chemotherapy- and radiation-induced esophageal stenosis under direct visualization. *Am J Otolaryngol.* 2007;28:98.

39. Langerman A, Stenson KM, Ferguson MK. Retrograde endoscopic-assisted esophageal dilation. *J Gastrointestinal Surg.* 2010;14(7):1186–1189.

40. Hirano M, et al. Dysphagia following various degrees of surgical resection for oral cancer. *Ann Otol Rhinol Laryngol.* 1992;101:138–141.

41. Zuydam AC, et al. Swallowing rehabilitation after oropharyngeal resection for squamous cell carcinoma. *Br J Oral Maxillofac Surg.* 2000;38:513–518.

42. Kao S, Peters M, Krishnan S, et al. Swallowing outcomes following primary surgical resection and primary free flap reconstruction for oral and oropharyngeal squamous cell carcinomas: a systematic review. *Laryngoscope.* 2016; 126(7):1572–1580.

43. Peng K, Kuan E, Unger L, et al. A swallow preservation protocol improves function for veterans receiving chemoradiation for head and neck cancer. *Otolaryngol Head Neck Surg.* 2015;152(5):863–867.

CHAPTER 16

Epiglottic Dysfunction

KARUNA DEWAN, MD • DINESH K. CHHETRI, MD

INTRODUCTION

The epiglottis is a leaf-shaped cartilaginous projection of the larynx above the glottis and is positioned vertically between the base of the tongue and the larynx. Its inferior attachment is to the larynx via the thyroepiglottic ligament just deep and inferior to the thyroid notch. The lower part of its anterior surface is connected to the hyoid bone by the hyoepiglottic ligament. The aryepiglottic folds are attached to the side of the epiglottis and extend to the arytenoid cartilages. Along with two other laryngeal valves—the true and false vocal folds—the epiglottis plays a role in preventing aspiration of liquids or food into the trachea during deglutition.[1] The dynamic function of the epiglottis is made possible by the flexibility of its structure, which is composed of elastic cartilage, and its muscular and ligamentous connections to the aryepiglottic folds and the true and false vocal cords that close the airway.[2] However, when it fails to retroflex it may become obstructive rather than protective. Abnormal epiglottic movement patterns such as immobility, prolonged inversion, horizontal tilt, or translocation with various etiologies, may cause swallowing and aspiration problems.[3,4]

Normal epiglottic inversion is one element of the airway protection mechanism during swallowing. During a normal swallow, the epiglottis moves from its vertical resting position to horizontal, and further to a complete downward tilt, covering the endolarynx, before returning to the resting upright position. The downward epiglottic tilt is a very rapid movement which takes 100 ms or less during a normal swallow.[5] Decreased and blunted epiglottic movement may cause incomplete laryngeal protection when the food bolus reaches the lower pharynx. Thyrohyoid approximation by laryngeal elevation and anterior displacement of the hyoid bone during swallowing produces the epiglottic tilt during swallowing. Airway protection during swallowing occurs by contact of the *epiglottic petiole* with the arytenoids, which closes the laryngeal

vestibule. Therefore, reduced epiglottic movement may also represent abnormal hyolaryngeal movement such as from pharyngeal weakness. The airway protection mechanisms activated upon initiation of oropharyngeal swallow consist of an *anterior-superior movement* of the hyoid bone, posterior retraction of the tongue base, closure of the supraglottic larynx by the aryepiglottic folds and the epiglottis, and adduction and closure of the vocal cords. Failure of one or more of those mechanisms may allow for laryngeal penetration and/or aspiration. On the other hand, failure of the epiglottis to invert can also create an obstacle for the food bolus leading to retention in the vallecula and dysphagia symptoms. This vallecular retention may result in cough, throat clearing, globus sensation, and even aspiration after the swallow.

PATHOPHYSIOLOGY

Elasticity and flexibility of the epiglottic cartilage play important roles in deglutition. The epiglottis is composed of cartilage and connective tissue in two layers. The superficial layer is composed of flattened chondrocytes, and the deep layer is composed of enlarged, round chondrocytes. The extracellular matrix increases with age in the superficial layer of the epiglottic cartilage, and the chondrocytes become more rounded. Kano et al. report that cartilage thickness significantly increased with age: calcium deposition in the lower level of the epiglottic cartilage was much higher than in the upper level, and superficially, the cartilage cell density was found to be significantly reduced in older age groups.[6] Elastic epiglottic cartilage calcifications show two patterns, diffuse and extensive calcium deposition. It has been shown that calcium deposition in the epiglottis has a tendency to increase with age.[7] However, it is difficult to describe the clinical importance, because of inadequate studies demonstrating that calcium accumulation in the lower sections of the epiglottis disrupt epiglottic function. Loss of retroflexion of the epiglottis can result in aspiration and consequently pneumonia. The reduction of absence of epiglottic retroflexion also leads to the attenuation of intrabolus pressures above the obstructing epiglottis. This results in vallecular residue. It is this vallecular residue that can also pose a potential aspiration risk.

The coexistence of a dysfunctional epiglottis in patients with dysphagia has been well described, often in association with aspiration. Garon et al. described the presence of *vallecular residue* of food as a strong indicator of abnormal epiglottic movement patterns and dysfunction.[1] *Nasal backflow* has also been described as an indicator of significant epiglottic dysfunction. Two major factors play a role in the development of epiglottic dysfunction: (1) narrowing of the anteroposterior diameter of the pharynx and (2) thickening and stiffening of the epiglottis. The dysfunctional epiglottis is unable to fully invert during a swallow for one or both of these reasons: either crowding of the pharynx or stiffening of the epiglottis. A common cause of such epiglottic thickening and stiffening is *radiation therapy to the neck* for treatment of head and neck cancer. A dysfunctional epiglottis leading to vallecular residue is observed[8] (Fig. 16.1).

Jamal et al. described a common finding of a stiff and thickened epiglottis on endoscopic evaluation in patients after radiation therapy that correlated with a lack of normal epiglottic deflection on modified barium swallow study (MBSS) (Fig. 16.2). They noted that this dysfunction results in an inefficient pharyngeal phase of swallow, with excessive vallecular residue that is difficult to clear even with behavioral maneuvers. Radiation therapy causes a narrowing of the circumference of the oropharynx, and this combined with the thickened radiated epiglottis leads to a relatively greater pharyngeal area occupied by the epiglottis that contributes to bolus obstruction. On average, the epiglottic to pharyngeal diameter is significantly increased in a radiated pharynx because the pharynx contracts and scars after radiation therapy.[8] Bleier et al. also found that patients who had undergone concomitant chemotherapy with radiation had a significantly increased incidence of chronic epiglottic changes manifesting as bulbous epiglottis, relative to those who had radiotherapy alone.[9]

Another cause of epiglottic dysfunction is reduction in the anteroposterior diameter of the pharynx leading to pharyngeal crowding. The most common cause of this is cervical spine pathology. Anterior cervical osteophytes are present in 10.6% of patients presenting with dysphagia[10] (Fig. 16.3). Pharyngeal-phase dysphagia caused by anterior cervical osteophytes is typically due

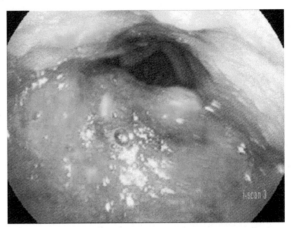

FIG. 16.1 Flexible endoscopic evaluation of swallowing in a patient with a history of radiation therapy for oropharyngeal squamous cell carcinoma, illustrating vallecular residue due to epiglottic thickening and stiffening, and narrowing of oropharyngeal diameter.

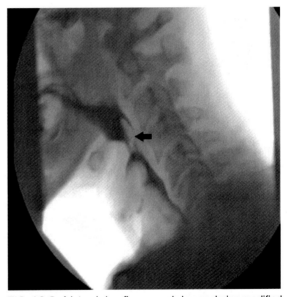

FIG. 16.2 A lateral view fluoroscopic image during modified barium swallow study from a patient after radiation therapy showing lack of normal epiglottic retroflexion.

to pharyngeal narrowing from a protuberant posterior pharyngeal wall with concurrent alteration of swallow physiology, including reduction or the absence of epiglottic inversion, leading to attenuation of intrabolus pressures above the obstructing epiglottis, and vallecular residue.[2–4] The same finding can be encountered in patients who have undergone cervical spine

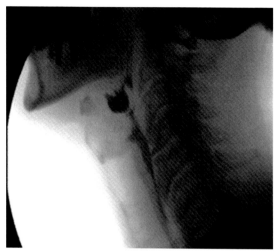

FIG. 16.3 Epiglottic dysfunction in a patient with cervical osteophytes and pharyngeal weakness.

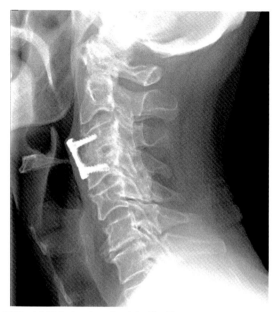

FIG. 16.5 Lateral neck plain film X-ray of the case from Fig. 16.4 reveals the relationship between the epiglottis and the spinal hardware.

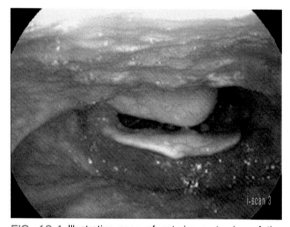

FIG. 16.4 Illustrative case of anterior protrusion of the posterior pharyngeal wall causing epiglottic dysfunction and vallecular residue on flexible endoscopic evaluation of swallowing.

surgery with hardware placement (Figs. 16.4 and 16.5). This hardware often causes thickening and protuberance of the posterior pharyngeal wall leading to narrowing of the anteroposterior diameter of the pharynx. Leonard and Belafsky reported significantly increased pharyngeal wall thickness in patients both early and late (>2 months) after anterior cervical discectomy and fusion surgery. Epiglottic inversion was either incomplete or absent in 84% of the patients <2 months after surgery and in 35% of individuals >2 months after C-spine hardware placement. The increased thickness of the posterior pharyngeal wall interfered with

epiglottic inversion and vallecular clearing.[11] In a study by Perlman et al. vallecular residue and epiglottic dysfunction were found to have the highest co-occurrence rate with aspiration, of all the parameters measured. The presence of residue has also been shown to have a prognostic value in predicting the outcome of rehabilitation for stroke patients with dysphagia.[4] Park et al. reported that stroke patients with greater residue in the valleculae and pyriform sinuses had poorer treatment outcomes following a rehabilitation protocol involving neuromuscular electrical stimulation.[12]

SYMPTOMS

Patients with epiglottic dysfunction can present with a wide range of symptoms including chronic cough, globus sensation, and throat clearing all of which can be secondary to vallecular residue. The most common presenting symptom of epiglottic dysfunction is solid food dysphagia. Vallecular residue is the most common finding associated with epiglottic dysfunction. Occasionally, epiglottic dysfunction may present with recurrent aspiration of retained food bolus that spills down from the vallecula, leading to aspiration pneumonia. In a retrospective analysis of 156 thin-liquid clearing swallows from patients with neurogenic dysphagia, Molfenter and Steele found that vallecular residue from the previous swallow was associated with double the risk of penetration—aspiration on the subsequent swallow.[13] Meaning, the more residue present from the previous swallow, the more likely the patient was to subsequently aspirate or penetrate. The association of reduced epiglottic movement with the risk of aspiration in patients with post-stroke dysphagia is demonstrated by Seo et al. in their quantitative measurements of epiglottic tilt during swallowing.[14] Patients with aspiration of vallecular residue were noted to have a decreased maximal tilt angle of the epiglottis as well as a decreased velocity of epiglottic movement. In epiglottic dysfunction, the vallecular residue may or may not clear with a liquid assist.

DIAGNOSIS

Three key methodologies play roles in the diagnosis of epiglottic dysfunction: fiberoptic laryngoscopy, flexible endoscopic evaluation of swallowing (FEES), and MBSS. On fiberoptic laryngoscopy one may see a thickened epiglottis with absent or reduced retroflexion while swallowing. When swallowing efficiency is impaired, saliva, secretions, and residue collects in the spaces of the pharynx including the valleculae and pyriform sinuses.

On FEES (see Chapter 8), there is notable stasis in the vallecula and often in the pyriform sinuses (Figs. 16.1 and 16.4). The pyriform sinus residue may represent distal spillage of the vallecular residue that occurs after the height of the swallow. The residues may or may not clear with a liquid assist. The free edge of the epiglottis is often displaced, pushed toward the back wall of the pharynx. This effectively narrows the anteroposterior diameter of the pharynx. Dysphagia due to epiglottic dysfunction is often improved with slight flexion of the head when swallowing.

Two distinct movements of epiglottic inversion are observed in MBSS studies (see Chapter 10). The first epiglottic movement positions the epiglottis in a horizontal position with the second epiglottic movement achieving full inversion. The first epiglottic movement is attributed to hyoid movement and hyolaryngeal approximation,[5,15] elevation of the hyoid and larynx,[16] and tongue base retraction.[17] Logemann et al. report that tongue base retraction underlies the second epiglottic movement, whereas Van Daele et al. conclude that the anterior hyoid movement and hyolaryngeal approximation, aided by lateral hyoepiglottic ligaments, completes the epiglottic inversion.[16,17] Pearson et al. report that reduced laryngeal elevation and reduced tongue base retraction, but not differences

in hyoid movement, underlie impaired epiglottic inversion in both the first and second epiglottic movements.[18] This suggests that the longitudinal pharyngeal muscles and styloglossus with hyoglossus are likely more important to the airway protection provided by the epiglottis than the suprahyoid or floor of the mouth muscles. The longitudinal pharyngeal muscles (stylopharyngeus, palatopharyngeus, and salpingopharyngeus) function as a posterior muscular sling to elevate the larynx. Epiglottic inversion correlates with the action of the pharyngeal constrictor muscles as well as laryngeal elevation and tongue base retraction.

TREATMENT

The treatment for epiglottic dysfunction is two pronged. It includes swallowing therapy and surgical intervention. In swallowing therapy, the purpose is to strengthen those muscles that are responsible for the inversion of the epiglottis, in an attempt to increase the efficiency of the swallow. Often times, in the case of swallow preservation therapy in head and neck cancer treatment, this can be preventive. Carroll et al. found that epiglottic inversion was maintained better in chemoradiation patients who participated in swallowing exercises.[19] Many of these exercises (tongue hold, tongue resistance, effortful swallow, and Mendelsohn maneuver) targeted muscle groups underlying hyoid movement, laryngeal elevation and tongue base retraction. Focused rehabilitation on particular muscle groups known to invert the epiglottis may encourage patient compliance and improve swallowing safety in dysphagia patients. Impaired epiglottic inversion is likely due to reduced laryngeal elevation and tongue base retraction.

Therapies that target the styloglossus, hyoglossus, and pharyngeal constrictor muscles may improve or preserve airway protection during swallowing.[19] Post-swallow residue is a potential source of subjective patient discomfort. It can be the irritation behind chronic cough, throat clearing, and globus sensation. It is also implicated as a potential risk for secondary aspiration. Nagy et al. demonstrated significant reductions in post-swallow measures of vallecular residue, particularly for thin and nectar-thick liquids with clinically effective resolution below a previously reported aspiration-risk threshold in 11%—29% of cases.[20] Thus, the head-turn-chin-down technique may be successful in reducing residue in patients with problematic and persistent vallecular residue. This is a compensatory maneuver that can be explored in patients displaying vallecular residue due to epiglottic dysfunction on MBSS or FEES.

Surgical intervention for epiglottic dysfunction involves the endoscopic CO_2 laser partial epiglottidectomy. This surgery may seem counterintuitive from a swallow standpoint since it is believed that the epiglottis plays a role in airway protection. However, it is likely a minor role. Numerous authors have described performing epiglottidectomies to treat benign supraglottic and hypopharyngeal obstruction.[21,22] These have been performed in cases of obstructive sleep apnea, laryngomalacia, and even globus pharyngeus. These patients experience improvement in their clinical symptoms without compromising swallowing. Leder et al. reported a case series of three adults who underwent isolated epiglottidectomy from three diverse causes: trauma, surgical resection for a supraglottic cancer, and malignant erosion of the entire epiglottis. The second patient reported odynophagia related to postoperative edema, but none of the patients had any other abnormalities of swallow, and none developed aspiration pneumonia. The authors concluded that patients can readily adapt to isolated epiglottidectomy and avoid aspiration.[23]

Partial epiglottidectomy can be considered in some patients with pharyngeal dysphagia following radiotherapy with or without chemotherapy for head and neck cancers. Posttreatment MBSS should be carefully reviewed for bolus obstruction due to epiglottic dysfunction, high levels of vallecular residue, and backflow from the vallecular space to the oral and/or nasal cavities in the setting of adequate tongue base contraction. The best candidates for epiglottidectomy are those patients who are able to retract the base of tongue to the posterior pharyngeal wall. Partial suprahyoid epiglottidectomy is performed via the transoral endoscopic approach under general anesthesia. A Dedo or Lindholm laryngoscope is used for exposure. The epiglottis is trimmed about halfway between the hyoepiglottic ligament and the tip of the epiglottis using a carbon dioxide laser. Any protruding or demucosalized portion of the epiglottic cartilage is gently ablated to prevent necrosis or infection in this area. Patients are typically discharged home the same day, on the diet they were previously tolerating. The time required to clear material through the pharynx and pharyngeal residue is expected to decrease postoperatively in this population. This results in greater ease and efficiency of swallowing, with the possibility for diet advancement. Occasionally, penetration to thin liquid may worsen in those with pharyngeal weakness and/or reduced pharyngeal sensation. This is managed

with swallow therapy and compensatory swallowing techniques and generally improves after surgical healing and pharyngeal strengthening.

CONCLUSION
Normal epiglottic inversion is a component of airway protection; however, when the normal function of the epiglottis is lost, it can become obstructive and a source of dysphagia. Radiation exposure, cervical spine surgery, and advanced age are all common factors in the development of epiglottic dysfunction. This condition can be managed with swallow therapy or surgery involving the endoscopic partial resection of the epiglottis in carefully selected patients. Those with residual adequate pharyngeal strength and sensation will do well following surgery, with marked improvement of dysphagia.

REFERENCES
1. Garon BR, Huang Z, Hommeyer M, Eckmann D, Stern GA, Ormiston C. Epiglottic dysfunction: abnormal epiglottic movement patterns. *Dysphagia.* 2002;17:57–68.
2. Mafee MF. CT of the normal larynx. *Radiol Clin N Am.* 1984;22:251–264.
3. Ekberg O. Epiglottic dysfunction during deglutition in patients with dysphagia. *Arch Otolaryngol.* 1983;109:376–380.
4. Perlman AL, Booth BM, Grayhack JP. Videofluoroscopic predictors of aspiration in patients with oropharyngeal dysphagia. *Dysphagia.* 1994;9:90–95.
5. Fink BR, Martin RW, Rohrmann CA. Biomechanics of the human epiglottis. *Acta Otolaryngol.* 1979;87:554–559.
6. Kano M, Shimizu Y, Okayama K, Igari T, Kikuchi M. A morphometric study of age-related changes in adult human epiglottis using quantitative digital analysis of cartilage calcification. *Cells Tissues Organs.* 2005;180:126–137.
7. Gunbey HP, Gunbey E, Sayit AT. A rare cause of abnormal epiglottic mobility and dyspagia: calcification of the epiglottis. *J Craniofac Surg.* 2014;25:e519–e521.
8. Jamal N, Erman A, Chhetri DK. Transoral partial epiglottidectomy to treat dysphagia in post-treatment head and neck cancer patients: a preliminary report. *Laryngoscope.* 2014;124:665–671.
9. Bleier BS, Levine MS, Mick R, et al. Dysphagia after chemoradiation: analysis by modified barium swallow. *Ann Otol Rhinol Laryngol.* 2007;116:837–841.
10. Lecerf P, Malard O. How to diagnose and treat symptomatic anterior cervical osteophytes? *Eur Ann Otorhinolaryngol Head Neck Dis.* 2010;127:111–116.
11. Leonard R, Belafsky P. Dysphagia following cervical spine surgery with anterior instrumentation: evidence from fluoroscopic swallow studies. *Spine (Phila Pa 1976).* 2011;36:2217–2223.

12. Park JM, Yong SY, Kim JH, et al. Cutoff value of pharyngeal residue in prognosis prediction after neuromuscular electrical stimulation therapy for dysphagia in subacute stroke patients. *Ann Rehabil Med.* 2014;38:612−619.

13. Molfenter SM, Steele CM. The relationship between residue and aspiration on the subsequent swallow: an application of the normalized residue ratio scale. *Dysphagia.* 2013; 28:494−500.

14. Seo HG, Oh BM, Han TR. Swallowing kinematics and factors associated with laryngeal penetration and aspiration in stroke survivors with dysphagia. *Dysphagia.* 2016;31: 160−168.

15. Ekberg O, Sigurjonsson SV. Movement of the epiglottis during deglutition. A cineradiographic study. *Gastrointest Radiol.* 1982;7:101−107.

16. Logemann JA, Rademaker AW, Pauloski BR, Ohmae Y, Kahrilas PJ. Normal swallowing physiology as viewed by videofluoroscopy and videoendoscopy. *Folia Phoniatr Logop.* 1998;50:311−319.

17. Vandaele DJ, Perlman AL, Cassell MD. Intrinsic fibre architecture and attachments of the human epiglottis and their contributions to the mechanism of deglutition. *J Anat.* 1995;186(Pt 1):1−15.

18. Pearson Jr WG, Taylor BK, Blair J, Martin-Harris B. Computational analysis of swallowing mechanics underlying impaired epiglottic inversion. *Laryngoscope.* 2016;126: 1854−1858.

19. Carroll WR, Locher JL, Canon CL, Bohannon IA, McColloch NL, Magnuson JS. Pretreatment swallowing exercises improve swallow function after chemoradiation. *Laryngoscope.* 2008;118:39−43.

20. Nagy A, Peladeau-Pigeon M, Valenzano TJ, Namasivayam AM, Steele CM. The effectiveness of the head-turn-plus-chin-down maneuver for eliminating vallecular residue. *Codas.* 2016;28: 113−117.

21. D'Agostino MA. Obstructive sleep apnea, diagnosis, management, and treatment. *Otolaryngol Clin N Am.* 2016;49: xiii−xiv.

22. Golz A, Goldenberg D, Westerman ST, et al. Laser partial epiglottidectomy as a treatment for obstructive sleep apnea and laryngomalacia. *Ann Otol Rhinol Laryngol.* 2000;109:1140−1145.

23. Leder SB, Burrell MI, Van Daele DJ. Epiglottis is not essential for successful swallowing in humans. *Ann Otol Rhinol Laryngol.* 2010;119:795−798.

CHAPTER 17

Cervical Osteophytes

MICHAEL I. ORESTES, MD • RICHARD W. THOMAS, MD, DDS, FACS •
SIDDHARTH U. SHETGERI, MD • LANGSTON T. HOLLY, MD •
DINESH K. CHHETRI, MD

INTRODUCTION

Osteophytes of the spine are bony outgrowths which are commonly seen in an elderly population.[1] Osteophytes are usually not symptomatic. However, in select locations of the cervical spine, these osteophytes can cause significant obstruction of swallowing, particularly in patients with an already compromised swallow function. Multiple etiologies have been reported, including trauma, cervical spondylosis, and most commonly, diffuse idiopathic skeletal hyperostosis (DISH).[2] Cervical spine osteophytes are present in approximately 10%–30% of the population[3,4]; however, it is estimated that they cause dysphagia in about 6%–30% of these cases.[3,5] Although frequently described as rare or uncommon, there are a large number of small case reports described in the literature. Through careful physical examination, radiological studies and evaluation of swallowing, the impact of cervical osteophytes can be determined and subsequently treated.

PATHOPHYSIOLOGY

Isolated Osteophytes

Abnormal bone formation can be found either at joint margins or at ligament/tendon insertions. Formations at the joint margins are known as osteophytes, while formations at the ligaments and tendons are called enthesophytes.[6] Both are associated with the cervical spine. Osteophytes are associated with aging and osteoarthritis and both frequently involve joint facets. Enthesophytes are more commonly seen at sites of repetitive muscle action such as the tibial tubercle and rotator cuff; however, they are more frequently seen in DISH.[6] An isolated osteophyte is seen in Fig. 17.1.

Osteophytes are mostly seen in the elderly and are due to osteoarthritis. Obesity is the most common cause, leading to increased stress on the spine. However, hypervitaminosis and oversecretion of bone morphogenetic factor can play a role.[5] In the cervical spine,

C5–C6 and C6–C7 are the most common sites due to their higher mobility and increased load from the head.[5] Other disorders such as ankylosing spondylitis can also cause cervical spine osteophytes.[7]

Diffuse Idiopathic Skeletal Hyperostosis

Osteophytes can present as either isolated foci or in a more diffuse fashion. When they present in the more diffuse fashion, this is known as DISH or Forestier's disease (Fig. 17.2). The underlying cause is thought to be flow ossification of the anterior longitudinal ligaments resulting in prolific and diffuse development of large osteophytes. DISH is a relatively common condition noted in 12%–28% of autopsies.[8] It is most common over the age of 50 years and has a strong male predominance. Nearly any region of the spine can be affected,

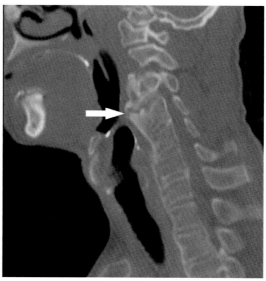

FIG. 17.1 Isolated osteophytes (arrow) seen on computed tomography scan neck, sagittal view.

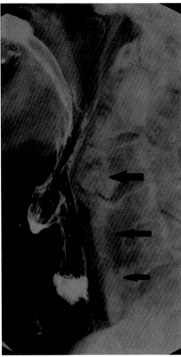

FIG. 17.2 Lateral view of the neck during barium esophagram in a patient with DISH. *Black arrows* point to multilevel osteophytes.

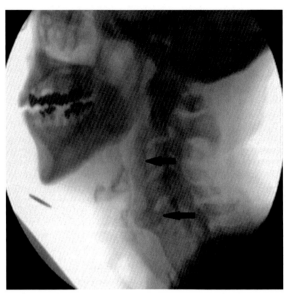

FIG. 17.3 Preoperative lateral fluoroscopic image of an 84-year-old male showing very large ventral osteophytes from the C2–C3 and C5–C6 levels. Osteophytes at C2–C3 (*upper arrow*) caused epiglottic dysfunction, and osteophytes at C5–C6 (*lower arrow*) obstructed passed of bolus through the upper esophageal sphincter.

though the thoracic spine appears to be the most common location. Despite being present in about 10% of people over the age of 50 years, it is not frequently diagnosed due to the lack of clinical symptoms in many of these patients.[9]

Early symptoms of DISH are typically associated with direct compressive effects resulting in dysphagia or dyspnea. Late-stage effects are often associated with instability of the spine leading to increased fractures.[9] Dysphagia is typically associated with cervical osteophytes and can result in aspiration,[9,10] while dyspnea can be associated with large cervical osteophytes with limitation of the vocal folds or upper airway or involvement of the sternum or ribs.[3,8,9]

The diagnosis of DISH is not well established; however, the following radiologic criteria has been proposed[11,12]: (1) flow ossification along the anterolateral aspect of at least four contiguous vertebral bodies, (2) relative preservation of intervertebral disk heights, and (3) the absence of apophyseal joint ankylosis and sacroiliac joint sclerosis to rule out inflammatory etiology.

SYMPTOMS

The effects of a cervical osteophyte on dysphagia are highly dependent on the location. A study by Seidler et al.[11] evaluated a series of 20 patients with osteophytes and dysphagia. They noted two distinct abnormalities in swallowing based on the level of the osteophytes: (1) osteophytes affecting the motion of the epiglottis, causing incomplete retroflexion of epiglottis, typically occurring at levels C3/4/5, and (2) osteophytes affecting the motion of the cricoid, causing incomplete elevation of the larynx and obstruction of the upper esophageal sphincter (UES), typically occurring at C5/6/7 (Fig. 17.3).

Furthermore, very large osteophytes can cause vocal fold mobility issues by restriction of vocal fold motion,[11] further impeding swallowing. Rarely, patients can exhibit a high degree of crowding of the level of the larynx that can result in respiratory stridor.[8] Papadopoulou et al.[13] proposed two other possible mechanisms for dysphagia in these patients: pain and spasm of the cricopharyngeus and inflammation around the esophagus. However, the exact mechanism for dysphagia is unclear and likely variable from case to case. As we know, formation of osteophytes along the spine is common and, in many cases, does not cause dysphagia.

DIAGNOSIS AND CLINICAL EVALUATION

Office Endoscopy

Office transnasal laryngoscopy can identify osteophytes from above C5 level. Examination of the oropharynx for higher osteophytes by laryngoscopy is sufficient in many cases. A characteristic bulging of the posterior pharyngeal wall is seen (Fig. 17.4). In contrast, osteophytes at or below the level of the cricoid (typically C5 and below) are difficult to visualize. Utilizing a transnasal esophagoscope can be useful to exclude other causes of dysphagia, but it is still difficult to visualize osteophytes in this region. In addition to being able to visualize oropharyngeal and hypopharyngeal osteophytes above the cricoid, office endoscopy is critical for examination of the interaction of the epiglottis with the osteophytes, along with the diagnosis of associated vocal fold disorders such as vocal fold immobility or paralysis.

Flexible Endoscopic Evaluation of Swallowing

Flexible endoscopic evaluation of swallowing (FEES) can be used to assess the effect of the pharyngeal osteophyte on swallowing as well as the obstructive effects of osteophytes at or just below the cricoid. For osteophytes above the cricoid, residue within the vallecula is frequently seen (Fig. 17.5). This is thought to be the result of a relative lack of retroflexion of the epiglottis caused by a combination of calcification of the epiglottic cartilage and protrusion of the anterior cervical spine due to the osteophyte.[14] There is generally a component of decreased pharyngeal strength as well. For patients with osteophytes at the level of the cricoid, solid food residue is more likely to be noted at the level of the piriform sinuses. In addition to visualizing the impact of food obstruction from the osteophytes, FEES is helpful in identifying additional swallowing problems such as decreased pharyngeal strength that is common in this population.[2,14] In general, FEES is most useful for identifying symptomatic cervical osteophytes above the cricoid.

Modified Barium Swallowing Study

Modified barium swallow study provides an excellent view of the anterior projection of the osteophytes along with the obstruction of a food bolus as it is swallowed. It is best for adequate visualization of osteophytes at or

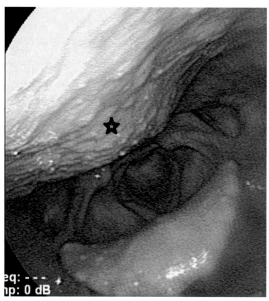

FIG. 17.4 Transnasal flexible laryngoscopy demonstrating a posterior pharyngeal bulge (*) due to an osteophyte.

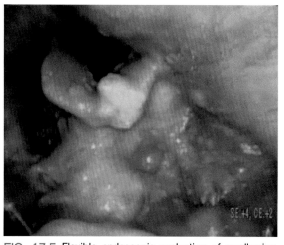

FIG. 17.5 Flexible endoscopic evaluation of swallowing demonstrating the effects of an osteophyte above the upper esophageal sphincter causing epiglottic dysfunction and vallecular residue of food.

below the cricoid which are not otherwise easily seen. It also allows for observation of swallowing during pharyngeal contraction which allows for assessment of pharyngeal strength and visualization of penetration and aspiration during the swallow.

Manometry

Esophageal manometry is not typically used in the evaluation of osteophytes specifically. However, it can be useful for evaluation of functional esophageal disorders and cricopharyngeal achalasia which is a common comorbid pathology in these patients. When significant osteophytes are present, the typical findings will be of increased intrabolus pressure in the area.[15,16] Interestingly, cervical osteophytes at the level of the cricopharyngeus may present with findings consistent with cricopharyngeal achalasia.[15] This demonstrates the need to correlate these findings with anatomic imaging of the neck.

TREATMENT

Swallow Therapy

The first step in medical management of a physical obstruction is diet modification. Typically, this involves cutting or thoroughly chewing foods to help in bypassing of the obstruction. In patients where aspiration is a concern, thickening the liquids and various swallowing maneuvers can be used to help control or prevent aspiration. In patients with poor dentition, semisoft foods or nutritional supplements can be useful along with improved hydration and oral hygiene.[17]

Medications

Some studies have indicated that analgesics, muscle relaxants, and nonsteroidal antiinflammatory drugs have improved dysphagia.[3] However, this is probably highly dependent on the location of the osteophytes. Some may impede the pharyngeal constrictors or portions of the larynx which can cause pain with swallowing.

Transoral Excision of Osteophytes

Originally reported by Saffouri and Ward,[18] transoral excision was performed by resection via blind placement of a osteotome into the mouth and truncating the offending osteophyte. This was effective but presented a hazard in terms of destabilization of the cervical spine. Furthermore, this could only be used if the osteophytes are present above the level of the cricoid. Advancements in technology and high-speed drills allow for more precise transoral excision, though there are no recent reported cases in the literature. With improvement in robotic technology and minimally invasive transoral techniques, it is likely that a transoral approach may be used more frequently in the future for both osteophytes above and below the cricoid. However, this approach is not commonly advocated.

Partial Epiglottidectomy

Originally proposed by Jamal et al.,[14] utilizing a transoral approach, the epiglottis can be selectively trimmed to avoid hitting the bulging of the epiglottis, allowing passage of the food bolus past the osteophyte. In older adults, the epiglottis typically stiffens. When combined with a narrowed posterior pharyngeal wall, the food bolus can be retained at the level of the vallecula (Fig. 17.6). After swallowing, the residual material trickles down to the level of the piriform sinus and can cause coughing or be aspirated. This approach of trimming of the epiglottis to allow for flexion and space for food bolus past the osteophyte can be curative with a lesser operation than osteophyte resection. In the small series by Jamal et al.,[14] all of the patients experienced marked improvement in swallowing with minimal morbidity. This approach may not be commonly used due to fear of aspiration; however, it is likely that the flexion over the epiglottis does not protect the larynx, but rather the opposition of the base of the epiglottis to the arytenoids which is not affected.[19]

Surgery is performed in the operating room under general anesthesia. After intubation with a laser-safe endotracheal tube, a tooth guard is placed and a large bore laryngoscope such as a Lindholm laryngoscope is used to expose the epiglottis. Cottonoids soaked in saline are placed to protect the endotracheal tube and the rest of the endolarynx in the path of the laser beam. A CO_2 laser is used to trim the superior half of the suprahyoid epiglottis (about halfway between the

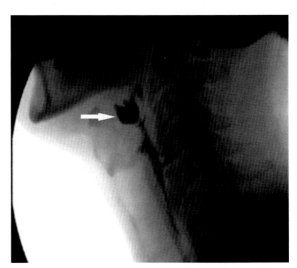

FIG. 17.6 Lateral view during video fluoroscopic swallow study demonstrating a lack of epiglottic retroflexion and resulting retention of barium in the vallecula (*arrow*).

hyoepiglottic ligament and the tip of the epiglottis), so that it retroflexes under the cervical osteophyte. A grasper can be used to estimate this position. In order to prevent issues with penetration and aspiration, only a third to half of the suprahyoid epiglottis should be resected. The aryepiglottic folds are left intact. Bleeding can be easily controlled by an endoscopic laryngeal suction cautery. In patients with a high risk of bleeding or if use of a laser is difficult or unavailable, a long harmonic scalpel can be used instead of the CO_2 laser.

Transcervical Excision

The most commonly used surgical technique for management of osteophytes, especially for the lower levels of the cervical spine, is the transcervical approach. There are multiple case reports describing improvement following resection, particularly in patients with DISH.[3,5,8] Further, the transcervical approach is the only effective method of management of osteophytes below the level of the cricoid.

The open approach to cervical osteophytes is similar to that used for exposure of the cervical spine for treatment of cervical radiculopathy or myelopathy. A transverse horizontal incision is created at the appropriate level of the neck as guided by lateral fluoroscopy and a metallic instrument. Three or more spinal levels commonly require a vertical incision. Either a right- or left-sided approach can be used depending on prior surgeries and the presence of preexisting vocal fold paralysis. Intervention is preferred on the side of preexisting vocal fold paralysis or can be performed on the nonoperated side if none exists. The left side is preferred by some surgeons for protection of the recurrent laryngeal nerve (RLN) which runs more medial than right; however, the right approach can be easier for right-handed surgeons. Most studies have not demonstrated a significantly different rate of RLN palsy between the left- or right-sided approaches.[20,21]

After skin incision, the platysma is incised and undermined. Branches of the external jugular vein may be seen and are either retracted or divided. The medial border of the sternocleidomastoid is dissected and retracted laterally. The strap muscles are identified and retracted medially. The omohyoid is identified and released as necessary. Access below the omohyoid is recommended for exposure of the inferior cervical levels and above for access to the superior cervical levels. The carotid artery is identified purely by digital palpation of the pulse, and careful blunt dissection medial to the carotid artery with a Kittner dissector is used to expose the retropharyngeal/esophageal space so as to not enter the carotid sheath. The laryngotracheal complex is retracted medially, the prevertebral muscles are dissected, and the osteophytes are exposed. Care must be taken at this stage to identify any adhesions that may have developed between the esophagus, the laryngotracheal complex, and osteophytes of large size, which must be released meticulously. The longus colli muscles are dissected off the lateral surfaces of the vertebral bodies either bluntly or with electrocautery. Blunt dissection is preferred to not violate the sympathetic chain. Spinal levels are then confirmed with lateral X-ray. Anterior cervical self-retaining retractor systems such as the Trimline, Shadowline, or black belt can then be placed underneath the longus colli muscles in the medial/lateral plane, with additional retraction placed in an offset manner for the craniocaudal plane. Not uncommonly, the longus coli muscles may be atrophied due to the longstanding presence of the osteophytes. In this circumstance, placement of the retractors may be more difficult and require additional finesse and effort. Partial boney resection may be needed just to place the retractor under the muscle, even before formal resection of the osteophyte begins.

Proper identification of the midline is essential for all anterior spinal surgery. In standard spinal decompression surgery, there are a few key anatomical structures which help the surgeon maintain orientation to the midline. Starting from more superficial to deep, these include the paired longus coli muscles, uncovertebral joints, and nerve roots. Large osteophytes can significantly alter the appearance and perceived location of the longus colli and uncovertebral joints, potentially leading the surgeon to become disoriented and lose track of the midline. Prevertebral osteophytes are commonly asymmetric and can actually lead the surgeon away from the more familiar midline anatomical plane (Fig. 17.7). A close study of the axial preoperative CT images, with active correlation to the observed intraoperative anatomy is usually the best method to maintain spatial orientation. Identification of more normal-appearing adjacent spinal levels can be quite helpful. Fluoroscopy, using both lateral and anterioposterior views is another option that can provide additional anatomical information.

Recognition of the anterior midline is particularly important at the C7 vertebral level due to the location of the vertebral artery. The vertebral artery is encased within the bony foramen transversarium at the cephalad spinal levels, yet it usually courses freely just lateral to the longus colli muscle at C7 prior to entering its bony confines. Asymmetrical osteophytes at the C7 level can direct the surgeon to the vertebral artery during the anatomical exposure, retractor placement,

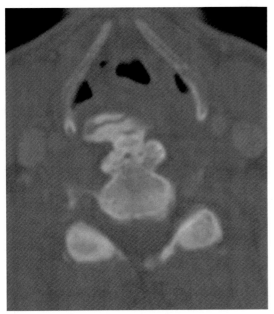

FIG. 17.7 Axial computed tomography scan of a 58-year-old male demonstrating a large ventral osteophyte asymmetrically pointed to the right side.

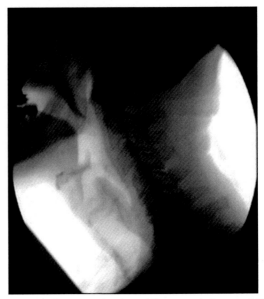

FIG. 17.8 Postoperative lateral fluoroscopic image of the same patient from Fig. 17.3, demonstrating resection of the osteophytes and normal contour of the ventral cervical spine.

or resection of the osteophytes, potentially leading to inadvertent vascular injury.

The location of the vertebral artery must always be considered during osteophyte resection surgery at this spinal level.

Once the exposure has been completed, and retractors are in place, coarse excision using Leksell rongeurs can be performed initially for reducing osteophytes of large size. In addition to being followed centrally, the osteophytes can be followed laterally symmetrically under the longus colli. Care must be taken to avoid exposure of the disk space and violation of the anterior annulus fibrosus. The resection can be discretely shaped using a high-speed drill with a fine tip such as an M8 or B27. In general, the main goal of the surgery is to remove the protruding osteophytes and create a smooth flat surface that reconstitutes the contour of the normal adjacent spinal levels. Neither the normal cortical vertebral body bone deep to the osteophytes nor disc spaces should be violated. Osteophyte removal can be associated with significant bone bleeding, yet this is easily controlled using bone wax or hemostatic agents.

Satisfactory osteophyte resection is confirmed using palpation, by direct visualization, and by comparing preoperative and postoperative fluoroscopic images (Fig. 17.8). The surgical bed is inspected for any sharp boney edges and then irrigated thoroughly with antibiotic saline. A suction drain may be placed below the platysma for multilevel surgeries or those involving excessive blood loss. Closure of the platysma and skin are then performed in the usual fashion. As this procedure does not destabilize the spine, neither rigid fixation nor a cervical orthosis is required.

Potential complications include hematoma for which elevating the head of bed postoperatively can assist in reducing venous hypertension, pharyngeal or esophageal perforation, infection, and damage to the branches of the vagus (the RLN and superior laryngeal nerve). However, most patients do well following the operation depending on their underlying swallowing dysfunction.

Outcomes of Osteophyte Resection

There are no controlled trials or large studies evaluating the long-term effects of osteophyte resection. However, in general, report results from case report and case series are good.[3,5,8] One of the largest studies by Miyamoto et al.[22] demonstrated a high rate of recurrence after 10–11 years. Given the low incidence of symptomatic osteophytes, it is unlikely that more controlled or larger studies would be performed.

CONCLUSION

Cervical osteophytes represent a cause of dysphagia in the elderly population via direct obstruction of bolus flow. The symptoms are highly dependent on the level of the osteophytes. With osteophytes at the level of the epiglottis causing epiglottic dysfunction, symptoms are typically pooling at the vallecula, penetration, and aspiration. Partial ossification of the epiglottis and pharyngeal weakness from aging and other etiologies contribute to the development of symptoms. At the level of the cricoid, symptoms are obstruction of the UES area due to the presence of two rigid structures (cricoid and spine) leading to pooling of secretions in the piriform sinuses and may seem similar to the cricopharyngeal achalasia. Other conditions leading to pharyngeal weakness such as stroke in this population can cause otherwise asymptomatic osteophytes to become major issues in swallowing. Medical management with swallow therapy should be started in all patients, particularly for those with comorbidities; however, surgical management is often required with large osteophytes. Partial epiglottic resection is preferred for osteophytes at the level of the epiglottis, while transcervical excision is preferred for those at the level of the cricoid.

REFERENCES

1. Kos MP, van Royen BJ, David EF, Mahieu HF. Anterior cervical osteophytes resulting in severe dysphagia and aspiration: two case reports and literature review. *J Laryngol Otol.* 2009;123:1169.
2. Moriwaki M, et al. Prolonged dysphagia due to a combination of cerebral hemorrhage and diffuse idiopathic skeletal hyperostosis: a case report. *NMC Case Rep J.* 2016;3:75–79.
3. Lecerf P, Malard O. How to diagnose and treat symptomatic anterior cervical osteophytes? *Eur Ann Otorhinolaryngol Head Neck Dis.* 2010;127:111–116.
4. Egerter AC, et al. Dysphagia secondary to anterior osteophytes of the cervical spine. *Glob Spine J.* 2015;5:78–83.
5. Klaassen Z, et al. Vertebral spinal osteophytes. *Anat Sci Int.* 2011;86:1–9.
6. Rogers J, Shepstone L, Dieppe P. Bone formers: osteophyte and enthesophyte formation are positively associated. *Ann Rheum Dis.* 1997;56:85–90.
7. Albayrak İ, Bağcacı S, Sallı A, Kucuksen S, Uğurlu H. A rare cause of dysphagia: compression of the esophagus by an anterior cervical osteophyte due to ankylosing spondylitis. *Korean J Int Med.* 2013;28:614.
8. Oppenlander ME, et al. Dysphagia due to anterior cervical hyperosteophytosis. *Surg Neurol.* 2009;72:266–270.
9. Mader R, et al. Diffuse idiopathic skeletal hyperostosis (DISH): where we are now and where to go next. *RMD Open.* 2017;3:e000472.
10. De Jesus-Monge WE, Cruz-Cuevas EI. Dysphagia and lung aspiration secondary to anterior cervical osteophytes: a case report and review of the literature. *Ethn Dis.* 2008;18:S2.
11. Seidler TO, Pèrez Àlvarez JC, Wonneberger K, Hacki T. Dysphagia caused by ventral osteophytes of the cervical spine: clinical and radiographic findings. *Eur Arch Otorhinolaryngol.* 2009;266:285–291.
12. Resnick D, Niwayama G. Radiographic and pathologic features of spinal involvement in diffuse idiopathic skeletal hyperostosis (DISH). *Radiology.* 1976;119:559–568.
13. Papadopoulou S, Exarchakos G, Beris A, Ploumis A. Dysphagia associated with cervical spine and postural disorders. *Dysphagia.* 2013;28:469–480.
14. Jamal N, Erman A, Chhetri DK. Transoral partial epiglottidectomy to treat dysphagia in post-treatment head and neck cancer patients: a preliminary report: transoral Epiglottidectomy for Dysphagia. *Laryngoscope.* 2014;124:665–671.
15. Lee TH, Lee JS. High-resolution manometry for oropharyngeal dysphagia in a patient with large cervical osteophytes. *J Neurogastroenterol Motil.* 2012;18:338–339.
16. Ozgursoy OB, Salassa JR, Reimer R, Wharen RE, Deen HG. Anterior cervical osteophyte dysphagia: manofluorographic and functional outcomes after surgery. *Head Neck.* 2010. https://doi.org/10.1002/hed.21226.
17. Ortega O, Martín A, Clavé P. Diagnosis and management of oropharyngeal dysphagia among older persons, state of the art. *J Am Med Dir Assoc.* 2017;18:576–582.
18. Saffouri MH, Ward PH. Surgical correction of dysphagia due to cervical osteophytes. *Ann Otol Rhinol Laryngol.* 1974;83:65–70.
19. Laitman JT, Crelin ES, Conlogue GJ. The function of the epiglottis in monkey and man. *Yale J Biol Med.* 1977;50:43–48.
20. Kilburg C, Sullivan HG, Mathiason MA. Effect of approach side during cervical discectomy and fusion on the incidence of recurrent laryngeal nerve injury. *J Neurosurg Spine.* 2006;4:273–277.
21. Beutler WJ, Sweeney CA, Connolly PJ. Recurrent laryngeal nerve injury with anterior cervical spine surgery risk with laterality of surgical approach. *Spine.* 2001;26:1337–1342.
22. Miyamoto K, Sugiyama S, Hosoe H, Iinuma N, Suzuki Y, Shimizu K. Postsurgical recurrence of osteophytes causing dysphagia in patients with diffuse idiopathic skeletal hyperostosis. *Eur Spine J.* 2009;18(11):1652–1658.

CHAPTER 18

Glottic Insufficiency

AARON J. FEINSTEIN, MD, MHS • JENNIFER L. LONG, MD, PHD

INTRODUCTION

Unilateral vocal fold paralysis (UVFP) occurs from dysfunction or injury of the recurrent laryngeal nerve (RLN), or its originating nerve, the vagus nerve (CN X). Clinically, it presents as immobility of one of the vocal folds. Classic presenting signs are dysphonia and dysphagia and impaired cough.[1] Among hospitalized patients with dysphagia referred for swallow evaluation, UVFP is identified in 5.6%, and among these patients, 44% demonstrate aspiration on fiberoptic endoscopic evaluation of swallowing (FEES).[2] While UVFP substantially impairs quality of life,[3] it is also known to recover spontaneously in 41%−77% of patients, including those with a history of neck or chest surgery.[4,5] Iatrogenic trauma during surgery is the leading cause of UVFP, accounting for about half of the cases.[6,7]

The term glottic insufficiency generally refers to any impaired closure of the vocal folds. It may refer to the presence of a persistent glottal gap, decreased closing forces, or increased open quotient of glottal vibration. Thus, some degree of glottal insufficiency is expected in uncorrected or uncompensated UVFP. It can also occur in a range of disorders including presbylarynges (age-related laryngeal weakness and atrophy), vocal fold paresis (unilateral weakness of RLN or superior laryngeal nerve [SLN] function with some motion preserved), postsurgical glottic tissue loss, radiation fibrosis, cricoarytenoid joint fixation, bilateral vocal fold paralysis (especially if fixed in the abducted position), deconditioning, and global neurodegenerative disorders. Glottic insufficiency itself can contribute to aspiration by impairing the normal glottic closure reflex.[8] However, because of heterogeneous pathophysiology and lack of uniform diagnostic criteria, generalizing findings in glottic insufficiency is difficult. This chapter will focus on UVFP, as it is better defined and the most studied in regard to the effects of treatment of glottic insufficiency on dysphagia.

PATHOPHYSIOLOGY

UVFP may be caused by cervical, thoracic, or intracranial surgery; cervical, thoracic, or intracranial malignancy; penetrating or blunt trauma; intubation; infection; autoimmune disease; or as an idiopathic process, frequently thought to be a postviral sequela.[7,9−11] Additional potential etiologies are described in Table 18.1. Surgical iatrogenic trauma to the RLN is the leading cause of UVFP, accounting for about half of all cases.[6,7] UVFP may occur in 15%−45% of thoracic and esophageal ablative procedures.[4,12,13] In a study by Spataro et al. of 938 cases over 10 years, the following etiologies of UVFP were found: postsurgical, 55.6%; malignancy, 17.8%; idiopathic, 13.2%; intubation, 6.2%; and trauma, 3.2%, with various rare etiologies representing the remainder.[7] Among the iatrogenic etiologies, thyroid/parathyroid surgery was the most frequent (16.8%) followed by thoracic (7.8%), cardiac (6.2%), and cervical spine surgery (5.1%). In a cohort of 5670 Medicare beneficiaries (age $\geq$ 65 years) undergoing thyroid surgery for well-differentiated thyroid cancer, UVFP was identified in 8.2% and bilateral vocal fold paralysis in 1.3%.[14]

The RLN is the primary nerve supplying the intrinsic laryngeal muscles (ILMs), including the thyroarytenoid, lateral cricoarytenoid, interarytenoid, and posterior cricoarytenoid. The cricothyroid muscle, however, is innervated by the external branch of the SLN. In addition to its critical motor role, the RLN also supplies sensory innervation to the mucosa of the vocal folds and subglottis, whereas the internal branch of the SLN innervates the supraglottic mucosa. The RLN also provides innervation to the cricopharyngeus muscle, in coordination with the pharyngeal plexus, which receives contributions from the pharyngeal branch of the vagus nerve (CN X), SLN, and glossopharyngeal nerve (CN IX). Thus, injury to the RLN results in injury to multiple components of the swallowing mechanism, including the protective structures of the glottis as well

TABLE 18.1
Etiology of Unilateral Vocal Fold Paralysis
Surgery
Thyroid
Cervical (including anterior spine approaches and carotid endarterectomy)
Thoracic
Intracranial
Malignancy
Laryngeal
Thyroid
Cervical (including lymphoma)
Thoracic
Intracranial
Others
Trauma
Intubation
Infection (including tuberculosis)
Autoimmune (including sarcoidosis)
Neurodegenerative diseases
Cerebrovascular accident
Diabetes
Malnutrition (including B12 deficiency)
Vinca alkaloids
Radiation therapy (including I-131)
Aortic arch aneurysm
Pulmonary hypertension
Mitral stenosis with left atrial dilatation (Ortner's syndrome)
Mitochondrial disorders
Porphyria
Familial hypokalemic periodic paralysis

as the musculature of the upper esophageal sphincter. Each of the separate laryngeal protective mechanisms is slowed, if not completely lost, by this injury. Because the glottic closure occurs in a delayed manner, liquid food dysphagia is quite common in these patients. Liquid does not maintain a cohesive bolus as it transits from the oral cavity into the pharynx, which means that small amounts of the liquid may more readily fall into the larynx and result in penetration and aspiration.

Vagus nerve (CN X) injury from intracranial and/or skull base neoplasms or surgery is a particularly difficult cause of UVFP to rehabilitate. In cases of high vagal paralysis, where vagal injury is located prior to the branching of the SLN, neural deficits include not only the RLN but both the SLN as well as the pharyngeal plexus of nerves. As mentioned earlier, the SLN provides afferent information from the supraglottic larynx while the RLN provides afferent sensation from the glottic and infraglottic larynx. The pharyngeal plexus provides motor innervation to the majority of the muscles involved in oropharyngeal swallow (see Chapter 3). In addition, all ipsilateral ILMs are paralyzed in these patients. Thus, this combined motor and sensory deficit affects such a large proportion of the swallowing apparatus that the incidence of dysphagia after vagal paralysis is quite high. Furthermore, many conditions that result in vagal paralysis may also affect adjacent nerves such as the glossopharyngeal (CN IX) and hypoglossal (CN XII) nerves. These cases of multiple cranial neuropathies are more devastating to the swallowing mechanism and make swallow rehabilitation particularly challenging. Similar outcomes occur from cerebrovascular accidents that cause injury to nerve cell bodies of the vagal nerve, as occurs in Wallenberg syndrome, which is caused by ischemic injury to the nerve cell bodies of CN IX and CN X in the lateral medulla oblongata in the brainstem. Fortunately, most cerebrovascular accidents affecting the motor cortex do not impair the lower cranial nerves because of bilateral inputs from the cerebral hemispheres to the brainstem nuclei.

UVFP can impact swallowing due to its effects on cough as well. Cough is a critical human reflex that prevents aspiration by expectorating penetrated or aspirated material.[15,16] Cough can be both volitional and reflexive and requires precise coordinated activity of the ILMs. The normal cough sequence consists of glottal opening during a slow inspiratory phase, a compression phase with closed glottis, and rapid glottal opening during the expiratory phase.[17] The compressive phase requires vocal fold adduction, via the ILMs, to allow the buildup of subglottic air pressure. The rapid expiratory phase is associated with initial vocal fold abduction via activation of the posterior cricoarytenoid muscles.[18,19] In patients with vocal fold paralysis, the glottic closure is inadequate, and this results in an impaired cough and pulmonary clearance.[20] One study found aspiration in over half of patients with acute postsurgical UVFP.[21] The combination of high aspiration risk and impaired pulmonary clearance places these patients at significant risk of pneumonia. A study of 259 patients undergoing thoracic aortic surgery found that UVFP resulted in increased rates of pneumonia (58% vs. 17%) and longer hospital stay (18 vs. 9 days) relative to patients without UVFP.[22] Similarly, pneumonia occurring after cardiac surgery is associated with worse patient outcomes. Patients in whom pneumonia develops have an estimated 2–6 times increased risk of death, approximately 3–6 times poorer scores on various rehabilitation measures, an average of 3 times longer stay in the hospital, and require higher levels of care after hospital discharge than those without pneumonia.[20]

SYMPTOMS

UVFP results in dysphonia and dysphagia and can also impair cough.[1] UVFP has a profound impact on quality of life. Acute voice impairment is nearly universal, and breathing and swallowing symptoms impact at least 76% and 66% of patients, respectively.[3]

Dysphagia is frequent in patients with UVFP. Francis et al. report a prevalence of 66%,[3] while Ollivere et al. report dysphagia in 56%.[1] Importantly, some patients complain of sensations related to swallow dysfunction, while others are unaware that they are aspirating due to sensory impairment. Objective evaluation of swallowing is thus of utmost importance in this population. Tabaee et al. reviewed 81 patients with UVFP undergoing flexible endoscopic evaluation of swallowing with sensory testing, wherein the etiology included iatrogenic (42%), malignancy (23%), and neurological (18%).[23] Aspiration was observed in 35% of patients during thin liquid trials and in 18% during puree trials. The laryngeal adductor reflex was absent in 34%.

Patients with UVFP may experience dysphagia for multiple reasons. Impairment in glottal closure produces an immediate impact on the main airway protective mechanism, which increases the likelihood for aspiration of foreign material. Domer et al. have also demonstrated that patients with UVFP of idiopathic or iatrogenic etiology have measurable pharyngeal muscle weakness.[24] Among 25 patients with UVFP undergoing a videofluoroscopic swallow study, the total pharyngeal transit time was increased and the pharyngeal constriction ratio was elevated relative to healthy controls. Aspiration was noted in 36% of these patients. Jang et al. had similar findings in their study of 28 patients with UVFP, where all patients had some degree of pharyngeal dysfunction as well as 46% of patients demonstrating oral phase abnormalities.[25]

DIAGNOSIS/EVALUATION

The diagnosis of UVFP requires laryngoscopy to assess vocal fold motion. Often the patient's history will

suggest the diagnosis; for example, in a patient with new onset hoarseness noted immediately following a cervical or thoracic operation. The history should always include a discussion of medical and surgical history, intubations, tobacco use, recent upper respiratory infection, and vocal habits and demands. Questions directed at autoimmune and neurologic disorders are useful as well. The physical exam should include careful search for neck masses and other cranial nerve deficits, as manifested by asymmetric facial motion, palate rise, or tongue protrusion. Laryngoscopy is then indicated in all patients.

While UVFP is easily diagnosed as absent abduction of one vocal fold, laryngoscopic findings of glottic insufficiency are far from standardized. A recent study sent videostroboscopic recordings to 20 fellowship-trained laryngologists, and among this group, only the following factors had even moderate agreement among reviewers: glottic insufficiency, vocal fold bowing, and salivary pooling.[26] Additional factors thought to be important in diagnosing UVFP, such as vocal fold tone, vocal fold shortening, and height mismatch, demonstrated poor to fair agreement among laryngologists. Patient-reported outcome measures, such as the Voice Handicap Index (VHI-10), may be collected at the initial evaluation. Objective assessment of swallowing, such as FEES, may be undertaken at this time to assess the severity of dysphagia. Patients with UVFP often have a sensory neuropathy concurrent with motor neuropathy that may preclude accurate insight into symptoms, which makes an objective assessment essential.

In cases with an obvious etiology, such as a known functioning vocal fold that becomes immobile postoperatively with surgeon confirmation of RLN resection, it is not mandatory to search for any further explanation. However, in the remainder of cases, it is imperative to obtain cross-sectional imaging from the skull base to aorta in order to assess the presence of any tumor that could be affecting the vagus or RLN. The utility of electromyography in the evaluation of patients with UVFP is beyond the scope of this chapter.

TREATMENT/CASE STUDIES

Patients with UVFP are typically treated for their dysphonia, where options include injection laryngoplasty, medialization thyroplasty, arytenoid adduction, RLN reinnervation with the ansa cervicalis nerve, and combinations of these procedures.[9,11,27–30] These procedures are known to improve dysphonia. The impact of these treatments on dysphagia will be reviewed herein. The comorbid impact of UVFP on cough aerodynamics remains unknown and is of great concern, especially in acute hospital inpatients who may be at a greater risk of pulmonary complications such as pneumonia or bronchial mucus plugging.[31]

Treatment of UVFP has been shown to improve dysphagia, although studies thus far are uncontrolled and variation exists in the reported degree of improvement. Kraus et al. reviewed 63 patients with UVFP due to intrathoracic malignancies.[32] Dysphagia was present in 15 and aspiration in 26 patients. Following medialization, dysphagia improved in 14 of 15 patients (93%), while aspiration improved in 24 of 26 patients (92%). Flint et al. performed medialization thyroplasty for 84 patients with UVFP, of whom 61% had dysphagia and 15% were dependent on feeding tubes.[33] Among these most severe cases, 9 of 13 returned to an oral diet after surgery, and an additional patient improved following cricopharyngeal myotomy. Bhattacharyya et al. reviewed 64 patients, of whom 31.3% and 23.4% experienced penetration and aspiration, respectively.[34] Among 23 surgically treated patients, there was no statistically significant change in the Penetration-Aspiration Scale score. Hendricker et al. found a dysphagia incidence of 50% in 113 patients with UVFP.[35] Among 47 patients undergoing modified barium swallow study (MBSS), 32 (68%) had penetration and/or aspiration. There were 20 patients with gastrostomy tubes preoperatively, of whom 11 (55%) were able to return to an oral diet. Cates et al. used patient-reported outcomes to assess improvement in dysphagia in 44 patients surgically treated for UVFP.[36] Patients answered the Eating Assessment Tool (EAT-10) pre- and postoperatively, and the authors reported an improvement in scores from 12.1 ± 11.1 to 7.7 ± 7.2 after medialization. These patients also had significant improvement in their dysphonia symptoms as quantified with the Voice Handicap Index (VHI-10). Barbu et al. reviewed 68 postoperative patients undergoing inpatient injection laryngoplasty for UVFP, 40 of whom were not yet taking oral intake.[37] 28 (70%) of those patients advanced to an oral diet within 5 days of the laryngoplasty; a noninjected cohort was not presented. The ease and safety of rapid injection laryngoplasty has led to difficulty designing controlled studies in an ethical manner, and the true impact of medialization on swallowing function therefore remains difficult to assess.

It remains to be answered if medialization can restore normal cough function in patients with numerous ongoing medical comorbidities affecting pulmonary function. The effect (if any) of the typical UVFP treatments on cough function is also unknown.

It has been proposed that very early vocal fold medialization (less than 3 days postoperatively) may promote more effective pulmonary hygiene by improving cough[31]; however, a physiologic link between this treatment and pulmonary effects has not been explored quantitatively. A study of three patients with glottal insufficiency deemed poor candidates for general anesthesia and treated with awake injection laryngoplasty demonstrated increased cough peak flow immediately after injection.[38] In patients with UVFP, medialization helps to partially overcome the impaired adductor function; however, the important role of the posterior cricoarytenoid in cough is not restored. Other factors also reduce cough airflow in hospitalized or acutely postoperative patients, such as pain, medications, and reduced chest wall compliance; those factors are independent of both UVFP and medialization.

Further work is warranted to define the optimal timing of treatment for UVFP. While voice outcomes clearly improve with early injection (usually defined as 1–2 weeks),[39] the value of very early postoperative injection (within 1–3 days) for the purpose of pulmonary hygiene remains unclear. Potential advantages to acute inpatient treatment remain, including patient convenience, rapid return to voicing, and reduced aspiration risk.[37] Zuniga et al. recently defined a protocol to provide inpatient injection laryngoplasty within 10 days to only those patients with UVFP presenting with an unsafe swallow as determined by FEES, while patients with a safe swallow deferred medialization to the outpatient setting.[40] Some patients with a safe swallow declined medialization at their outpatient visit, and there was no significant increase in pulmonary morbidity. Inpatient treatment for acutely ill patients has not been prospectively compared to delayed outpatient treatment for otherwise rehabilitated patients.

CONCLUSIONS

The larynx is a complex organ with critical roles in respiration, speech, swallowing, and prevention of aspiration. Neuromuscular dysfunction such as UVFP results in an incompetent larynx and not only causes dysphonia but also dysphagia. The diagnosis of UVFP requires laryngoscopy to assess vocal fold motion, and objective assessment of swallowing with FEES and/or MBSS is indicated. If aspiration occurs, it may lead to major consequences such as aspiration pneumonia and contribute to significant morbidity and mortality. Thus, treatment of glottic insufficiency plays an important role in the management of the patient with dysphagia. Vagus nerve (CN X) injury from intracranial and/or skull base neoplasms or surgery is a particularly difficult cause of UVFP to rehabilitate. Treatment options include injection laryngoplasty, medialization thyroplasty, arytenoid adduction, RLN reinnervation with the ansa cervicalis nerve, and combinations of these procedures and appropriate treatment is expected to improve dysphagia in the majority of patients.

REFERENCES

1. Ollivere B, Duce K, Rowlands G, Harrison P, O'Reilly BJ. Swallowing dysfunction in patients with unilateral vocal fold paralysis: aetiology and outcomes. *J Laryngol Otol.* 2006;120(1):38–41.
2. Leder SB, Ross DA. Incidence of vocal fold immobility in patients with dysphagia. *Dysphagia.* 2005;20(2):163–167; discussion 168–169.
3. Francis DO, McKiever ME, Garrett CG, Jacobson B, Penson DF. Assessment of patient experience with unilateral vocal fold immobility: a preliminary study. *J Voice.* 2014;28(5):636–643.
4. Baba M, Natsugoe S, Shimada M, et al. Does hoarseness of voice from recurrent nerve paralysis after esophagectomy for carcinoma influence patient quality of life? *J Am Coll Surg.* 1999;188(3):231–236.
5. Joo D, Duarte VM, Ghadiali MT, Chhetri DK. Recovery of vocal fold paralysis after cardiovascular surgery. *Laryngoscope.* 2009;119(7):1435–1438.
6. Merati AL, Shemirani N, Smith TL, Toohill RJ. Changing trends in the nature of vocal fold motion impairment. *Am J Otolaryngol.* 2006;27(2):106–108.
7. Spataro EA, Grindler DJ, Paniello RC. Etiology and time to presentation of unilateral vocal fold paralysis. *Otolaryngol Head Neck Surg.* 2014;151(2):286–293.
8. Sasaki CT, Hundal JS, Kim Y-H. Protective glottic closure: biomechanical effects of selective laryngeal denervation. *Ann Otol Rhinol Laryngol.* 2005;114(4):271–275.
9. Rubin AD, Sataloff RT. Vocal fold paresis and paralysis. *Otolaryngol Clin North Am.* 2007;40(5):1109–1131. viii–ix.
10. Vikram HR, Dhaliwal G, Saint S, Simpson CB. Clinical problem-solving. A recurrent problem. *N Engl J Med.* 2011;364(22):2148–2154.
11. Misono S, Merati AL. Evidence-based practice: evaluation and management of unilateral vocal fold paralysis. *Otolaryngol Clin North Am.* 2012;45(5):1083–1108.
12. Nishimaki T, Suzuki T, Suzuki S, Kuwabara S, Hatakeyama K. Outcomes of extended radical esophagectomy for thoracic esophageal cancer. *J Am Coll Surg.* 1998;186(3):306–312.
13. Hulscher JB, van Sandick JW, Devriese PP, van Lanschot JJ, Obertop H. Vocal cord paralysis after subtotal oesophagectomy. *Br J Surg.* 1999;86(12):1583–1587.
14. Francis DO, Pearce EC, Ni S, Garrett CG, Penson DF. Epidemiology of vocal fold paralyses after total thyroidectomy for well-differentiated thyroid cancer in a Medicare population. *Otolaryngol Head Neck Surg.* 2014;150(4):548–557.
15. Irwin RS, Madison JM. The diagnosis and treatment of cough. *N Engl J Med.* 2000;343(23):1715–1721.
16. Pitts T. Airway protective mechanisms. *Lung.* 2014;192(1):27–31.
17. Leden von H, Isshiki N. An analysis of cough at the level of the larynx. *Arch Otolaryngol.* 1965;81:616–625.
18. Hillel AD. The study of laryngeal muscle activity in normal human subjects and in patients with laryngeal dystonia using multiple fine-wire electromyography. *Laryngoscope.* 2001;111(4 Pt 2 suppl 97):1–47.
19. Chhetri DK, Neubauer J, Sofer E. Posterior cricoarytenoid muscle dynamics in canines and humans. *Laryngoscope.* 2014;124(10):2363–2367.
20. Kulnik ST, Rafferty GF, Birring SS, Moxham J, Kalra L. A pilot study of respiratory muscle training to improve cough effectiveness and reduce the incidence of pneumonia in acute stroke: study protocol for a randomized controlled trial. *Trials.* 2014;15(1):123.
21. Morpeth JF, Williams MF. Vocal fold paralysis after anterior cervical diskectomy and fusion. *Laryngoscope.* 2000;110(1):43–46.
22. Lodewyks CL, White CW, Bay G, et al. Vocal cord paralysis after thoracic aortic surgery: incidence and impact on clinical outcomes. *Ann Thorac Surg.* 2015;100(1):54–58.
23. Tabaee A, Murry T, Zschommler A, Desloge RB. Flexible endoscopic evaluation of swallowing with sensory testing in patients with unilateral vocal fold immobility: incidence and pathophysiology of aspiration. *Laryngoscope.* 2005;115(4):565–569.
24. Domer AS, Leonard R, Belafsky PC. Pharyngeal weakness and upper esophageal sphincter opening in patients with unilateral vocal fold immobility. *Laryngoscope.* 2014;124(10):2371–2374.
25. Jang YY, Lee SJ, Lee SJ, Jeon JY, Lee SJ. Analysis of video fluoroscopic swallowing study in patients with vocal cord paralysis. *Dysphagia.* 2012;27(2):185–190.
26. Rosow DE, Sulica L. Laryngoscopy of vocal fold paralysis: evaluation of consistency of clinical findings. *Laryngoscope.* 2010;120(7):1376–1382.
27. Chhetri DK, Jamal N. Percutaneous injection laryngoplasty. *Laryngoscope.* 2014;124(3):742–745.
28. Bielamowicz S, Berke GS, Gerratt BR. A comparison of type I thyroplasty and arytenoid adduction. *J Voice.* 1995;9(4):466–472.
29. Chhetri DK, Gerratt BR, Kreiman J, Berke GS. Combined arytenoid adduction and laryngeal reinnervation in the treatment of vocal fold paralysis. *Laryngoscope.* 1999;109(12):1928–1936.

30. Paniello RC, Edgar JD, Kallogjeri D, Piccirillo JF. Medialization versus reinnervation for unilateral vocal fold paralysis: a multicenter randomized clinical trial. *Laryngoscope.* 2011;121(10):2172–2179.

31. Bhattacharyya N, Batirel H, Swanson SJ. Improved outcomes with early vocal fold medialization for vocal fold paralysis after thoracic surgery. *Auris Nasus Larynx.* 2003;30(1):71–75.

32. Kraus DH, Ali MK, Ginsberg RJ, et al. Vocal cord medialization for unilateral paralysis associated with intrathoracic malignancies. *J Thorac Cardiovasc Surg.* 1996;111(2):334–339; discussion 339–341.

33. Flint PW, Purcell LL, Cummings CW. Pathophysiology and indications for medialization thyroplasty in patients with dysphagia and aspiration. *Otolaryngol Head Neck Surg.* 1997;116(3):349–354.

34. Bhattacharyya N, Kotz T, Shapiro J. Dysphagia and aspiration with unilateral vocal cord immobility: incidence, characterization, and response to surgical treatment. *Ann Otol Rhinol Laryngol.* 2002;111(8):672–679.

35. Hendricker RM, deSilva BW, Forrest LA. Gore-Tex medialization laryngoplasty for treatment of dysphagia. *Otolaryngol Head Neck Surg.* 2010;142(4):536–539.

36. Cates DJ, Venkatesan NN, Strong B, Kuhn MA, Belafsky PC. Effect of vocal fold medialization on dysphagia in patients with unilateral vocal fold immobility. *Otolaryngol Head Neck Surg.* 2016;155(3):454–457.

37. Barbu AM, Gniady JP, Vivero RJ, Friedman AD, Burns JA. Bedside injection medialization laryngoplasty in immediate postoperative patients. *Otolaryngol Head Neck Surg.* 2015;153(6):1007–1012.

38. Ruddy BH, Pitts TE, Lehman J, Spector B, Lewis V, Sapienza CM. Improved voluntary cough immediately following office-based vocal fold medialization injections. *Laryngoscope.* 2014;124(7):1645–1647.

39. Grant JR, Hartemink DA, Patel N, Merati AL. Acute and subacute awake injection laryngoplasty for thoracic surgery patients. *J Voice.* 2008;22(2):245–250.

40. Zuniga S, Ebersole B, Jamal N. Inpatient injection laryngoplasty for vocal fold immobility: when is it really necessary? *Am J Otolaryngol.* 2017;38(2):222–225.

CHAPTER 19

Cricopharyngeal Dysphagia

ANDREW VAHABZADEH-HAGH, MD • DINESH K. CHHETRI, MD

INTRODUCTION

The inferior pharyngeal constrictor (IPC) is the thickest and best developed of the three pharyngeal constrictors. Its most caudal portion is commonly referred to as the cricopharyngeus (CP) muscle. This muscle forms the majority of the upper esophageal sphincter (UES). Although the UES is often described as a 2- to 4-cm zone of high pressure encompassing the IPC, CP, and the upper esophagus, in practice, the UES and CP are interchangeable (see Chapter 5 for full description of the UES). The CP originates from the cricoid anteriorly just posterior to the insertion of the cricothyroid muscles and extends posteriorly to interdigitate with the midline raphe and transverse (circular) esophageal muscle layer inferiorly. Anterolaterally, at the junction of the CP and esophageal muscle also known as the Killian–Jamieson area, the neurovascular bundle including the recurrent laryngeal nerve (RLN) and the inferior laryngeal artery, a branch of the thyrocervical trunk of the subclavian vessels, enters the larynx. The CP muscle is primarily composed of the slow-twitch (type I) striated muscle fibers. It receives motor innervation from the vagus nerve (CN X) via the pharyngeal plexus and the RLNs. There are likely sensory contributions from the superior laryngeal and the glossopharyngeal nerves, and the sympathetic nerve fibers from the cervical ganglia, also via the pharyngeal plexus.[1]

Unlike the constrictor muscles, the CP is tonically contracted at rest, allowing it to serve its sphincteric function as the UES. During a swallow, vagal tone is inhibited and sphincter pressure falls about 200 ms prior to its opening.[2] This is followed by anterosuperior hyolaryngeal elevation and the generation of a pharyngeal constrictor and tongue base propulsive force, which drives UES opening. Failure of the UES to open leads to dysphagia symptoms and risk for aspiration. Many neuromuscular diseases such as amyotrophic lateral sclerosis, polymyositis, myasthenia gravis, multiple sclerosis, Parkinson's disease (PD), and cerebrovascular accidents result in reduced CP relaxation. These conditions also lead to reduced pharyngeal contraction and hyolaryngeal elevation from muscular weakness and compound the reduced UES opening. CP achalasia, failure of CP relaxation, may also be idiopathic or result from gastroesophageal reflux disease among other etiologies.

Cricopharyngeal dysfunction refers broadly to poor compliance of the UES or pharyngoesophageal segment resulting in reduced or absent opening during swallowing. It may result from primary neuromuscular dysfunction, mechanical obstruction or stenosis of the UES, or from discoordination of the UES opening with the rest of the swallow. Depending on the severity of dysfunction, symptoms may be absent or patients may complain of dysphagia, regurgitation, cough, aspiration, weight loss, dysphonia, and/or globus.[2] Misdirection of the food bolus or penetration of the laryngeal vestibule may lead to cough, choking, and/or aspiration. Globus, which is experienced by many patients with UES dysfunction, has also been uniquely correlated with hyperdynamic respiratory UES pressure fluctuations as well as higher residual UES pressures on average when compared to nondysphagic controls (2.6 mmHg vs. 0.6 mmHg).[3,4]

CAUSES OF DYSFUNCTION

Bolus transit through the UES may be slowed by (1) restricted UES opening, (2) reduced pharyngeal driving pressures, and (3) impaired hyolaryngeal elevation.[2] The most common causes of CP dysfunction are neurological disorders and the consequences, directly or indirectly, of head and neck cancer. Aging results in reduced CP compliance, strength, and muscle mass. Oral, pharyngeal, and esophageal dysfunction also affect UES function, sometimes making it difficult to specify the role of UES dysfunction in dysphagia.

Gastroesophageal Reflux Disease

Extraesophageal reflux (EER) and UES function have a complex relationship that has been a topic of much debate. With air insufflation of the esophagus, the UES relaxes to permit belching, while instillation of water leads to UES contraction, a protective reflex against gastroesophageal reflux.[5] In patients with EER symptoms, this UES contractile reflex is impaired, unlike in controls or those with gastroesophageal reflux without extraesophageal symptoms.[6] Thus, decreased UES contractile reflex might contribute to laryngopharyngeal reflux and its signs and symptoms. On the other hand, when this reflex loop is intact, the CP muscle will tighten in response to slow esophageal exposure to acid reflux. As such, these patients may present with cricopharyngeal achalasia secondary to gastroesophageal reflux disease.[7]

Radiation Fibrosis

Up to 50% of patients treated for head and neck cancer will report some degree of posttreatment dysphagia. A major cause of this posttreatment dysphagia is poor cricopharyngeal opening due to CP fibrosis from radiation technique, dose, and/or the concurrent use of chemotherapy.[8] Intensity-modulated or conformal radiotherapy may allow sparing radiation dose to the pharyngeal constrictors and cricopharyngeus muscle. Studies show that those undergoing intensity-modulated radiotherapy instead of conventional radiotherapy have improved oropharyngeal swallow, bolus transit times, greater UES opening, and better airway protection.[9] Damage to the pharyngoesophageal segment includes muscle atrophy, denervation, fibrosis, and permanent muscle contracture.

Neurogenic and Systemic Illness

Impaired UES opening diameter, pharyngeal constriction, and resultant aspiration is reported at greater frequencies in patients with iatrogenic or idiopathic unilateral vocal fold paralysis.[10] Other neurogenic and/or infectious causes include polio, neuritis, and muscular dystrophy. Although CP achalasia has been described in PD, a more recent standardized look at the swallowing features of PD has failed to identify CP achalasia as a prominent feature.[11] Systemic sclerosis or scleroderma patients have a high incidence of dysphagia related to oral leakage, retention, penetration, mild or moderate aspiration, and UES incoordination. Additionally, 80% of those with scleroderma exhibit esophageal dysmotility.[12] UES dysfunction may also be a consequence of exaggerated changes to cricopharyngeal compliance with the natural aging process. Reduced excursion of hyolaryngeal elevation with aging results in reduced anteroposterior opening of the UES. Additionally, for a given UES cross-sectional area,

intrabolus pressures have been found to be higher in the elderly when compared to their younger counterparts suggesting that the UES becomes stiffer with age. Shaker et al. found that increases in intrabolus pressure seen in the elderly were related to smaller UES openings during deglutition.[13–15]

ASSESSMENT

Any clinical assessment of a chief complaint always begins with a history and physical exam. Evaluation of dysphagia for possible UES dysfunction is no exception and a lot can be gathered from a focused history and physical exam. Patients with UES dysfunction will often describe combined solid food and liquid dysphagia and can often localize their dysphagia to the neck as opposed to lower in the chest. On physical exam, poor hyolaryngeal elevation during dry swallows may predict for poor UES opening. Additionally, repeated swallows or throat clearing after solid or liquid intake may suggest hypopharyngeal residue from UES dysfunction and/or pharyngeal weakness.[16] To adequately evaluate CP dysphagia, one may use some combination of the following clinical and/or radiographic tools.

Flexible Endoscopic Evaluation of Swallowing

Flexible endoscopic evaluation of swallowing (FEES) allows for thorough assessment of the oropharyngeal anatomy and swallowing function as well as the integrity of afferent sensation and motor strength of the laryngopharynx (see Chapter 8). UES dysfunction is often suggested by hypopharyngeal and postcricoid pooling of secretions with intact pharyngeal strength as assessed by the pharyngeal squeeze maneuver; for example, patient providing a forceful and sustained "eee" during phonation demonstrating intact lateral hypopharyngeal wall contraction.[16] In the absence of adequate pharyngeal squeeze, demonstrating pharyngeal weakness, conclusions about UES dysfunction are more ambiguous.

Modified Barium Swallow Study

The modified barium swallow study (MBSS) is a videofluoroscopic procedure designed to evaluate the passage of food and/or liquid through the mouth and pharynx and into the esophagus (see Chapter 10). Analysis of the oral and pharyngeal stages of swallow allows for the identification of aspiration, the detection of any oral or oropharyngeal residue following the swallow, and lastly to identify treatment strategies to improve the safety and efficiency of the patient's swallow. The oral phase of swallowing transitions to the pharyngeal phase with relaxation of the UES. UES opening requires first the relaxation of the CP muscle and subsequent hyolaryngeal elevation. Once the food bolus enters the pharynx, it normally takes only about 1 s to pass through the pharynx and UES. The MBSS uniquely allows for the simultaneous assessment of UES opening, hyolaryngeal elevation, and pharyngeal and tongue base contraction. With increasing bolus volume, the UES has been shown to open wider, sooner, and stay open longer to accommodate the larger bolus.[17] With aging beyond 65 years, the UES opening has been shown to be reduced. Leonard et al. established normative data in 60 healthy adult volunteers. They showed a statistically significant direct correlation with bolus size and UES opening and a lack of correlation between UES opening and sex, height, weight, or body mass index.[18] For 1, 3, and 20 cc bolus sizes, they found the UES opening to be 0.39, 0.51, and 0.89 cm, respectively, on average.[18] Usage of larger bolus sizes (15–20 cc) may be necessary during an MBSS to provide maximal UES distention to better highlight pharyngoesophageal luminal abnormalities.

A hallmark of UES dysfunction on MBSS is the posterior indentation at the pharyngoesophageal junction, typically between C4 and C6 vertebrae (Fig. 19.1A).[19] This is commonly known as the cricopharyngeal bar or prominence. However, this is not necessarily diagnostic of UES dysfunction as Leonard et al. found that a mild, moderate, or marked cricopharyngeal bar may be present in up to 30% of nondysphagic elderly patients.[19] Therefore, although these patients have reduced maximum upper esophageal opening as seen on lateral view, the functional consequence of this is not always clear. The clinician must look for further evidence of bolus obstruction proximal to the UES. Some parts of this assessment are very subjective and require experience with patient symptom assessment and the degree of dysfunction seen (which may be a combination of the characteristics of the CP bar, how narrow the esophageal inlet gets in the middle of bolus movement through the CP area, how much residue remains above the CP bar, and the overall efficiency of bolus flow through the pharyngoesophageal segment). Early CP dysfunction in nonobstructive CP bars may be even harder to pin down. Sometimes, a dilation of the pharynx above the UES ("Cobra sign") is seen to corroborate the suspicion. This is best appreciated on the anteroposterior view with the barium within the pharynx forming a dilated silhouette (Fig. 19.1B). Additionally, a CP bar may be of functional consequence to bolus flow when present in the setting of poor nutrition, regurgitation, history of choking episodes, or an early Zenker's diverticulum.

Barium Esophagram

The barium esophagram is a key diagnostic test for the evaluation of anatomic and physiologic esophageal abnormalities (see Chapter 11). These may include inflammatory or neoplastic disease, hiatal hernias, lower esophageal rings or strictures, gastroesophageal reflux disease, various types of esophagitis, and esophageal motility disorders. In addition to highlighting pathophysiology centered on the gastroesophageal junction, the barium esophagram may also highlight the UES and provide further insight into possible UES dysfunction.

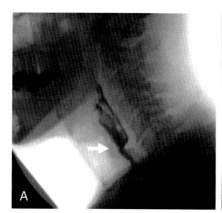 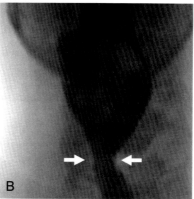

FIG. 19.1 **Modified Barium Swallow Study Views of the Upper Esophageal Sphincter Region. (A)** Lateral view highlights (*white arrow*) a cricopharyngeus bar. **(B)** Anteroposterior view demonstrates an apparent narrowing at the level of the upper esophageal sphincter (*white arrows*) with reflexive proximal pharyngeal dilation ("Cobra sign").

Transnasal Esophagoscopy

Since its introduction in 1994, unsedated transnasal esophagoscopy has become embraced by many otolaryngologists for its utility in the diagnostic work-up of reflux, dysphagia, head and neck cancer, and esophageal pathology (see Chapter 5).[20] Transnasal esophagoscopy (TNE) can be used to appreciate cricopharyngeal hyperfunction based on resistance encountered intubating the esophagus. Although a useful insight, this is a subjective assessment and can be swayed by the anxiety or discomfort of the patient, the skill of the operator, and the angle by which the CP is entered and timing of esophageal cannulation with swallow. Thus, we do not rely solely on TNE to assess CP dysfunction. However, TNE is invaluable in defining other pathologies that exist in this area and present as CP dysfunction, such as stenosis and webs. In addition, TNE is invaluable in assessing the UES region for abnormalities when radiologic studies show "UES dysfunction" (i.e., the UES opening is absent or reduced) in the setting of severe pharyngeal weakness.

High-Resolution Manometry

High-resolution manometry (HRM) has contributed substantially to understanding UES function (see Chapter 12). It involves the use of a solid-state manometric catheter, 4.2 mm in outer diameter with 36 circumferential sensors spaced 1 cm apart, capable of circumferential pressure detection. The catheter is placed transnasal, taped in place, and positioned to record from the hypopharynx to stomach. Basal sphincter pressures are measured as well as pressure changes following ten 5-mL water swallows. Recordings should begin once the spontaneous swallow rate falls to about once per minute. In addition to the 5-mL water swallows in the recumbent position, it is advised to also have the patient practice dry swallows and to repeat these exercises with the patient sitting upright. A change in position may help to reduce anxiety and detract from too much mental focus on the tasks at hand.[21]

Many HRM systems provide automated analysis and measurement of UES basal pressure, relaxation duration, recovery time, and peak pharyngeal pressures. Studies have established an inverse association of UES opening diameter with UES residual pressure, making HRM a good device to assess UES dysfunction.[22,23] However, many factors may complicate the interpretation of UES pressures on HRM and one must take caution when relying on its findings. The complex anatomy, asymmetry, and laterality of the UES must be considered when looking at HRM readings as slight changes in the placement or lie of the HRM sensors within the pharyngoesophageal segment can mean large changes in the output. Additionally, possible external factors modifying UES pressures must be considered. It has been shown that factors such as emotional stress, speech, crying, and coughing may have dramatic effects on the UES basal pressure.[24-26] The upper limit of basal UES pressures is less than 100–150 mmHg. Values greater than this may be indicative of myotonic or myopathic abnormalities. UES inhibition durations range from 200 to 500 ms, with the deglutition nadir of UES pressures reaching 10–15 mmHg. There are many potential causes of elevated residual UES pressures. These include impaired deglutitive UES relaxation, impaired anterior traction on the UES, reduced pharyngoesophageal distensibility, elevated downstream pressures, swallow of a larger or more viscous bolus, extreme cervical angulation during swallow, or a calibration drift in the HRM sensor.[21] With the aforementioned limitations and difficulties with interpretation, HRM provides a useful, but not sufficient, tool for the assessment of UES dysfunction.

TREATMENT

Treatment options depend on the underlying cause of UES dysfunction but typically are geared toward reducing sphincter tone, or mechanically enhancing the UES opening through myotomy and/or dilation, or improving swallowing function and UES opening with swallowing therapy and exercises. As a last resort in cases of intractable aspiration, diverting the UES via nonoral feeding or separation of airway from the digestive tract is necessary. Medical, or nonsurgical, management of UES dysfunction may include dietary modifications to a thin, less viscous, and moist diet. In patients where gastroesophageal reflux symptoms are present and perhaps implicated in UES hypertrophy and dysfunction, one may treat with empiric reflux therapy including proton pump inhibitors and/or an H2 blocker.[16] Kahrilas et al. suggest that in a select population, swallow therapy or modified biofeedback can be used to volitionally augment UES opening. Videofluoroscopy and manometry were used to evaluate the biomechanics of UES opening in eight normal subjects. These subjects were taught the Mendelsohn maneuver, a technique to prolong the anterosuperior displacement of the larynx at mid-swallow. Using this technique, subjects were able to significantly delay UES closure by approximately 200 ms.[27]

Botulinum Toxin Injection

Botulinum toxin (Botox) injection to the UES was originally described in 1994 as an alternative to the more invasive CP myotomy.[28] Botox provides chemodenervation and temporary muscle paralysis by inhibiting the presynaptic release of acetylcholine. Botox has reported response rates ranging from 43% to 100%, yet a recent Cochrane review determined that there was insufficient evidence for the use of Botox to the UES to inform clinical practice.[29] A retrospective of review of 49 patients with UES dysfunction treated with Botox showed symptomatic improvement in 65% of patients although many patients complained of a temporary worsening of dysphagia following CP Botox administration. There is a wide variation in the dose and technique used. A range of 5−100 units has been reported. Botox can be administered in the outpatient setting via transcutaneous transcervical electromyographic guided technique or in the operating room via direct suspension laryngoscopy and rigid esophagoscopy. The overall complication rate was minimal, with one patient requiring hospitalization for worsening dysphagia and inability to eat orally.[30] The effects of Botox may be appreciated within a couple weeks and may last for 5−6 months.

Further work is needed to better understand the dose, route, injection location(s), and patient characteristics to predict which patients will benefit. There is a real concern for diffusion of Botox to surrounding tissue causing *worsening* of dysphagia. Small volumes and high concentration (e.g., 50 units per mL) with injection into the posterior midline CP muscle is recommended.

Dilation

Esophageal dilation dates back to the 17th century with esophageal dilation performed using a whale bone. In the past several decades, UES dilation using bougie dilators was performed. Fixed-diameter wire guided dilators such as the Savary dilators have been used with efficacy and are safer due to wire guidance of the bougie. Most dilations currently are performed using controlled radial expansion (CRE) balloon dilators, primarily due to the ease of dilation using this technology. A large published series of 46 patients showed that two-thirds of patients experienced improvement in their swallow that lasted at least 2 years.[31] A large meta-analysis showed success rates ranging from 65% to 100% with recurrence seen in 0%−50% of patients.[32] In general, CP dilations are typically temporary procedures for nonfibrotic UES and have a higher incidence of recurrence of symptoms.

In our practice, endoscopic cricopharyngeal myotomy is the preferred treatment for CP achalasia, as it can be performed with minimal morbidity. Patients are informed about the option of balloon dilation as

well, and this modality is occasionally chosen by patients. Although UES balloon dilation can be performed in the clinic using TNE and transnasal insertion of the balloon catheter, we prefer to perform initial dilation in the operating room, so that the UES region can be examined, CP muscle palpated, and the largest balloon possible used for dilation. As mentioned previously, although we have multiple tools to evaluate for UES dysfunction preoperatively, none of these tools provide a definitive functional diagnosis. Therefore, sometimes the findings in the operating room may differ from what the preoperative work-up suggested. The UES and CP is exposed using a Dedo laryngoscope placed in the postcricoid area just above the CP. This places the CP under slight tension. A thin caliber rigid suction is then used to palpate the CP to get an impression of how hypertrophic and/or spastic it might be. A complete flexible esophagoscopy is then performed using the TNE scope through the Dedo scope for assessment of the entire esophagus. Balloon dilation is then typically performed with a CRE esophageal balloon dilator to 20 mm for 30−60 s. The balloon is deflated and repeat esophagoscopy performed to assess for any mucosal trauma or significant esophageal laceration and to confirm easier passage through the UES.

Myotomy

The first CP myotomy (CPM) was performed by Samuel Kaplan in 1949 using an open transcervical approach under local anesthesia in a 28-year-old postpoliomyelitis patient.[33] The patient's bulbar poliomyelitis resulted in multiple unilateral cranial neuropathies including nerves 7, 9, 12, and what is described but not specifically stated as 10. Within months of CPM, the patient's gastrostomy tube was removed. Today, surgical CPM is the gold-standard treatment for UES dysfunction, ideally situated to treat those with focal neurologic deficits or those with isolated UES dysfunction. Improvements following CPM in patients with central neurological diseases such as amyotrophic lateral sclerosis or PD are less predictable. CPM may be performed via the traditional transcervical open approach or via the endoscopic laser-assisted approach.

Open CPM is performed under general anesthesia. It should always begin with a direct laryngoscopy and esophagoscopy to evaluate the cricopharyngeus muscle and to rule out the presence of an early diverticulum. Then, under direct visualization, an endotracheal tube, Maloney dilator, or bougie may be placed within the esophagus to provide moderate distension of the pharyngoesophageal segment. This helps the identification of the upper esophageal sphincter, the division of its fibers, and the evaluation of the appropriate myotomy depth. A transcervical incision is made at the level of the cricoid cartilage within a neck crease from the sternocleidomastoid muscle (SCM) edge on the left side to just across midline. Subplatysmal flaps are elevated from the level of the thyroid notch to 2–3 cm below the cricoid cartilage. The medial border of the SCM is skeletonized to open the carotid triangle. As the omohyoid comes into view, this is retracted inferiorly or can be divided. The larynx can be rotated to the right using a single hook anchored to its lateral border. The inferior cornu of the thyroid cartilage is used as a landmark for the level of the CP muscle. A CPM is then performed using a No. 15 blade in the posterior midline from distal to proximal for a length of at least 2.5 cm to up to 6 cm. The incision should be carried slightly into the inferior constrictor proximally at the level of the mid-thyroid cartilage and into the muscle fibers of the cervical esophagus distally. Upon completion of the myotomy, the mucosa should be clearly seen without any overlying muscle fibers. One must inspect for and repair any luminal injuries immediately. We typically repair such injuries with interrupted 3-0 vicryl mattress sutures followed by a sternothyroid or omohyoid onlay muscle flap. The wound is then irrigated copiously, hemostasis is obtained, and the placement of a 7 mm flat Jackson–Pratt drain is often used. Multilayer closure is then performed.

Endoscopic CPM is most often performed with the Dedo laryngoscope. For early or established Zenker's diverticuli, a bivalve diverticuloscope (Weerda) is used. The patient is induced under general anesthesia and intubated with a 5-0 laser safe endotracheal tube. The UES and CP is exposed using a Dedo laryngoscope placed in the postcricoid area just above the CP and suspension adjusted so the distal esophageal introitus can be appreciated (see Case 1 below, Fig. 19.2A). Esophagoscopy is then performed to evaluate for any esophageal pathology or sequela from possible reflux. Saline-soaked pledgets are placed within the esophageal lumen, and slight tension is placed on the pledget strings pulling the cephalad from the CP sling (Fig. 19.2B). The tails of the strings are taped to the handle of the laryngoscope to keep them in place and to maintain their tension. Routine laser precautions are taken. The operating microscope with the line-of-sight carbon dioxide laser is used. The laser is then used to incise the mucosa at the midline of the CP, and continued through the horizontal muscle fibers until separation of the muscle fibers with ablation is no longer appreciated and the pharynx is flush with the esophageal lumen (Fig. 19.2C). Following myotomy,

a CRE balloon may be used to obtain full division of the muscle fibers (CRE balloon 15-18 mm is typically used). This helps complete the myotomy if there are any residual intact muscle fibers. Hemostasis is achieved with cocaine-soaked pledgets or endoscopic suction cautery. The mucosa is left to heal by secondary intention in all cases.

In the absence of an inadvertent pharyngotomy postoperative care of a patient following open versus endoscopic CPM is similar with the exception of surgical drain management. Both are admitted overnight to a monitored bed. If the patient appears stable and without subcutaneous emphysema, they are started on ice chips in the evening of surgery day. For an uncomplicated course a soft diet is started on postoperative day 1 and maintained for 1–2 weeks. Discharge medications include antibiotics and pain medications. Open myotomy patients are kept as inpatients until neck drain is removed. In cases of an inadvertent pharyngotomy and repair during open myotomy, a nasogastric tube (NG) is placed and the patient kept nil per os for a minimum of 3 days. After 3 days, the NG tube is pulled and a gastrograffin esophagram is performed to rule out any contrast leak. Diet is advanced if no leak is found and drain removed the following day if output remains low.

Outcome comparisons between open and endoscopic CPM have all been retrospective. Dauer et al. looked at the outcomes of 14 patients who underwent endoscopic laser CPM compared to 8 patients who underwent open transcervical CPM. The endoscopic group had shorter operative times and hospital stays, with less major complications, while both groups demonstrated measurable functional improvement.[32,34] A more recent and larger retrospective review by Huntley et al. compared the outcomes of 38 open versus 41 endoscopic CPM cases and found lesser surgical time and improved symptomatic outcomes in the endoscopic group.[35] Given these reported benefits and our experience, we consider endoscopic laser-assisted CPM as the gold standard and preferred technique.

CASES

Case 1

A 90-year-old woman with lumbar spine disease presents with 3 months of dysphagia following a ground level fall. Prior to the fall, she noted occasional dysphagia to solids. This became worse after her fall to the point that she could not tolerate oral intake and a gastrostomy tube was placed. FEES and MBSS were consistent with CP achalasia. She underwent

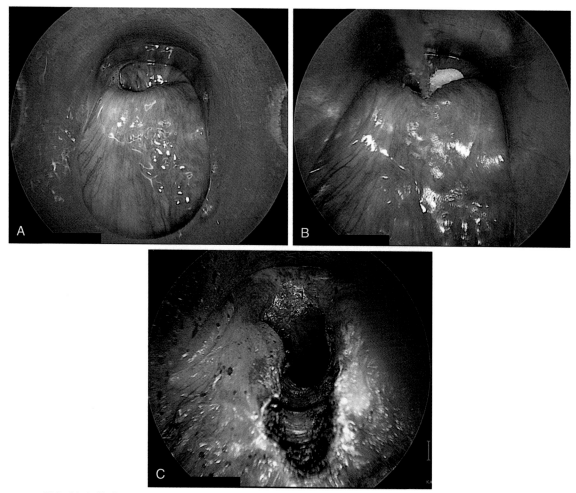

FIG. 19.2 **Endoscopic Carbon Dioxide Laser Cricopharyngeal Myotomy.** **(A)** The cricopharyngeus (CP) is exposed with a Dedo laryngoscope in the postcricoid region placing CP under tension. **(B)** Placement of saline-soaked pledget(s) into esophageal inlet under slight tension to enhance exposure and reduce laser injury distally. **(C)** Completion of laser CP myotomy showing direct view into the esophageal lumen.

endoscopic cricopharyngeal myotomy. Fig. 19.2A–C detail exposure, setup, and completion of endoscopic CPM using the Dedo laryngoscope and Lumenis line-of-sight carbon dioxide laser. Postoperative course was without complications. Postoperative MBSS demonstrated resolution of CP bar. The patient was started on a mechanical soft diet with advancement to regular food shortly after. One month following her surgery her gastrostomy tube was removed.

Case 2

A 57-year-old woman who underwent prolonged hospitalization following complications of breast cancer chemotherapy presents with progressive dysphagia to solids and occasionally liquids. On further questioning, she reveals a history of esophageal dilations and neurologic evaluation for oculopharyngeal muscular dystrophy. FEES demonstrated mild pooling of saliva in postcricoid region, pyriform fossa, and vallecula. Transnasal esophagoscopy failed to delineate any stricture or CP bar. The MBSS showed pharyngeal weakness, epiglottic dysfunction, and a prominent CP bar (Fig. 19.3A). She underwent endoscopic cricopharyngeal myotomy. Postoperative swallowing revealed no obstruction at the level of the UES (Fig. 19.3B).

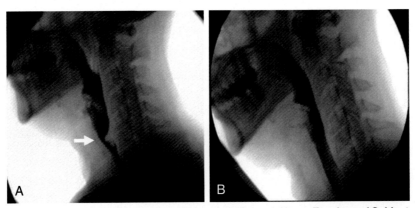

FIG. 19.3 **Modified Barium Swallow Study of Bolus Flow Through Upper Esophageal Sphincter Region Before and After Cricopharyngeus Myotomy.** **(A)** Pre-op modified barium swallow study (MBSS) showing prominent cricopharyngeus (CP) bar (white arrow) and narrowing of lumen at the level of C6. **(B)** Postoperative MBSS showing resolution of CP bar and improved bolus flow.

REFERENCES

1. Sivarao DV, Goyal RK. Functional anatomy and physiology of the upper esophageal sphincter. *Am J Med.* 2000;108(suppl 4a):27s–37s.
2. Allen JE. Cricopharyngeal function or dysfunction: what's the deal? *Curr Opin Otolaryngol Head Neck Surg.* 2016; 24(6):494–499.
3. Kwiatek MA, et al. Hyperdynamic upper esophageal sphincter pressure: a manometric observation in patients reporting globus sensation. *Am J Gastroenterol.* 2009; 104(2):289–298.
4. Peng L, et al. Assessment of upper esophageal sphincter function on high-resolution manometry: identification of predictors of globus symptoms. *J Clin Gastroenterol.* 2015;49(2):95–100.
5. Babaei A, et al. Response of the upper esophageal sphincter to esophageal distension is affected by posture, velocity, volume, and composition of the infusate. *Gastroenterology.* 2012;142(4):734–743.e7.
6. Babaei A, et al. Impaired upper esophageal sphincter reflexes in patients with supraesophageal reflux disease. *Gastroenterology.* 2015;149(6):1381–1391.
7. Horvath OP, et al. Esophageal complications of gastroesophageal reflux disease: consequences or defensive reactions? *Orv Hetil.* 2017;158(20):763–769.
8. Dawe N, et al. Targeted use of endoscopic CO_2 laser cricopharyngeal myotomy for improving swallowing function following head and neck cancer treatment. *J Laryngol Otol.* 2014;128(12):1105–1110.
9. Pauloski BR, et al. Comparison of swallowing function after intensity-modulated radiation therapy and conventional radiotherapy for head and neck cancer. *Head Neck.* 2015;37(11):1575–1582.
10. Domer AS, Leonard R, Belafsky PC. Pharyngeal weakness and upper esophageal sphincter opening in patients with unilateral vocal fold immobility. *Laryngoscope.* 2014; 124(10):2371–2374.
11. Ellerston JK, et al. Quantitative measures of swallowing deficits in patients with Parkinson's disease. *Ann Otol Rhinol Laryngol.* 2016;125(5):385–392.
12. Montesi A, et al. Oropharyngeal and esophageal function in scleroderma. *Dysphagia.* 1991;6(4):219–223.
13. Kern M, et al. Comparison of upper esophageal sphincter opening in healthy asymptomatic young and elderly volunteers. *Ann Otol Rhinol Laryngol.* 1999;108(10):982–989.
14. Shaw DW, et al. Influence of normal aging on oral-pharyngeal and upper esophageal sphincter function during swallowing. *Am J Physiol.* 1995;268(3 Pt 1):G389–G396.
15. Shaker R, et al. Effect of aging and bolus variables on pharyngeal and upper esophageal sphincter motor function. *Am J Physiol.* 1993;264(3 Pt 1):G427–G432.
16. Kuhn MA, Belafsky PC. Management of cricopharyngeus muscle dysfunction. *Otolaryngol Clin N Am.* 2013;46(6): 1087–1099.
17. Kendall KA, et al. Timing of events in normal swallowing: a videofluoroscopic study. *Dysphagia.* 2000;15(2):74–83.
18. Leonard RJ, et al. Structural displacements in normal swallowing: a videofluoroscopic study. *Dysphagia.* 2000;15(3): 146–152.
19. Leonard R, Kendall K, McKenzie S. UES opening and cricopharyngeal bar in nondysphagic elderly and nonelderly adults. *Dysphagia.* 2004;19(3):182–191.
20. Shaker R. Unsedated trans-nasal pharyngoesophagogastroduodenoscopy (T-EGD): technique. *Gastrointest Endosc.* 1994;40(3):346–348.
21. Shaker R, et al. *Manual of Diagnostic and Therapeutic Techniques for Disorders of Deglutition.* New York: Springer; 2012.
22. Omari TI, et al. Upper esophageal sphincter impedance as a marker of sphincter opening diameter. *Am J Physiol Gastrointest Liver Physiol.* 2012;302(9):G909–G913.
23. Lan Y, et al. The correlation between manometric and videofluoroscopic measurements of the swallowing function in brainstem stroke patients with Dysphagia. *J Clin Gastroenterol.* 2015;49(1):24–30.

24. Cook IJ, Dent J, Collins SM. Upper esophageal sphincter tone and reactivity to stress in patients with a history of globus sensation. *Dig Dis Sci.* 1989;34(5):672−676.

25. Omari T, et al. Measurement of upper esophageal sphincter tone and relaxation during swallowing in premature infants. *Am J Physiol.* 1999;277(4 Pt 1):G862−G866.

26. Cook IJ, et al. Measurement of upper esophageal sphincter pressure. Effect of acute emotional stress. *Gastroenterology.* 1987;93(3):526−532.

27. Kahrilas PJ, et al. Volitional augmentation of upper esophageal sphincter opening during swallowing. *Am J Physiol.* 1991;260(3 Pt 1):G450−G456.

28. Schneider I, et al. Treatment of dysfunction of the cricopharyngeal muscle with botulinum A toxin: introduction of a new, noninvasive method. *Ann Otol Rhinol Laryngol.* 1994;103(1):31−35.

29. Regan J, et al. Botulinum toxin for upper oesophageal sphincter dysfunction in neurological swallowing disorders. *Cochrane Database Syst Rev.* 2014;(5):Cd009968.

30. Kelly EA, et al. Botulinum toxin injection for the treatment of upper esophageal sphincter dysfunction. *Ann Otol Rhinol Laryngol.* 2013;122(2):100−108.

31. Clary MS, et al. Efficacy of large-diameter dilatation in cricopharyngeal dysfunction. *Laryngoscope.* 2011;121(12): 2521−2525.

32. Ashman A, Dale OT, Baldwin DL. Management of isolated cricopharyngeal dysfunction: systematic review. *J Laryngol Otol.* 2016;130(7):611−615.

33. Kaplan S. Paralysis of deglutition, a post-poliomyelitis complication treated by section of the cricopharyngeus muscle. *Ann Surg.* 1951;133(4):572−573.

34. Dauer E, et al. Endoscopic laser vs open approach for cricopharyngeal myotomy. *Otolaryngol Head Neck Surg.* 2006;134(5):830−835.

35. Huntley C, Boon M, Spiegel J. Open vs. endoscopic cricopharyngeal myotomy; is there a difference? *Am J Otolaryngol.* 2017;38(4):405−407.

CHAPTER 20

Zenker's Diverticulum

NAUSHEEN JAMAL, MD • JONATHAN HAROUNIAN, MD •
HILARY YANKEY, BS • DINESH K. CHHETRI, MD

INTRODUCTION

Upper gastrointestinal diverticula fall under two broad categories: pulsion or traction diverticula. Pulsion diverticula form as a result of increased pressure in the lumen, causing protrusions of the mucosal layer without a muscularis propria layer. Traction diverticula form by traction forces that lead to outpouching of all three layers of the esophagus.[1]

Zenker's diverticulum (ZD), a pulsion diverticulum, is the most common upper gastrointestinal diverticulum. It is an acquired herniation of the mucosal and submucosal layers through the posterior wall of the pharyngoesophageal junction, known as Killian's triangle. Killian's triangle is a pharyngeal weak point formed between the horizontal fibers of the cricopharyngeus (CP) muscle and the oblique fibers of the inferior pharyngeal constrictors (IPCs) and is also known as *Killian's dehiscence*. Occasionally, other diverticula, such as a Killian–Jamieson (KJ) diverticulum, may be found in a lateral or posterolateral aspect of the upper esophageal wall and must be distinguished from ZD because treatment approaches for the two are different.[2]

ZD was first reported in 1769 as an incidental finding during an autopsy by Dr Abraham Ludlow, who described an abnormal dilation of the posterior pharynx in a deceased patient who had complained of dysphagia. In 1877, German pathologists Zenker and von Ziemsen characterized this disease and elucidated that the diverticulum formed due to "forces within the lumen acting against restriction" after their work on 34 patients who had the disease. Dr Gustav Killian, a surgeon in the early 1900s, described the underlying anatomy of what is now commonly known as Killian's triangle.[3]

ZD is typically found in patients in their seventh and eighth decades of life, with a prevalence ranging from 0.01% to 0.11%. The annual incidence is about 1–2 per 100,000. This rare condition has a preponderance for affecting males more often than females, with a 1.5:1.0 ratio. The true incidence and prevalence of ZD is unknown; many diverticula may remain asymptomatic, as many older patients with minimal symptoms may not seek medical help. Geographically, ZD is more common in the northern parts of Europe. The reported incidence of cancer in association with ZD is about 0.5% and is likely a result of chronic irritation and inflammation.[4,5]

PATHOPHYSIOLOGY

While considerable debate exists with respect to the mechanism of ZD development, a dysfunctional CP muscle is most often implicated. The most widely accepted theory is that incoordination of the IPC muscle with an abnormally functioning CP muscle leads to increased intraluminal pressure, resulting in gradual, progressive mucosal herniation at the site of the inherently weak Killian's triangle.[6] Cook et al. suggested CP dysfunction occurs due to muscle fiber degeneration and replacement with fibroadipose tissue. Histological analysis of CP muscle biopsies from 14 patients with ZD obtained at the time of diverticulectomy to 10 controls obtained via autopsy revealed abundant fibrosis within the CP muscle of ZD patients.[7] Additionally, Venturi et al. noted an increased collagen to elastin ratio in the CP muscle in ZD patients. It is thought that these structural changes are responsible for reduced upper esophageal sphincter (UES) opening during deglutition in ZD patients.[8] Nevertheless, whether these histological changes are the etiology or the result of ZD is unknown.

Several authors have noted an association between gastroesophageal reflux disease (GERD) and ZD since the early 1970s.[9] Early studies report an increased incidence of hiatal hernia and GERD in ZD patients.[10] Resouly et al. found that nearly all of their patients with ZD had GERD.[11] Mulder et al. further supported this association with findings of the presence of Barrett's esophagus, a known complication of GERD, in approximately 15%–20% of ZD patients.[12] Though these studies suggest a possible relationship, no direct causal association has been identified. Proposed causal explanations for GERD include persistently elevated CP tone or spasms secondary to reflux, or that acid-induced esophageal shortening results in a gap between the constrictors and the CP, allowing for herniation caudal to the pharyngeal constrictors.[13]

Manometric pressure recordings in patients with ZD have revealed abnormalities of the UES during swallowing. Cook et al. found that UES opening was significantly reduced and intrabolus pressures significantly increased in patients with ZD compared to controls.[14] However, the technical difficulties of manometric studies of the UES have proven to be substantial and limiting. The process of collecting measurements stimulates the swallowing reflex, resulting in catheter displacement and loss of data. Furthermore, results are often confounded by the inherent asymmetry of the UES.[15] Manometric studies evaluating UES function and pressure have been inconsistent, and it stands to reason that these technical challenges account for the varied results.[16]

In summary, the pathophysiology of ZD is complex and likely to be multifactorial, with contributions from the multiple processes described above.

SYMPTOMS/PRESENTATION

Progressive oropharyngeal dysphagia is the leading symptom in patients with ZD, occurring in greater than 90% of presenting patients. Transient dysphagia may be noted early in the course of ZD development.[17] The duration of symptoms may span from a few weeks to many years.[12] The diverticular aperture is often aligned with the superior–inferior pharyngeal axis so that food is preferentially diverted into the diverticulum. When the diverticular sac becomes large enough to retain contents such as mucus, sputum, and food, symptoms of pulmonary aspiration, halitosis, cough, throat gurgling, and regurgitation may begin to develop. Other symptoms include noisy swallowing, belching, choking, hoarseness, chest pain, globus sensation, recurrent respiratory infections, and weight loss, depending on the severity of dysphagia.

External physical examination findings are often normal in patients with ZD. If present, findings may include audible regurgitation sounds, emaciation, dehydration, and, rarely, a Boyce sign—a swelling in the neck that gurgles on palpation due to air passage from the sac rostrally.[18]

DIAGNOSIS

Diagnosis of Zenker's may be suspected based on history of dysphagia and regurgitation. Radiologic swallow evaluation such as modified barium swallow study (see Chapter 10) or an esophagram can reveal a posteriorly based pouch and confirm the diagnosis (Fig. 20.1).[19] Esophagopharyngeal reflux, or regurgitation of swallowed food from pouch back into the pharynx, may be seen on flexible endoscopic evaluation of swallowing within a few seconds after the swallowed bolus disappears below the hypopharynx and is generally a pathognomonic sign for ZD (Fig. 20.2).[18] Other confirmatory tests include esophageal endoscopy, for example, a transnasal esophagoscopy, which can be easily performed in the office (Fig. 20.3). It is not uncommon for ZD to be initially encountered incidentally during upper endoscopy as part of a workup for the patient with dysphagia.[20]

MANAGEMENT

Curative treatment of ZD is surgery. Different types of surgical approaches have evolved over the decades, with modifications focusing on the potential for reduced intraoperative or postoperative complications and overall morbidity. Surgery is indeed not necessary in the asymptomatic patient; nevertheless, long-term monitoring is indicated and patients should be counseled as such. Surgical treatment is performed via a transoral endoscopic approach or a transcervical open

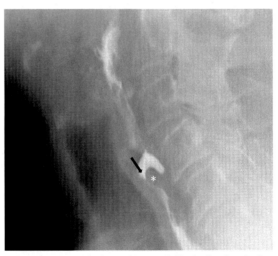

FIG. 20.1 Lateral view of a small Zenker's diverticulum on an esophagram. *Arrow* indicates esophageal opening; * indicates cricopharyngeal bar.

surgery. Transoral rigid endoscopy with cricopharyngeal myotomy has become the most popular treatment method for ZD because it is less invasive, shortens hospital stay, decreases anesthesia time, and has fewer complications compared to the open approach.[3,21] Endoscopic approaches using a flexible endoscope have been described more recently but have not yet reached the popularity of the rigid approach.[22–24]

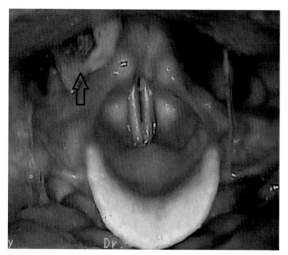

FIG. 20.2 Esophagopharyngeal reflux seen on flexible fiberoptic evaluation of swallowing. *Arrow* points to slow reflux of food from the Zenker's diverticulum into the right hypopharynx.

The Transoral Rigid Endoscopic Technique

Transoral endoscopic treatment of ZD was first described by Mosher in 1917. Mosher's method divided the cricopharyngeal wall between the esophagus and the diverticulum, functionally connecting the diverticulum and the esophagus. He utilized a scissor punch through the operative window of the rigid esophagoscope to divide the common party wall. However, his technique carried a risk of mediastinitis, which proved fatal in one of his seven patients.[25] The endoscopic approach was thus abandoned until Dohlman improved upon Mosher's technique. In his publication of this method in 1960, he described using a bivalved endoscope and electrocautery to divide the party wall. In his report of 100 patients, he recorded no cases of mediastinitis and a low 7% recurrence rate, which, according to Dohlman, were easily treated via revision endoscopic surgery. Additionally, Dohlman's endoscopic esophagodiverticulostomy and myotomy resulted in decreased operative time, decreased recovery time, and, more importantly, decreased morbidity. Dohlman was a pioneer in safe, endoscopic treatment of ZD.[26]

Improvising on Dohlman's technique, in 1984, van Overbeek used a carbon dioxide (CO_2) laser instead of electrocautery to divide the common wall. Kuhn and Bent attempted refinement of the technique with the use of the potassium titanyl phosphate (KTP) laser in 1992. However, the endoscopic technique was still not commonly practiced until 1996, when Scher and Richtsmeier introduced the use of the endoscopic stapler to divide the party wall.[25] Subsequently,

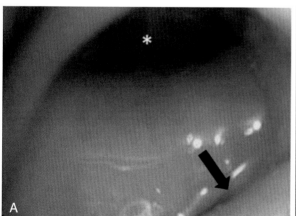
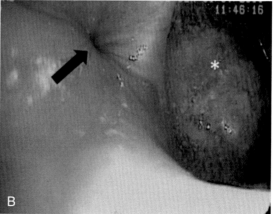

FIG. 20.3 Office transnasal endoscopic view of **(A)** Zenker's diverticulum (ZD) versus **(B)** Killian–Jamieson diverticulum (KJ). In ZD, the esophageal opening (*arrow*) is anterior to the ZD (*star*) and the cricopharyngeal (CP) bar is in-between. In KJ, the esophageal opening (*arrow*) is medial to the KJ (*star*) and CP bar is absent.

endoscopic stapling became widely adopted, its popularity due to the ability to concurrently transect the diverticular wall and seal the edges of the cut party wall, thus providing "peace of mind" in regard to potential postoperative leak-related complications.[27] However, because endoscopic stapling leaves a small residual bar with potential recurrence risk, CO_2 laser surgery for ZD has become popular again, as it is possible to more fully divide the party wall with the latter technique and no adverse events compared to stapling have been encountered. Both the CO_2 laser and the endoscopic stapler techniques remain popular in endoscopic ZD surgery today.[28]

The rigid endoscopic approach is performed with the patient supine and the head and neck placed in a "sniffing" position under general anesthesia. A bivalved diverticuloscope (Weerda Scope, Karl Storz, Tuttlingen, Germany) is inserted through the mouth and advanced to the hypopharynx and slowly passed into the esophageal inlet. The common party wall—the CP bar—is visualized and the diverticulum exposed with the anterior tine of the scope into the esophagus and the posterior tine into the ZD pouch (Fig. 20.4). A rigid 0-degree Hopkins rod telescope may be used to further visualize anatomy and contents of the pouch and esophageal inlet. Some surgeons have described placing retraction sutures at the lateral margins of the common wall to allow for tension and facilitate stapler positioning, but this is not necessary. Either the CO_2 laser or the

endoscopic stapler can then be used to divide the party wall. In dividing the common wall, a cricopharyngeal myotomy is achieved, and the diverticulum contents are then able to drain easily into the esophageal lumen during swallowing. With the stapler, as described above, a small remnant of the party wall is left behind. In addition, in patients with diverticula less than 2 cm in depth, CP myotomy is not possible due to the inability of the stapler to pass deep enough to perform a complete myotomy. In such cases, CO_2 laser should be used.[3] With the laser, incision is made starting at the midline of the party wall and extended to the bottom of the pouch, but the underlying buccopharyngeal fascia is not exposed. One way to avoid excessive surgery is to limit the laser incision to division of the muscle fibers only (Fig. 20.5).

In some cases, an endoscopic approach to diverticulotomy can be particularly challenging, usually due to difficulty attaining exposure. The most common reason for difficult exposure is a small or triangular mandible. Other major anatomic constraints for exposure include a large tongue and full dentition. In other cases, the diverticuloscope can be advanced to the pouch but the esophagus cannot be cannulated with the anterior tine of the scope because of excessive CP spasm or poor angle to the esophageal inlet (Fig. 20.6). In these cases, the Weerda diverticuloscope should be advanced to the postcricoid space in the closed position and advanced to the CP bar if possible. If the diverticuloscope tip is entirely within the pouch, it should be slowly withdrawn until the party wall is visualized. If it is too proximal without visualizing the party wall, the tines should be opened and the diverticuloscope placed into suspension. A 0-degree rigid telescope may then be advanced

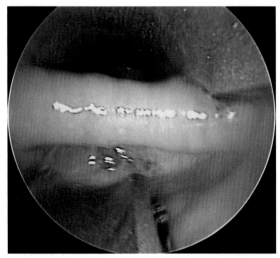

FIG. 20.4 Endoscopic exposure of Zenker's diverticulum using a bivalved diverticuloscope. Anterior tine (top) is in the esophageal lumen and the posterior tine (bottom) is in the diverticulum.

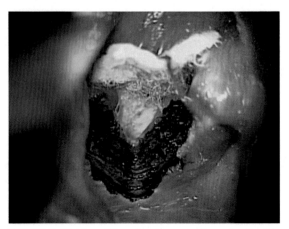

FIG. 20.5 Division of the cricopharyngeal bar using the CO_2 laser.

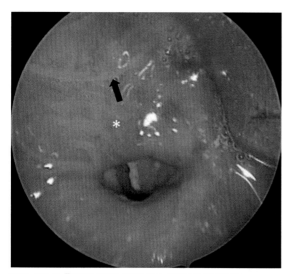

FIG. 20.6 Endoscopic view of a difficult surgical exposure of the Zenker's diverticulum. The esophageal opening (*arrow*) is difficult to cannulate with the anterior tine of the diverticuloscope due to a spasmodic cricopharyngeal bar and/or poor angle.

for a close-up view to identify the party wall. Alternatively, an ultraslim flexible esophagoscope can be used to confirm the esophageal entry point, and the scope itself or a guidewire can be used to guide the diverticuloscope. If the CP muscle is under excessive spasm and the esophageal lumen still cannot be cannulated, a controlled radial expansion balloon dilation up to 15–18 mm may be performed. Then, the anterior tine of the diverticuloscope is often easily advanced into the esophagus. In cases with significant pharyngeal narrowing, such as in the case of cervical spine osteophytes, the narrower Dohlman diverticuloscope or a Benjamin Hollinger scope may be more easily passed.

After endoscopic surgery, patients are admitted for overnight observation and may start on ice chips or small sips of water on the day of surgery if there is no crepitus or subcutaneous emphysema and discharged on a soft diet on the first or second postoperative day. Antibiotics and pain medications are given intravenously while in the hospital.

Swallowing outcomes after endoscopic repair are generally excellent, with greater improvement in dysphagia and regurgitation scores and a lower rate of symptomatic recurrence with CO_2 laser treatment compared to stapler.[28,29] A recent meta-analysis revealed no differences in nil per os duration, length of hospitalization, dental complications, major complications (mediastinitis, pharyngoesophageal stenosis, or

requiring other operative intervention), or revision surgery. However, there were significantly greater incidence of subcutaneous emphysema without mediastinitis or bleeding noted in the CO_2 group.[30] Definitive conclusions from this meta-analysis are limited by the quality of studies included, as only seven nonrandomized, retrospective case series were identified.

The rigid endoscopic method carries the additional risk of gingival/mucosal laceration, tongue numbness, and dental injury, inherent in the use of a modified suspension laryngoscope. Patients should be counseled about these risks preoperatively. There are also limitations of the endoscopic stapling technique that are worth mentioning. Visual intraoperative exposure of the diverticulum may prove challenging due to patient factors such as kyphosis, mandibular tori, or limited oropharyngeal opening.

Flexible Endoscopic Technique

Flexible endoscopic treatment of ZD was introduced in 1995. Rigid endoscopy may not be feasible in patients with limited neck extension, prominent teeth, retrognathia, rigid cervical kyphosis, and severe temporomandibular joint disease. These limitations can affect rigid endoscopy and lead to a conversion to an open surgery, which may have more complications.[31] In addition, many patients who have ZD are older adults, potentially malnourished, and stand a higher risk for perioperative adverse events from general anesthesia. Flexible endoscopic treatment can more easily access the ZD and theoretically avoid general anesthesia, although most procedures to date have been performed under general anesthesia.[32,33] While the goals are the same as in rigid endoscopy, the myotomy can be accomplished by electrocautery, or alternatively, with argon plasma coagulation. Division technique is chosen based on the preference and experience of the physician performing it.[3,24] Some endoscopists maintain the use of a nasogastric tube (passed via a guidewire) to maximize endoscopic visual exposure of the cricopharyngeal septum, in addition to helping protect the anterior esophageal wall during incision. The decision to remove or leave the tube postoperatively is based on the surgeon's preference.[23]

The flexible endoscopic approach is still novel and holds some promise, especially for high-risk older patients who are poor surgical candidates and would benefit from a shorter procedure without the need for general anesthesia and neck extension. Nevertheless, most surgeons in the United States are not trained in flexible endoscopic approach and the learning curve is unknown.[22]

Open (External) Technique

The management of ZD in late 19th century was very risky due to the high incidence of mediastinitis. Thus, surgical treatment often meant fistulization of the pouch, either externally or internally.[34] In 1886, Wheeler was the first to successfully perform open surgery. His first approach was a diverticulectomy, which was further modified into a diverticulectomy plus myotomy in 1936 by Aubin after a meta-analysis that highlighted the various failures of a diverticulectomy alone.[34] In 1962, Sutherland successfully treated two patients by performing a myotomy alone, leading to the realization that myotomy may be sufficient in certain cases. A few years later in 1966, Belsey advocated for cricopharyngeal myotomoy with diverticulopexy as an improvement over Schmid's previous diverticulopexy in 1912.[35,36]

Upper esophageal dysfunction is implicated in the development of ZD, and CP myotomy is necessary to normalize the opening size of the UES, reduce resting UES pressure, and decreasing intrabolus pressure. Cricopharyngeal myotomy is performed via a left cervical incision and the CP muscle divided close to the posterior midline encompassing a small amount of IPC and esophageal muscles above and below the muscle. Myotomy as a sole treatment has been reported to result in good clinical outcomes.[37–39] On the other hand, a comparative study by Gutschow et al. in 2002 reported there was no difference in symptomatic outcomes when comparing diverticulectomy alone with other approaches with a myotomy. However, the study also noted that diverticulectomy without myotomy may predispose one to fistula formation and recurrence of ZD.[34,40]

The extent of the myotomy is something that has not been agreed upon, with research showing the length of myotomy to range from 2 to 6 cm.[34,41] Adequate CP myotomy (commonly believed to be 4–5 cm) is considered an important procedure to prevent early recurrence.[41] In a recent systematic review investigating 93 studies evaluating the effect of the surgical intervention for ZD, 2526 out of 2826 patients received either a myotomy alone or a myotomy plus other approaches.[34] Interestingly, the largest available case series, involving 888 patients, did not show any advantage or improvement following the addition of myotomy to a diverticulectomy.[42] One major concern regarding myotomy, that of aspiration pneumonia, was found to be rare (9/2826 = 0.3%).[34] It is important to note that the systematic review, though containing a sizeable sample size, lacked the inclusion of randomized controlled trials.

How to Manage the Diverticulum

Management of the diverticular sac in open surgery, whether to resect, suspend, or invert the diverticulum, has been a matter of great debate. Diverticulectomy (resection) requires identifying the diverticulum, dissecting any adhesions of connective tissues to the diverticular opening, resecting the pouch, and repairing the esophageal wall by stapling or division and suturing to close the diverticulotomy.[43] Diverticulopexy (suspension) involves mobilizing then suspending the diverticulum superiorly to the prevertebral fascia or the pharyngeal musculature such that the orifice of the diverticulum is facing away from the hypopharynx, thus preventing the accumulation of debris. Inversion involves the placing of a purse-string suture around the neck of the diverticulum, inverting the diverticulum through the suture, and then ligating it.[3] The main advantages of diverticulopexy (suspension) and inversion over diverticulectomy is that the mucosal wall is not divided thus the possibility for fistula formation and mediastinitis is significantly reduced. Other minor advantages include shorter antibiotic treatment, shorter hospital stay, and earlier resumption of oral feeding.[34] However, stapler diverticulectomy is the currently preferred technique in open resection.

Comparing the Options Within Open Surgery

In a comparative study by Gutschow et al. of 169 patients, those who had received a diverticulectomy without a myotomy had the longest median postoperative stay of 11 days (range: 8–61 days), followed by 9 days (range: 7–43 days) for a diverticulectomy with a myotomy, 3 days (range: 1–6 days) for a myotomy alone, and 1.5 days (range: 0–26 days) for a diverticulopexy with myotomy. The postoperative fasting period followed a similar trend, with 7 days (range: 5–55 days) after a diverticulectomy alone and 1 day (range 0–4 days) after myotomy alone. The fistula rates in diverticulectomy alone, diverticulectomy with myotomy, myotomy alone, and diverticulopexy with myotomy were 1/12, 0/10, 0/8, and 1/42, respectively.[40] Simic et al. compared a diverticulectomy combined with myotomy (n = 14), myotomy alone (n = 2), and diverticulopexy with myotomy (n = 36). This study observed no fistulas in any of the surgical options, however, diverticulectomy with myotomy had the longest postoperative stay and fasting period. Four of 36 of the diverticulopexy with myotomy patients and 2/14 of the diverticulectomy with myotomy patients had a recurrence of dysphagia within a 6-month period, but eventually became symptom free within a year.[44]

Morton and Bartley compared 15 cases of diverticulectomy with 18 cases of inversion and showed lower complication rates (0%–6% vs. 0%–21%), shorter operation time (90 min vs. 130 min), and shorter postoperative stays (0–4 days vs. 5 to more than 21 days) in the diverticular inversion cases. Additionally, cases of inversion were free of recurrence after 56 months of follow-up, whereas diverticulectomy with myotomy had a 5.7% recurrence. Common complications in inversion, extracted from literature before this study, were recurrent nerve injury (1.3%), fistula (1.3%), wound infections (2.7%), and death (1.3%). In the study, however, there was only one incident of infection and one case of death.[45] A systematic review by Verdonck and Morton of over 70 studies compared the various transcervical techniques and showed that the rate of fistulas and length of hospital stay was the highest in diverticulectomy (4% and 9.5 days) compared to diverticular inversion (1% and 6.2 days) and diverticulopexy (1% and 5.4 days).[46]

Due to a lack of randomized controlled trials, it is virtually impossible to ascertain the optimal open surgical approach with certainty. A review of recent trends, however, does reveal that diverticulectomy with myotomy has gained widespread popularity in the last 20 years, making up 56.4% of all open surgical procedures.[34]

Comparing Open Surgery to Endoscopic

The overall data identified in a review of 93 studies by Yuan et al. comparing open surgery and endoscopic procedures showed that open surgery can resolve symptoms in 90%–95% of patients, with a morbidity of 10.5% and a mortality of 0.6%. The most common complications in open surgery were recurrent nerve injury (3.3%), leak or perforation (3.3%), cervical infection (1.8%), and hematoma (1%). Respiratory infection, stenosis, mediastinitis, and other complications had a rate of <1%. Endoscopic surgery resolved symptoms in 63%–100% of patients, with a morbidity of 8.7% and a mortality of 0.2%. The most common complications in endoscopic surgery were cervical or mediastinal emphysema (2.2%), perforation (1.4%), dental injury (1.1%), and bleeding (0.9%). Mediastinitis, leak, respiratory infection, stenosis, recurrent nerve injury, and neck abscesses were all complications happening at a rate of <1%.[34]

Verdonck and Morton's systematic review showed an overall higher complication rate in open surgery than endoscopic surgery (11% vs. 7%). Surgery-related deaths were infrequent in both groups (0.9% for the open approach vs. 0.4% for endoscopic techniques).

The mean reported postoperative stay is shorter in endoscopic surgery than open (3.9 days vs. 8.4 days). Recurrence after endoscopic treatment (especially stapling endoscopy) was higher for endoscopic surgery than for open (18.4% vs. 4.2%); however, many believe that re-operation via the endoscopic approach is usually successful and straightforward, with low complication and morbidity rate. Overall, open surgeries appear to have higher success rates than endoscopic approaches, but they also have more complications (7.9% vs. 4.3%). Deaths were infrequent in the two groups but potentially more frequent in open surgery (0.9% vs. 0.4%).[46]

NOVEL MODALITIES

A review of the recent literature shows a focus on optimization of the flexible endoscopic approach. Flexible endoscopy is slowly becoming an acceptable treatment option for ZD. One emerging instrument currently being investigated is the soft diverticuloscope. While this device is not yet available in the United States, in Europe it has shown promise in reducing the complication rate in flexible endoscopy. The soft diverticuloscope is a "V" shaped tube that is inserted into the mouth to protect the anterior esophageal wall and posterior diverticular wall, thereby exposing, stretching, and fixing the septum in place to allow for maximal visualization.[47] Due to concerns of adverse events such as perforation, some endoscopists are adopting a clip-assisted technique, in which prior to cutting the septum, two endoclips are placed on either side of the septum.[48] Referred to as the "clip and cut," this technique decreases the risk of perforation, but it has not yet been proven in a clinical trial.

Conventional flexible endoscopic techniques involve incision of both the muscularis and mucosal layers that form the diverticular septum, and thereby introduce the risk of perforation and leak, the most feared complications during the procedure. A recently published endoscopic technique, the submucosal tunneling endoscopic septum division (STESD) technique,[49] incorporates a submucosal tunneling technique, popularized by per-oral endoscopic myotomy, to accomplish complete muscular septum dissection while preserving the mucosal integrity, so as to reduce the risk of perforation and mediastinitis. With this approach, a 1.5- to 2.0-cm longitudinal mucosal incision is performed to create a submucosal longitudinal tunnel between the muscular and mucosal layers. Under direct endoscopic visualization, CP muscle fibers of the septum are dissected down to the base of the diverticulum and further into the normal esophageal muscle.[50] After hemostasis is achieved, the mucosal incision site is closed with several hemostatic clips. Any mucosal injury is also clipped. A promising treatment modality, the STESD technique is currently under trial.

CONCLUSION

Zenker's diverticulum is a pulsion diverticulum that forms in the Killian's triangle, with an annual incidence of 1–2 per 100,000. CP muscle dysfunction is the most implicated etiology, and thus CP myotomy is an essential component of ZD surgery. Affected patients typically present with dysphagia, and the diagnosis may be established with an esophagram or endoscopy. Management of ZD is mainly surgical, via either an endoscopic or open approach, with these different approaches evolving since the 18th century. Currently, the rigid endoscopic approach is the most common approach in the United States, although there has been growing interest in the flexible endoscopic technique in recent years. An open/external technique, while performed with less frequency than the endoscopic technique, still plays a role in specific circumstances, such as very large ZD or difficult endoscopic exposure. Overall, the endoscopic approach is less invasive, has decreased anesthesia time, shorter hospital stays, faster time to per *oral* intake and recovery, and fewer major complications. The main disadvantage is a higher recurrence rate, which is till low and can usually be treated endoscopically again. Open surgery appears to have higher success rate (i.e., fewer recurrences) but more major complications, and longer surgical time and hospital stay. Currently, novel modalities focus on the optimization of the operative exposure and reduction of the risk for perforation and major complications.

REFERENCES

1. Tanaka S, Toyonaga T, Ohara Y, et al. Esophageal diverticulum exposed during endoscopic submucosal dissection of superficial cancer. *World J Gastroenterol*. 2015;21(10): 3121–3126.
2. Nehring P, Krasnodebski IW. Zenker's diverticulum: aetiopathogenesis, symptoms and diagnosis. Comparison of operative methods. *Prz Gastroenterol*. 2013;8(5):284–289.
3. Dzeletovic I, Ekbom DC, Baron TH. Flexible endoscopic and surgical management of Zenker's diverticulum. *Expert Rev Gastroenterol Hepatol*. 2012;6(4):449–465; quiz 466.
4. Klockars T, Makitie A. Case report of Zenker's diverticulum in identical twins: further evidence for genetic predisposition. *J Laryngol Otol*. 2010;124(10):1129–1131.
5. Beard K, Swanstrom LL. Zenker's diverticulum: flexible versus rigid repair. *J Thorac Dis*. 2017;9(suppl 2): S154–S162.
6. Allen MS. Pharyngoesophageal diverticulum: technique of repair. *Chest Surg Clin N Am*. 1995;5(3):449–458.
7. Cook IJ, Blumbergs P, Cash K, Jamieson GG, Shearman DJ. Structural abnormalities of the cricopharyngeus muscle in patients with pharyngeal (Zenker's) diverticulum. *J Gastroenterol Hepatol*. 1992;7(6):556–562.
8. Venturi M, Bonavina L, Colombo L, et al. Biochemical markers of upper esophageal sphincter compliance in patients with Zenker's diverticulum. *J Surg Res*. 1997;70(1): 46–48.
9. Feussner H, Siewert JR. Zenker's diverticulum and reflux. *Hepatogastroenterology*. 1992;39(2):100–104.
10. Hunt PS, Connell AM, Smiley TB. The cricopharyngeal sphincter in gastric reflux. *Gut*. 1970;11(4):303–306.
11. Resouly A, Braat J, Jackson A, Evans H. Pharyngeal pouch: link with reflux and oesophageal dysmotility. *Clin Otolaryngol Allied Sci*. 1994;19(3):241–242.
12. Mulder CJ, Costamagna G, Sakai P. Zenker's diverticulum: treatment using a flexible endoscope. *Endoscopy*. 2001; 33(11):991–997.
13. Sasaki CT, Ross DA, Hundal J. Association between Zenker diverticulum and gastroesophageal reflux disease: development of a working hypothesis. *Am J Med*. 2003; 115(suppl 3A):169s–171s.
14. Cook IJ, Gabb M, Panagopoulos V, et al. Pharyngeal (Zenker's) diverticulum is a disorder of upper esophageal sphincter opening. *Gastroenterology*. 1992;103(4): 1229–1235.
15. Fulp SR, Castell DO. Manometric aspects of Zenker's diverticulum. *Hepatogastroenterology*. 1992;39(2):123–126.
16. Sen P, Kumar G, Bhattacharyya AK. Pharyngeal pouch: associations and complications. *Eur Arch Otorhinolaryngol*. 2006;263(5):463–468.
17. Chang CY, Payyapilli RJ, Scher RL. Endoscopic staple diverticulostomy for Zenker's diverticulum: review of literature and experience in 159 consecutive cases. *Laryngoscope*. 2003;113(6):957–965.
18. Veivers D. Pharyngeal pouch: which technique? *J Laryngol Otol*. 2015;129(suppl 3):S30–S34.
19. Bergeron JL, Long JL, Chhetri DK. Dysphagia characteristics in Zenker's diverticulum. *Otolaryngol Head Neck Surg*. 2013;148(2):223–228.
20. Wilmsen J, Baumbach R, Stuker D, et al. New flexible endoscopic controlled stapler technique for the treatment of Zenker's diverticulum: a case series. *World J Gastroenterol*. 2017;23(17):3084–3091.
21. Koch M, Mantsopoulos K, Velegrakis S, Iro H, Zenk J. Endoscopic laser-assisted diverticulotomy versus open surgical approach in the treatment of Zenker's diverticulum. *Laryngoscope*. 2011;121(10):2090–2094.
22. Friedrich DT, Scheithauer MO, Greve J, et al. Application of a computer-assisted flexible endoscope system for transoral surgery of the hypopharynx and upper esophagus. *Eur Arch Otorhinolaryngol*. 2017;274(5):2287–2293.

23. Ishaq S, Hassan C, Antonello A, et al. Flexible endoscopic treatment for Zenker's diverticulum: a systematic review and meta-analysis. *Gastrointest Endosc.* 2016;83(6): 1076−1089.e1075.

24. Peretti G, Piazza C, Del Bon F, Cocco D, De Benedetto L, Mangili S. Endoscopic treatment of Zenker's diverticulum by carbon dioxide laser. *Acta otorhinolaryngol Ital.* 2010; 30(1):1−4.

25. Scher RL, Richtsmeier WJ. Endoscopic staple-assisted esophagodiverticulostomy for Zenker's diverticulum. *Laryngoscope.* 1996;106(8):951−956.

26. Hillel AT, Flint PW. Evolution of endoscopic surgical therapy for Zenker's diverticulum. *Laryngoscope.* 2009;119(1): 39−44.

27. Adam SI, Paskhover B, Sasaki CT. Revision Zenker diverticulum: laser versus stapler outcomes following initial endoscopic failure. *Ann Otol Rhinol Laryngol.* 2013;122(4): 247−253.

28. Adam SI, Paskhover B, Sasaki CT. Laser versus stapler: outcomes in endoscopic repair of Zenker diverticulum. *Laryngoscope.* 2012;122(9):1961−1966.

29. Pollei TR, Hinni ML, Hayden RE, Lott DG, Mors MB. Comparison of carbon dioxide laser-assisted versus stapler-assisted endoscopic cricopharyngeal myotomy. *Ann Otol Rhinol Laryngol.* 2013;122(9):568−574.

30. Parker NP, Misono S. Carbon dioxide laser versus stapler-assisted endoscopic Zenker's diverticulotomy: a systematic review and meta-analysis. *Otolaryngol Head Neck Surg.* 2014;150(5):750−753.

31. Keck T, Rozsasi A, Grun PM. Surgical treatment of hypopharyngeal diverticulum (Zenker's diverticulum). *Eur Arch Otorhinolaryngol.* 2010;267(4):587−592.

32. de la Morena Madrigal EJ, Perez Arellano E, Rodriguez Garcia I. Flexible endoscopic treatment of Zenker's diverticulum: thirteen years' experience in Spain. *Rev Espanola Enfermedades Dig.* 2016;108(6):297−303.

33. Jones D, Aloraini A, Gowing S, et al. Evolving management of Zenker's diverticulum in the endoscopic Era: a North American experience. *World J Surg.* 2016;40(6):1390−1396.

34. Yuan Y, Zhao YF, Hu Y, Chen LQ. Surgical treatment of Zenker's diverticulum. *Dig Surg.* 2013;30(3):207−218.

35. Crescenzo DG, Trastek VF, Allen MS, Deschamps C, Pairolero PC. Zenker's diverticulum in the elderly: is operation justified? *Ann Thorac Surg.* 1998;66(2):347−350.

36. Bock JM, Van Daele DJ, Gupta N, Blumin JH. Management of Zenker's diverticulum in the endoscopic age: current practice patterns. *Ann Otol Rhinol Laryngol.* 2011;120(12): 796−806.

37. Ellis Jr FH, Schlegel JF, Lynch VP, Payne WS. Cricopharyngeal myotomy for pharyngo-esophageal diverticulum. *Ann Surg.* 1969;170(3):340−349.

38. Schmit PJ, Zuckerbraun L. Treatment of Zenker's diverticula by cricopharyngeus myotomy under local anesthesia. *Am Surg.* 1992;58(11):710−716.

39. Zuckerbraun L, Bahna MS. Cricopharyngeus myotomy as the only treatment for Zenker diverticulum. *Ann Otol Rhinol Laryngol.* 1979;88(Pt 1):798−803.

40. Gutschow CA, Hamoir M, Rombaux P, Otte JB, Goncette L, Collard JM. Management of pharyngoesophageal (Zenker's) diverticulum: which technique? *Ann Thorac Surg.* 2002;74(5):1677−1682; discussion 1682−1673.

41. Lerut T, van Raemdonck D, Guelinckx P, Dom R, Geboes K. Zenker's diverticulum: is a myotomy of the cricopharyngeus useful? How long should it be? *Hepatogastroenterology.* 1992;39(2):127−131.

42. Payne WS. The treatment of pharyngoesophageal diverticulum: the simple and complex. *Hepatogastroenterology.* 1992;39(2):109−114.

43. Constantin A, Mates IN, Predescu D, Hoara P, Achim FI, Constantinoiu S. Principles of surgical treatment of Zenker diverticulum. *J Med Life.* 2012;5(1):92−97.

44. Simic A, Radovanovic N, Stojakov D, et al. Surgical experience of the national institution in the treatment of Zenker's diverticula. *Acta Chirurgica Iugosl.* 2009;56(1): 25−33.

45. Morton RP, Bartley JR. Inversion of Zenker's diverticulum: the preferred option. *Head Neck.* 1993;15(3):253−256.

46. Verdonck J, Morton RP. Systematic review on treatment of Zenker's diverticulum. *Eur Arch Otorhinolaryngol.* 2015; 272(11):3095−3107.

47. Aggarwal N, Thota PN. Are there alternatives to surgery for Zenker diverticulum? *Clevel Clin J Med.* 2016;83(9): 645−647.

48. Bizzotto A, Iacopini F, Landi R, Costamagna G. Zenker's diverticulum: exploring treatment options. *Acta otorhinolaryngol Ital.* 2013;33(4):219−229.

49. Cai M, Xu M, Li Q, et al. Preliminary results of submucosal tunneling endoscopic septum division in the treatment of esophageal diverticulum. *(Zhonghua wei chang wai ke za zhi) Chin J Gastrointest Surg.* 2017;20(5):530−534.

50. Brieau B, Leblanc S, Bordacahar B, et al. Submucosal tunneling endoscopic septum division for Zenker's diverticulum: a reproducible procedure for endoscopists who perform peroral endoscopic myotomy. *Endoscopy.* 2017; 49(6):613−614.

CHAPTER 21

Dysphagia Following Laryngectomy

HEATHER STARMER, MA

OVERVIEW

Laryngeal cancer and the treatments utilized to address it may lead to substantial changes in the swallowing mechanism. Dysphagia may be related to structural changes (anatomic) or changes in swallowing function (physiologic); and often is the result of the combination of both. Such dysphagia may impact both the safety and the efficiency of the swallow and may lead to pulmonary and nutritional complications as well as detrimental impact on quality of life. Hence, consideration of dysphagia in individuals with laryngeal cancer is a critical aspect of patient care.

Treatment for laryngeal cancer may include surgery, radiation, and chemotherapy, either as single- or multimodality treatment. In general, the potential for dysphagia increases with treatment involving more than one modality.[1] Unfortunately, laryngeal cancer survival rates have remained relatively stable over the past 40 years, despite treatment advances, suggesting that de-intensification of laryngeal cancer treatment may not be a feasible strategy to minimize toxicities such as dysphagia.[2] Treatment-related dysphagia thus remains a major concern for individuals diagnosed with larynx cancer. This chapter will focus on the description of swallowing disorders associated with surgical management of laryngeal cancer, outline strategies for the management of such dysphagia, and highlight the importance of multidisciplinary treatment of these patients for optimal outcomes.

Surgical Management of Laryngeal Cancer

Primary surgical intervention is associated with relatively predicable swallowing outcomes based on the extent and location of resection. Surgical procedures may include limited laryngeal resection, partial laryngectomy, and total laryngectomy (TL), each of which may result in varied severity and characteristics of dysphagia. From a functional perspective, the larynx can be anatomically divided into three regions: the supraglottis, glottis, and subglottis. Each functional region of the larynx has an important role in maintaining safe and efficient swallow function.

Supraglottic laryngeal tumors are typically surgically managed with supraglottic or supracricoid laryngectomy.[3,4] Alternatively, they may be treated with radiation and/or chemotherapy.[5] Surgical resection of the supraglottic larynx may include resection of parts of the hyoid bone, epiglottis, aryepiglottic folds, and false (ventricular) vocal folds. These structures each play an important role in achieving full closure of the laryngeal vestibule during the swallow. Laryngeal vestibule closure is critical to airway protection and relies on narrowing of the supraglottic region through anterior/superior excursion of the hyoid bone, epiglottic retroflexion, approximation of the arytenoids to the epiglottis, and adduction of the false vocal folds (see Chapter 4). As a result, surgical resection of the supraglottic region may impair airway protection, leading to aspiration and its associated risks.

The most common site of laryngeal cancer is the glottic larynx.[6] Glottic primary tumors may require minimally invasive surgery, vertical hemilaryngectomy, TL, or radiation-based treatment.[7] While supraglottic airway narrowing contributes greatly to airway protection, glottic closure is the final level of defense against aspiration. As such, surgery at the level of the glottis may lead to aspiration as well as reduced cough efficiency when aspiration occurs.

Cancers arising from or extending to the subglottic larynx will often require TL and/or radiation-based treatment. TL is typically associated with reduced swallowing efficiency due to surgical separation of the trachea and esophagus. This is related to reduced pharyngeal propulsive forces due to disruption of the pharyngeal constrictors, lack of hyolaryngeal excursion, and diminished opening of the upper esophageal sphincter (UES). Thus, while aspiration is not a concern for patients following TL, it is quite common for swallowing disorders to exist following TL. For limited resections of the subglottic larynx, swallowing deficits may be related to changes in sensory innervation of the subglottic mechanoreceptors critical for cough response when aspiration does occur.

Partial Laryngectomy and Swallowing

Partial laryngectomy procedures may be utilized as an alternative to radiation-based treatment for advanced stage larynx cancer.[8] Successful swallowing rehabilitation following partial laryngectomy depends on careful patient selection. Patient factors such as age, comorbidity, pulmonary reserve, motivation, and baseline swallow function should all be taken into consideration prior to proceeding with partial laryngectomy procedures.[9,10] In addition to patient factors, treatment factors such as extent of resection, site of resection, and the need for postoperative radiation therapy may influence swallowing outcomes.[11–13] Supraglottic and supracricoid laryngectomy are the most common partial laryngectomy procedures employed for management of laryngeal cancer.

Supraglottic laryngectomy involves removal of structures above the level of the glottis including the false vocal folds, aryepiglottic folds, and epiglottis. Therefore, the true vocal folds, arytenoids, and tongue base are the only remaining structures that can be used to achieve airway closure. Supraglottic laryngectomy can be accomplished through open surgical approaches through the neck or minimally invasive transoral endoscopic/laser resections. Following open supraglottic laryngectomy, patients may initiate limited oral intake within 1 month of surgery, but often require several months to return to a full oral diet.[14,15] More extensive surgeries, higher T-stage, and need for postoperative radiation are associated with prolonged recovery and more severe dysphagia.[14,16]

In contrast to open surgical approaches, endoscopic laser resection of supraglottic tumors is associated with more rapid return to oral intake and more favorable long-term swallowing outcomes.[17,18] This may be related to less tissue disruption as well as the preservation of the superior laryngeal nerve (SLN). The SLN is critical for maintenance of laryngeal sensation, which modulates the glottic closure reflex. In patients undergoing endoscopic supraglottic laryngectomy, the glottic closure reflex was observed in most patients within 72 h of surgery, while the majority of patients undergoing open surgery never recovered full function.[18] Newer robotic approaches also may provide additional minimally invasive approaches to partial laryngectomy.[19–21] In a series of 84 patients undergoing transoral robotic surgery for supraglottic laryngectomy, 24% initiated an oral diet by post-op day 1.[22] For the remainder of patients, median duration of tube feeding was only 8 days. It should be noted, however, that nearly 10%

of patients required long-term enteral feeding and 23% of patients developed aspiration pneumonia during post-op recovery. Thus, while these minimally invasive approaches may be preferable to open procedures, aspiration and dysphagia should be anticipated, particularly in the early post-op phase of recovery.

Aspiration due to lack of laryngeal vestibular closure is the primary swallowing deficit associated with supraglottic laryngectomy. Aspiration is most common in those undergoing Type IV supraglottic resection, which includes resection of the ventricular fold, and potentially the arytenoid.[23] Extended resections including the hyoid bone and tongue base may further impact bolus transit, increasing the presence of residue after the swallow as well as penetration/aspiration before and after the swallow. Thus, there are a complex of physiologic and anatomic changes that may be anticipated based on the extent of surgical resection.

Supracricoid laryngectomy includes the removal of the true and false vocal folds bilaterally, the entire thyroid cartilage, and at times the epiglottis and/or one arytenoid (cricohyoidepiglottopexy). Rehabilitation relies on apposition of the arytenoid to the epiglottis or base of tongue to achieve airway protection. While essentially all patients have dysphagia immediately after surgery, many series have reported recovery of swallowing function within 3 months of surgery for the majority of patients[24] (see Figs. 21.1 and 21.2). In fact, late complications such as aspiration pneumonia, feeding tube dependence, and transition to functional TL have been infrequently reported.[24] However,

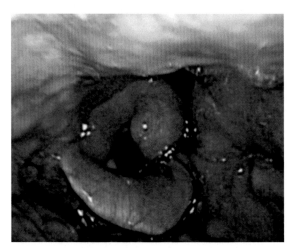

FIG. 21.1 Initial fiberoptic endoscopic evaluation of swallowing 2 weeks following supracricoid partial laryngectomy. Note poor pharyngeal clearance and infiltration of blue contrast in the laryngeal vestibule.

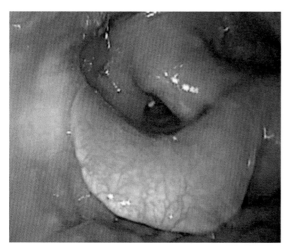

FIG. 21.2 Follow-up fiberoptic endoscopic evaluation of swallowing 3 months following supracricoid partial laryngectomy. Note improved pharyngeal clearance and lack of laryngeal penetration.

Simonelli et al.[25] reported an aspiration rate of 38% in patients >3 years post-op suggesting there may be a need to monitor these patients over time for the impact of progressive fibrosis or aging.

Total Laryngectomy and Swallowing

TL involves the surgical removal of the larynx and establishment of tracheal stoma on the neck skin, thus permanently separating the airway and swallowing. As a result of the division of these systems, airway protection is no longer a concern; however, swallowing efficiency is often impaired. In a 2002 report by Ward et al.,[26] only 58% of patients undergoing TL and 50% of those undergoing total laryngopharyngectomy were able to enjoy a normal diet in 3 years following surgery. Maclean et al.[27] surveyed 110 laryngectomees in Australia regarding swallowing function. Their data demonstrated that 71% self-reported some degree of dysphagia following TL. Swallowing complaints included food sticking in the throat daily, longer time required to swallow, and tightness in the throat daily. Social eating was reportedly avoided in 57% of those reporting dysphagia. Those patients reporting dysphagia were more likely to have depression, anxiety, and stress in comparison to those who did not report dysphagia after TL. Patients with dysphagia following TL may report an increased sense of social isolation due to the combined impact of their communication and swallowing difficulties.[28] Thus, while aspiration may not be a concern after TL, dysphagia may still have significant implications.

The assessment of dysphagia following TL requires direct visualization of the swallowing passage to ascertain the exact etiology. The videofluoroscopic swallowing study (VFSS) is the most effective method for evaluating swallowing following TL. The VFSS is preferred in this population as it allows for visualization of the UES and cervical esophagus as well as assessment of bolus flow through the neopharynx. It should be emphasized that the intent of the VFSS with laryngectomees is not to evaluate for aspiration but rather to assess for other factors such as postoperative fistulas, strictures, efficiency of bolus clearance, and pseudoepiglottis and pseudovallecula. The VFSS can also be used to assess the cervical esophagus in relation to tracheoesophageal voice prosthesis issues. With the rising incidence of salvage laryngectomy following radiation-based treatment in contrast to primary laryngectomy,[29] the VFSS is increasingly used following surgery to assess healing and identifying potential complications such as pharyngocutaneous fistula. Historically, pharyngocutaneous fistula was uncommon and impacted less than 20% of patients; however, in the era of salvage surgery, rates have risen to nearly 30%.[30,31] The presence of a postoperative fistula will delay initiation of oral intake. A prolonged nil per os (NPO) status may result in issues such as atrophy, fibrosis, and stricture leading to further delays in diet advancement. While pharyngocutaneous fistula has a marked impact on oral intake, it is typically a transient condition expected to resolve over time.

Disruption of typical pharyngeal physiologic function is anticipated following laryngectomy; however, unlike pharyngocutaneous fistula, these issues do not typically resolve with time. Thus, the swallowing problems associated with changes in the pharyngeal swallow apparatus are likely to persist over time and are likely to be of greater severity in patients undergoing salvage laryngectomy.[32,33] One common issue impacting the efficiency of bolus clearance is related to the removal of the hyolaryngeal complex. The elevation and anterior excursion of the hyolaryngeal complex is responsible for the traction forces that pull open the UES. Thus, disruption of this force may result in decreased bolus clearance into the esophagus. Driving pressures behind the bolus are also important for pharyngeal clearance and bolus entry into the esophagus. Disruption of the pharyngeal constrictors will result in lower bolus driving pressures, thus impacting both pharyngeal stripping and UES opening. Typically, a myotomy will be performed during TL to reduce resistance at the level of the UES.[34]

In addition to the alteration of muscular influences leading to reduced traction of and pressure against the

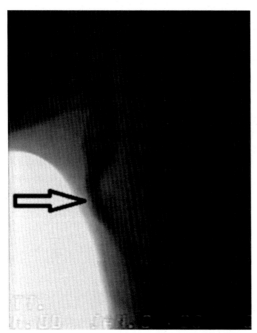

FIG. 21.3 Demonstration of narrowing at the esophageal inlet on videofluoroscopy following total laryngectomy (TL) despite completion of myotomy (*arrow*). This is a common finding explaining elevated intrabolus pressure following TL.

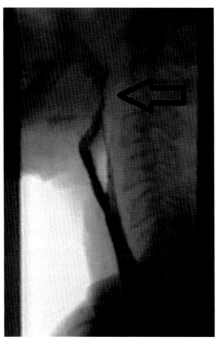

FIG. 21.4 Demonstration of poor pharyngeal propulsive forces (*arrow*) on videofluoroscopy following total laryngectomy. Poor pharyngeal clearing forces may lead to pharyngeal residue, increased effort with swallowing, and/or regurgitation into the oral and nasal passages.

UES, stricture may further restrict bolus flow into the esophagus. Stricture is a common challenge after TL with incidence rates ranging from ∼19% to 39%.[35,36] Strictures are particularly common in patients undergoing salvage surgery with hypopharyngeal primary tumors, closed primarily rather than with free tissue transfer, in females and in those requiring extended laryngectomy.[37–39] Dilation or stretching of the region of stricture has been the primary treatment approach; however, in order to adequately manage stricture, dilation may need to be repeated multiple times.[40]

Manometric assessment has contributed greatly to our understanding of pressure changes following TL. Most notably, manometry has demonstrated that intrabolus pressures are consistently high following laryngectomy and that higher intrabolus pressure is associated with worse patient perceived dysphagia.[40] This suggests that despite the typical practice of myotomy during laryngectomy, there remains obstruction of bolus flow at the level of the UES (see Fig. 21.3). Additionally, hypopharyngeal peak contraction is typically lower in patients following laryngectomy in comparison to controls, although not associated with increasing dysphagia severity[40,41] (see Fig. 21.4).

Another possible contributor to postlaryngectomy dysphagia is the formation of a pseudoepiglottis/pseudovallecula. This is a structural byproduct of vertical closure and looks much like a normal epiglottis/vallecula on videofluoroscopy[36] (see Fig. 21.5). In Davis' series, all patients with vertical closure and two-thirds of patients with T-closure had pseudoepiglottis following TL. As the pseudoepiglottis is an immobile structure, foods and liquids may build up in the pseudovallecular space, potentially backflowing into the oral or nasal passages. If warranted, laser resection may be offered to eliminate this problem.

TREATMENT OF DYSPHAGIA FOLLOWING LARYNGECTOMY

Dysphagia management in patients with laryngeal cancer often requires a multidisciplinary approach. While surgical strategies may be necessary in some cases, behavioral rehabilitation also plays a critical role. Optimal outcomes can be anticipated when the multidisciplinary team provides collaborative care.[42] Behavioral intervention is typically provided by speech

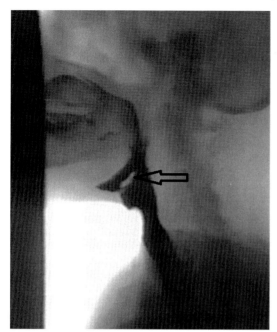

FIG. 21.5 Demonstration of a pseudoepiglottis and pseudovallecula on videofluoroscopy following total laryngectomy.

language pathologists (SLPs) while surgical intervention is typically provided by otolaryngologists and/or gastroenterologists. Other members of the multidisciplinary team may include dieticians, nursing staff, and the patient's caregivers.

Behavioral Treatment

Behavioral treatment of dysphagia after treatment for laryngeal cancer may include compensatory postures and strategies, diet modifications, and therapeutic exercise. Treatments should be selected based on comprehensive assessment of the specific nature of the swallowing deficits. SLPs working with patients with laryngeal cancer need to have a firm and comprehensive understanding of swallowing physiology and the structures impacted by treatment in order to devise an appropriate treatment plan. In the absence of clinical trials demonstrating superiority of particular exercises, the SLP must enlist their knowledge and expertise to select the most appropriate exercises.

Following partial laryngectomy procedures, the most common therapeutic target is establishing alternative methods of airway protection. The supraglottic and super-supraglottic swallowing maneuvers are commonly employed following supraglottic laryngectomy. These

techniques aim to facilitate glottal airway closure prior to and while the bolus remains within the pharynx. The swallow is followed by a throat clear prior to inspiration to expel any residual material on the superior aspect of the vocal folds.[43] The super-supraglottic swallow adds an increase in effort in order to further narrow the laryngeal inlet through apposition of the tongue base to the arytenoids. For patients undergoing supracricoid laryngectomy, airway closure is typically accomplished when the arytenoid(s) appose against the remnant epiglottis or tongue base. This is often accomplished by asking the patient to hold their breath and bear down. Ideally, patients will be trained in these compensatory maneuvers prior to surgery to facilitate the ease of use following surgery. Following surgery, training these new mechanisms of airway closure is often slow and stepwise, starting with managing secretions and subsequently advancing slowly from thicker items like purees to thinner liquids. Endoscopic biofeedback can be quite beneficial for patients learning new methods of swallowing.

Additional compensations may be chosen to impact bolus flow properties. For example, a chin tuck posture may be employed to minimize the potential of airway infiltration prior to the swallow response. In cases where there is asymmetry, a head turn to the impaired side may assist with bolus diversion to the intact side. The use of diet modifications such as thicker liquids and avoidance of mixed consistencies may also be employed to increase swallowing safety.

In addition to swallowing maneuvers, the SLP should utilize therapeutic exercise to address physiologic deficits noted from the instrumental swallowing study. Commonly, for patients with laryngeal cancer, exercises may include effortful swallow, the Mendelsohn maneuver, the Masako maneuver, and the Shaker exercises. The effortful swallow has been shown to result in increased duration of laryngeal vestibular closure, increased hyoid excursion, and longer duration of pharyngeal pressure.[44] The Mendelsohn maneuver is associated with increased pharyngeal contraction, hyolaryngeal excursion, and duration of cricopharyngeal opening.[45] The Masako maneuver is associated with higher pressure between the tongue base and the posterior pharyngeal wall.[46] The Shaker exercise targets the suprahyoid musculature in an attempt to increase extent and duration of UES opening.[47]

While structural changes following TL are typically not impacted by behavioral intervention, the SLP working with laryngectomees should consider therapeutic intervention and compensatory strategies that may help improve bolus flow. Swallowing exercises targeting tongue strength and base of tongue retraction may improve bolus clearance and reduce the severity of dysphagia. Compensations are commonly recommended by the SLP and may include alternating liquids and solids and the avoidance of problematic food items.

While the focus of this chapter is on surgical swallowing outcomes, it must be acknowledged that many patients undergoing laryngeal resection will also require radiation and/or chemotherapy. Interventions should be applied prior to the onset of radiation to minimize the potential for disuse atrophy and fibrosis. A number of studies have supported the importance of prophylactic swallowing exercises in individuals undergoing radiation-based therapy for head and neck cancers.[48-50] Further, there is evidence that avoidance of NPO status during radiation is associated with more favorable swallowing outcomes.[51,52] Thus, it is critical that the SLP be an active team member in the care of patients with laryngeal cancer through all stages of treatment.

Unfortunately, despite the important role of the SLP in assessing pre- and posttreatment swallowing function, administering pre-and rehabilitative exercises, and prescribing compensatory strategies and dietary modifications, patients with laryngeal cancer may have limited interaction with the SLP over the course of their care. In a study using Medicare Surveillance, Epidemiology, and End Result data to evaluate the use and impact of SLP care on patients with laryngeal cancer over the age of 65 years in the United States, only 6% were seen by SLPs between diagnosis and 6 months following completion of primary therapy.[53] Further, less than a quarter of patients were seen by an SLP at some point between cancer diagnosis and 5 years later. However, patients were most likely to consult with SLPs during the initial treatment phase if undergoing TL or if presenting with dysphagic symptoms. Long-term SLP care was seen most in individuals with dysphagia, TL, tracheostomy, or salvage surgery. Yet, when SLP care was provided, it significantly reduced the risk of stricture, weight loss, dysphagia, and aspiration pneumonia. Finally, SLP care was associated with reduced risk of death. These data collectively support the value of the SLPs in not only caring for the patient with laryngeal cancer but also in highlighting the underutilization of SLPs in older patients with laryngeal cancer posttreatment outcome.

Surgical Treatment

Preventive surgical measures may be considered to minimize the potential for postoperative dysphagia. These primarily include strategies to reduce resistance

at the level of the UES in order to facilitate pharyngeal clearance. Cricopharyngeal myotomy is commonly employed during partial and TL procedures to optimize swallowing outcomes.[54] However, there is conflicting evidence as to the extent of benefit it yields, which may suggest that in some cases of failed UES opening treated with myotomy, muscular tonicity was not the primary cause of failed UES opening.[55-57] Hence, careful consideration of the underlying mechanism of failed UES opening is critical to determining surgical candidacy. Cricopharyngeal myotomy can also be completed independent of ablative surgery if dysphagia is associated with cricopharyngeal hypertonicity. In addition to cricopharyngeal myotomy, laryngeal suspension is frequently utilized to optimize swallowing safety in individuals undergoing partial laryngectomy.[58] This technique tucks the exposed glottic larynx under the tongue base to facilitate airway protection and may facilitate UES opening due to anterior traction of the cricopharyngeus muscle.

Additionally, reconstructive options following TL may influence swallowing outcomes. Patients receiving mucosa—muscle closure have been shown to have more favorable peak pharyngeal pressures and pharyngeal clearance than patients receiving mucosal-only closure.[59] Patients receiving pectoralis major flaps appear to be at higher risk for stricture-associated dysphagia than patients receiving free flap reconstruction.[60,61] Thus, when appropriate, free tissue transfer reconstruction appears to have more favorable swallowing outcomes following TL.

Stricture is one of the common causes of dysphagia following laryngeal cancer treatment requiring surgical management. It is important to determine the length of the stenotic site during videofluoroscopy as strictures longer than 2—5 cm are typically less responsive to minimally invasive dilation strategies and may require more extensive surgical management.[62] In a recent systematic review of the literature regarding dilation in head and neck cancer patients, the success rate for dilation was estimated to be 72.9%, though the methods utilized to measure success varied widely among studies.[63] Commonly, patients require multiple dilations to maintain a patent swallowing tract.[63,64] It should be noted, that across series, complication rates were estimated at ~ 10% suggesting that the devascularized, fibrotic tissue often seen following radiation therapy may result in elevated risk of esophageal tears or perforations. The clinician treating radiation-induced strictures must remain mindful of this elevated risk. Botulinum toxin has also played a role in the management of cricopharyngeal spasm following partial laryngectomy and TL, and may, however, require repeated injections to maintain efficacy.[65,66]

SUMMARY

Patients with laryngeal cancer undergoing partial laryngectomy and TL can be expected to have significant changes in their swallowing function. Changes may impact both the safety and efficiency of swallowing leading to medical, nutritional, and psychosocial consequences. The multidisciplinary swallowing team plays a pivotal role in the evaluation of the underlying nature of the dysphagia as well as the determination of the most appropriate treatment strategies including behavioral therapies and medical/surgical intervention.

REFERENCES

1. Burnip E, Owen SJ, Barker S, Patterson JM. Swallowing outcomes following surgical and non-surgical treatment for advanced laryngeal cancer. *J Laryngol Otol*. 2013;127:1116−1121.
2. Howlader N, Noone AM, Krapcho M, et al., eds. *SEER Cancer Statistics Review, 1975-2014*. Bethesda, MD: National Cancer Institute; April 2017. https://seer.cancer.gov/csr/1975_2014/. Based on November 2016 SEER data submission, posted to the SEER web site.
3. Spriano G, Antognoni P, Piantanida R, et al. Conservative management of T1-T2N0 supraglottic cancer: a retrospective study. *Am J Otolaryngol*. 1997;18:229−305.
4. Ferlito A, Silver CE, Howard DJ, et al. The role of partial laryngeal resection in current management of laryngeal cancer: a collective review. *Acta Otolaryngol*. 2000;120:456−465.
5. Meyers EN, Alvi A. Management of carcinoma of the supraglottic larynx: evolution, current concepts, and future trends. *Laryngoscope*. 1996;106:559−567.
6. Chu EA, Kim Y. Laryngeal cancer: diagnosis and preoperative work-up. *Otolaryngol Clin N Am*. 2008;41(4):673−695.
7. Hartl DM. Evidence-based practice: management of glottic cancer. *Otolaryngol Clin N Am*. 2012;45:1143−1161.
8. Harris BN, Bhuskute AA, Rao S, Farwell DG, Bewley AF. Primary surgery for advanced-stage laryngeal cancer: a stage and sub-site specific survival analysis. *Head Neck*. 2016;38:1380−1386.
9. Benito J, Holsinger FC, Perez-Martin A, et al. Aspiration after supracricoid partial laryngectomy: incidence, risk factors, management, and outcomes. *Head Neck*. 2011;33(5):679−685.
10. Tufano R. Organ preservation for laryngeal cancer. *Otolaryngol Clin N Am*. 2002;35:1067−1080.
11. Breunig C, Benter P, Seidl RO, Coordes A. Predictable swallowing function after open horizontal supraglottic partial laryngectomy. *Auris Nasus Larynx*. 2016;43(6):658−665.
12. Bussu F, Galli J, Valenza V, et al. Evaluation of swallowing function after supracricoid laryngectomy as a primary or salvage procedure. *Dysphagia*. 2015;30(6):686−694.
13. Clayburgh DR, Graville DJ, Palmer AD, Schindler JS. Factors associated with supracricoid laryngectomy functional outcomes. *Head Neck*. 2013;35(10):1397−1403.
14. Lazarus CL. Management of swallowing disorders in head and neck cancer patients: optimal patterns of care. *Semin Speech Lang*. 2000;21:293−309.
15. Logemann JA, Gibbons P, Rademaker AW, et al. Mechanisms of recovery of swallow after supraglottic laryngectomy. *J Speech Hear Res*. 1994;37:965−974.
16. Wasserman T, Murry T, Johnson JT, Myers EN. Management of swallowing in supraglottic and extended supraglottic laryngectomy patients. *Head Neck*. 2001;23:1043−1048.
17. Jepsen MC, Gurushanthaiah D, Roy N, et al. Voice, speech, and swallowing outcomes in laser-treated laryngeal cancer. *Laryngoscope*. 2003;113:923−928.
18. Sasaki CT, Leder SB, Acton LM, Maune S. Comparison of the glottic closure reflex in traditional "open" versus endoscopic laser supraglottic laryngectomy. *Ann Otol Rhinol Laryngol*. 2006;115:93−96.
19. Park YM, Byeon HK, Chung HP, Choi EC, Kim SH. Comparison of treatment outcomes after transoral robotic surgery and supraglottic partial laryngectomy: our experience with seventeen and seventeen patients respectively. *Clin Otolaryngol*. 2013;38(3):270−274.
20. Mendelsohn AH, Remacle M, Van Der Vorst S, Bachy V, Lawson G. Outcomes following transoral robotic surgery: supraglottic laryngectomy. *Laryngoscope*. 2013;123(1):208−214.
21. Ozer E, Alvarez B, Kakarala K, et al. Clinical outcomes of transoral robotic supraglottic laryngectomy. *Head Neck*. 2013;35(8):1158−1161.
22. Razafindranaly V, Lallemant B, Aubry K, et al. Clinical outcomes with transoral robotic surgery for supraglottic squamous cell carcinoma: experience of a French evaluation cooperative subgroup of GETTEC. *Head Neck*. 2016;38:E1097−E1101.
23. Piazza C, Barbieri D, Del Bon F, et al. Functional outcomes after different types of transoral supraglottic laryngectomy. *Laryngoscope*. 2016;126:1131−1135.
24. Lips M, Speyer R, Zumach A, Kross KW, Kremer B. Supracricoid laryngectomy and dysphagia: a systematic literature review. *Laryngoscope*. 2015;125(9):2143−2156.
25. Simonelli M, Ruoppolo G, de Vincentiis M, et al. Swallowing ability and chronic aspiration after supracricoid partial laryngectomy. *Otolaryngol Head Neck Surg*. 2010;142(6):873−878.
26. Ward EC, Bishop B, Frisby J, Stevens M. Swallowing outcomes following laryngectomy and pharyngolaryngectomy. *Arch Otolaryngol Head Neck Surg*. 2002;128(2):181−186.
27. Maclean J, Cotton S, Perry A. Dysphagia following a total laryngectomy: the effect on quality of life, functioning, and psychological well-being. *Dysphagia*. 2009;24:314−321.

28. Doyle PC. *Foundations of Voice and Speech Rehabilitation Following Laryngeal Cancer.* San Diego, CA: Singular Publishing Group; 1994.

29. Maddox PT, Davies L. Trends in total laryngectomy in the era of organ preservation: a population-based study. *Otolaryngol Head Neck Surg.* 2012;147(1):85–90.

30. Paydarfar JA, Birkmeyer NJ. Complications in head and neck surgery: a meta-analysis of postlaryngectomy pharyngocutaneous fistula. *Arch Otolaryngol Head Neck Surg.* 2006;132:67–72.

31. Hasan Z, Dwivedi RC, Gunaratne DA, et al. Systematic review and meta-analysis of the complications of salvage total laryngectomy. *Eur J Surg Oncol.* 2017;43:42–51.

32. Arinaz BB, Pendelton H, Westin U, Rydell R. Voice and swallowing after total laryngectomy. *Acta Otolaryngol.* 2017;5:1–5.

33. Robertson SM, Yeo JC, Dunnet C, Young D, Mackenzie K. Voice, swallowing, and quality of life after total laryngectomy: results of the west of Scotland laryngectomy audit. *Head Neck.* 2012;34(1):59–65.

34. Horowitz JB, Sasaki CT. Effect of cricopharyngeus myotomy on postlaryngectomy pharyngeal contraction pressures. *Laryngoscope.* 1993;103:138–140.

35. Sweeny L, Golden JB, White HN, et al. Incidence and outcomes of stricture formation postlaryngectomy. *Otolaryngol Head Neck Surg.* 2012;146(3):395–402.

36. Davis R, Vincent M, Shapshay S, Strong M. The anatomy and complications of "T" closure versus vertical closure of the hypopharynx after laryngectomy. *Laryngoscope.* 1982;92:16–22.

37. Vu KN, Day TA, Gillespie MB, et al. Proximal esophageal stenosis in head and neck cancer patients after total laryngectomy and radiation. *ORL J Otorhinolaryngol Realt Spec.* 2008;70:229–235.

38. Nyquist GG, Hier MP, Dionisopoulos T, Black MJ. Stricture associated with primary tracheoesophageal puncture after pharyngolaryngectomy and free jejunal interposition. *Head Neck.* 2006;28:205–209.

39. Wulff NB, Kristensen CA, Andersen E, et al. Risk factors for postoperative complications after total laryngectomy following radiotherapy or chemoradiation; a 10-year retrospective longitudinal study in Eastern Denmark. *Clin Otolaryngol.* 2015;40:662–671.

40. Zhang T, Szczeniak M, Maclean J, et al. Biomechanics of pharyngeal deglutitive function following total laryngectomy. *Otolaryngol Head Neck Surg.* 2016;155:295–302.

41. Lippert D, Hoffman MR, Britt CJ, et al. Preliminary evaluation of functional swallow after total laryngectomy using high-resolution manometry. *Ann Otol Rhinol Laryngol.* 2016;125(7):541–549.

42. Starmer HM, Ayoub N, Byward C, et al. The impact of developing a speech and swallow rehab program: impact of multidisciplinary care. *Laryngoscope.* 2017;127(11):2578–2581.

43. Ohmae Y, Logemann JA, Kaiser P, Hanson DG, Kahrilas PJ. Effects of two breath-holding maneuvers on oropharyngeal swallow. *Ann Otol Rhinol Laryngol.* 1996;105:123–131.

44. Hind JA, Nicosia MA, Roecker EB, et al. Comparison of effortful and noneffortful swallows in healthy middle-aged and older adults. *Arch Phys Med Rehabil.* 2001;82:1661–1665.

45. Boden K, Hallgren A, Witt Hedstrom H. Effects of three different swallow maneuvers analyzed by videomanometry. *Acta Radiol.* 2006;47:628–633.

46. Lazarus CL, Logemann JA, Song CW, et al. Effects of voluntary maneuvers on tongue base function for swallowing. *Folia Phoniatr Logop.* 2002;54:171–176.

47. Easterling C, Kern M, Nitschke T, et al. A novel rehabilitative exercise for dysphagia patients: effect on swallow function and biomechanics. *Gastroenterology.* 1998;114:A747.

48. Carroll WR, Locher JL, Canon CL, et al. Pretreatment swallowing exercises improve swallow function after chemoradiation. *Laryngoscope.* 2008;118:39–43.

49. Kotz T, Federman AD, Kao J, et al. Prophylactic swallowing exercises in patients with head and neck cancer undergoing chemoradiation: a randomized trial. *Arch Otolaryngol Head Neck Surg.* 2012;138:376–382.

50. Carnaby-Mann G, Crary MA, Schmalfus I, Amdur R. "Pharyngocise": randomized control trial of preventative exercises to maintain muscle structure and swallowing function during head and neck chemoradiotherapy. *Int J Radiat Oncol Bio Phys.* 2012;83:210–219.

51. Langmore S, Krisciunas GP, Miloro KV, Evans SR, Cheng DM. Does PEG cause dysphagia in head and neck cancer patients? *Dysphagia.* 2012;27:251–259.

52. Hutcheson KA, Bhayani MK, Beadle BM, et al. Eat and exercise during radiotherapy or chemoradiotherapy for pharyngeal cancers. Use it or lose it. *JAMA Otolaryngol Head Neck Surg.* 2013;139:1127–1134.

53. Starmer HM, Quon H, Simpson M, et al. Speech-language pathology care and short- and long-term outcomes of laryngeal cancer treatment in the elderly. *Laryngoscope.* 2015;125:2756–2763.

54. Hirano M, Tateishi M, Kurita S, Matsuoka H. Deglutition following supraglottic horizontal laryngectomy. *Ann Otol Rhinol Laryngol.* 1987;96:7–11.

55. Jacobs JR, Logemann J, Pajak TF, et al. Failure of cricopharyngeal myotomy to improve dysphagia following head and neck cancer surgery. *Arch Otolaryngol Head Neck Surg.* 1999;125(9):942–946.

56. Knigge MA, Thibeault SL. Swallowing outcomes after cricopharyngeal myotomy: a systematic review. *Head Neck.* October 30, 2017;40(1):203–212.

57. Yip HT, Leonard R, Kendall KA. Cricopharyngeal myotomy normalizes the opening size of the upper esophageal sphincter in cricopharyngeal dysfunction. *Laryngoscope.* 2006;116:93–96.

58. Calcaterra TC. Laryngeal suspension after supraglottic laryngectomy. *Arch Otolaryngol.* 1971;94(4):306–309.

59. Maclean J, Szczesniak M, Cotton S, et al. Swallowing outcomes following laryngectomy and pharyngolaryngectomy. *Arch Otolaryngol Head Neck Surg.* 2011;144:21–28.
60. Piazza C, Taglietti V, Nicolai P. Reconstructive options after total laryngectomy with subtotal or circumferential hypopharyngectomy and cervical esophagectomy. *Curr Opin Otolaryngol Head Neck Surg.* 2012;20(2): 77–88.
61. Nguyen S, Thuot F. Functional outcomes of fasciocutaneous free flap and pectoralis major flap for salvage total laryngectomy. *Head Neck.* 2017;39(9):1797–1805.
62. Sullivan CA, Jaklitsch MT, Haddad R, et al. Endoscopic management of hypopharyngeal stenosis after organ sparing therapy for head and neck cancer. *Laryngoscope.* 2004;14:1924–1931.
63. Moss WJ, Pang J, Orosco RK, et al. Esophageal dilation in head and neck cancer patients: a systematic review and meta-analysis. *Laryngoscope.* May 12, 2017;128(1):111–117.
64. Harris RL, Grundy A, Odutoye T. Radiologically guided balloon dilatation of neopharyngeal strictures following total laryngectomy and pharyngolaryngectomy: 21 years' experience. *J Laryngol Otol.* 2010;124(2):175–179.
65. Crary MA, Glowasky AL. Using botulinum toxin A to improve speech and swallowing function following total laryngectomy. *Arch Otolaryngol Head Neck Surg.* 1996; 122:760–763.
66. Ashan SF, Meleca RJ, Dworkin JP. Botulinum toxin injection of the cricopharyngeal muscle for the treatment of dysphagia. *Otolaryngol Head Neck Surg.* 2000;122: 691–695.

CHAPTER 22

Esophageal Dysphagia

IAN T. MACQUEEN, MD • DAVID CHEN, MD

INTRODUCTION

Esophageal dysphagia may be defined as dysphagia caused by a structural or functional abnormality of the esophagus, lower esophageal sphincter (LES), or cardia of the stomach. It is characterized by impaired swallowing that occurs several seconds after initiating a swallow. These symptoms may occur in isolation or in a widely variable constellation of associated symptoms. The pathophysiologic causes of esophageal motility similarly vary broadly and comprise a range of primary and secondary (i.e., as the result of another local or systemic disease process) disorders. The majority of pathologic processes causing esophageal dysphagia are manifested in middle age, though some such as esophageal and esophagogastric junction (EGJ) cancers occur more commonly in the elderly.[1]

PATHOPHYSIOLOGY

Causes of esophageal dysphagia can be divided into primary disorders of motility, secondary effects of systemic or infiltrative processes, and structural abnormalities. Structural etiologies are further divided into benign and malignant causes. These broad groups and the causes specific to each are discussed below.

Esophageal Dysmotility

Esophageal dysmotility refers to impaired or ineffective esophageal contraction. As with esophageal dysphagia in general, causes may be primary or secondary. Primary disorders of esophageal motility include *achalasia*, distal *esophageal spasm* (DES), and *hypercontractile* esophagus (jackhammer esophagus).

Achalasia is characterized by abnormal peristalsis and impaired relaxation of the LES, preventing transit of swallowed bolus at that site. Achalasia may be primary or idiopathic, or may occur secondary to other disease processes, most notably *Chagas disease*, which is caused by the parasite *Trypanosoma cruzi*. Additionally, it is known to be one of the manifestations of *Allgrove disease*, along with adrenal insufficiency and alacrima.

The pathophysiology of achalasia is poorly understood, but impaired relaxation is thought to be caused by inflammatory degradation of neurons in esophageal myenteric plexuses.[2,3] Achalasia is clinically divided into subcategories based on the results of esophageal manometry[4]: Type I (classic achalasia), achalasia with no esophageal pressurization; Type II, achalasia with panesophageal pressurization; Type III (spastic achalasia), achalasia with spastic esophageal contraction. Pseudoachalasia or EGJ outflow obstruction (Fig. 22.1) is a related disorder with abnormally high relaxation pressures at the LES but is distinguished from achalasia by the presence of normal peristalsis.

Hypercontractile or jackhammer esophagus is characterized by high amplitude, coordinated contraction propagated through the esophagus. It may occur through the entire esophagus or segmentally.[4] This terminology has replaced the previously described phenomenon of hypertensive peristalsis or nutcracker esophagus.[5] The pathophysiology of this condition is mediated by a hyperactive response to excitatory innervation on the smooth muscle of the esophagus.[6]

DES (sometimes referred to by the less accurate term, "diffuse esophageal spasm"[7]) is characterized by premature and disordered esophageal contractions, with or without the presence of normal peristalsis. The underlying pathophysiologic cause is poorly understood

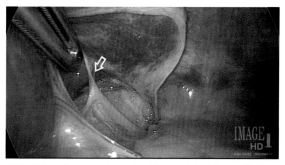

FIG. 22.1 Scarring (*arrow*) with herniated fundoplication causing esophageal outlet obstruction.

but is thought to be associated with impaired inhibitory innervation.[8,9] The result is premature contractions and abnormally high contraction propagation velocity in the distal esophagus.

Infiltrative and Systemic Causes

A wide range of infiltrative and systemic conditions can have secondary effects on the esophagus, causing esophageal dysphagia. The following description is not an exhaustive list but covers some of the more common causes.

Scleroderma and systemic sclerosis have wide-reaching systemic effects, and upward of 70% of patients may have esophageal manifestations of their disease.[10,11] Systemic sclerosis affects the microvasculature, nervous system, and immune system, leading to organ dysfunction and ultimately to fibrosis. In the esophagus, this leads to muscular atrophy and fibrosis in the distal two-thirds of the esophageal body and in the LES. These changes result in hypotensive peristalsis and impaired bolus transit in the affected region, as well as incompetence of the LES and gastroesophageal reflux.

Eosinophilic esophagitis may result from gastroesophageal reflux disease (GERD), infection, diet, or medications, or it may be idiopathic (see Chapter 23). It is characterized by predominantly eosinophilic inflammatory infiltration of the esophagus in the presence of clinical symptoms frequently including dysphagia, odynophagia, and food impaction.

Infectious esophagitis can similarly cause dysphagia and odynophagia. Infectious esophagitis is uncommon in immune competent patients but occurs more frequently in the setting of immune compromise. Common pathogens include herpes simplex virus (HSV), cytomegalovirus, and candida.

Caustic ingestion can cause esophageal dysphagia through direct immediate injury and through the sequalae of healing. Injury severity is related to the caustic properties, volume, and concentration of the ingested substance, and to the duration of contact with the esophageal surface. Alkali ingestions, as compared to acid ingestions, are more likely to cause esophageal injury.[12] Alkali causes rapid liquefactive necrosis of the mucosa and esophageal wall and may extend transmurally if enough of the substance is ingested. Acid ingestion causes a superficial coagulation necrosis, in which the coagulation and consolidation of mucosa and superficial tissues have a protective effect on the underlying structures of the esophageal wall.[13,14] In either scenario, life-threatening complications are possible. Even in the absence of severe progression or complications, the resulting inflammatory state persists

and may cause dysphagia and odynophagia for weeks. Healing from these injuries often results in esophageal stricture, which may additionally contribute to dysphagia as discussed below.

Benign Mechanical Causes

Structural abnormalities may cause dysphagia via partial or total obstruction of the esophagus, or by disruption of normal motility. The following discussion of mechanical sources of esophageal dysphagia is not exhaustive.

Esophageal stricture is a common benign mechanical cause of esophageal dysphagia. Strictures are the result of fibrosis, the underlying causes of which may include GERD (most common cause), eosinophilic esophagitis, radiation exposure, caustic ingestion, surgical anastomosis, and external compression from fibrosing processes of the mediastinum (e.g., secondary to tuberculosis).

Esophageal rings refer to concentric bands of tissue protruding into the esophageal lumen. Rings may be mucosal in composition or may less frequently involve the muscle of the esophagus. The pathogenesis of these rings is unclear, with separate hypotheses suggesting that they are the result of chronic GERD and that they are congenital in origin. The most common esophageal ring is the *Schatzki ring*, which occurs at the squamocolumnar junction.

Hiatal and paraesophageal hernias may contribute to esophageal dysphagia. A hiatal hernia is present when the EGJ is displaced proximally above the diaphragm into the thorax. A paraesophageal hernia is present when the gastric fundus (or other intraabdominal organ) herniates through a localized defect in the phrenoesophageal membrane (Fig. 22.2). These hernias may be present independently or in combination. Dysphagia may result as a secondary effect of GERD, most common with isolated hiatal hernia, or from external compression by hernia contents on the esophagus.

Gastric volvulus is characterized by rotation of the stomach along its longitudinal or transverse axis. When this occurs chronically, it may cause mechanical obstruction at the EGJ, resulting in esophageal dysphagia. Gastric volvulus may occur independently or in the setting of hiatal or paraesophageal hernia (Fig. 22.2).

Benign esophageal neoplasms are a mechanical cause of esophageal dysphagia. The most common benign neoplasms occurring in the esophagus are *leiomyomas* (Fig. 22.3). These are submucosal mesenchymal tumors and usually occur in the mid or distal esophagus.

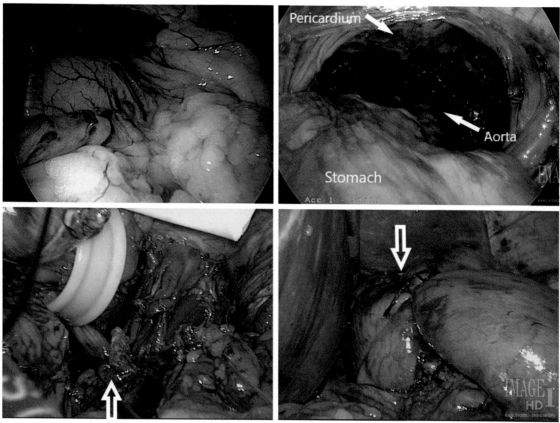

FIG. 22.2 Paraesophageal hernia. Giant paraesophageal hernia viewed from the abdomen, with gastric volvulus and intrathoracic stomach (*upper left*; hernia most easily seen as dark area at the top of the image); reduced hiatal hernia with visible aorta and pericardium (*upper right*); Posterior hiatal repair (*lower left*; penrose around esophagus, repair marked by *arrow*); Nissen fundoplication (*lower right*, *arrow marks* fundus sutured around esophagus).

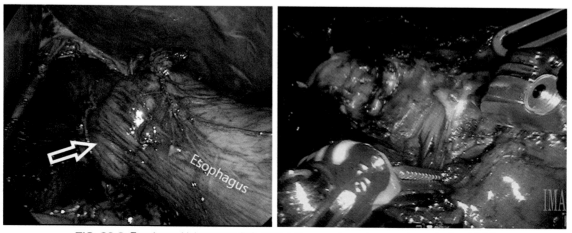

FIG. 22.3 Esophageal leiomyoma (*left*, marked by *arrow*); myotomy and enucleation (*right*).

Dysphagia occurs typically only when one of these tumors grows to large size.

Malignant Mechanical Causes

Esophageal and gastric cancers are an important cause to consider in patients with esophageal dysphagia. Cancers arising from the esophagus and cardia of the stomach may cause mechanical obstruction or motility disruption leading to dysphagia. Relevant malignancies include squamous cell carcinoma (SCC), adenocarcinoma, and gastrointestinal stromal tumor (GIST). Representative examples are shown in Fig. 22.4.

Esophageal cancer can arise anywhere along the length of the esophagus. Malignant tumors in the proximal and mid esophagus tend to be SCC, while those in the distal third of the esophagus are more commonly

adenocarcinoma. Esophageal SCC is associated with exposures to tobacco, alcohol, extremely hot drinks, and betel nut.[15,16] Adenocarcinoma of the esophagus or EGJ is associated with tobacco, obesity, and GERD, especially after progression to Barrett's esophagus.[17–19] EGJ cancers occur in three subtypes. The first is adenocarcinoma of the distal esophagus, as described above. The second type is true gastric cardia cancer, adenocarcinoma arising from the epithelium of the gastric cardia. The third type is subcardial gastric adenocarcinoma, originating distal to the EGJ and invading from below.

GISTs of the esophagus or proximal stomach may cause esophageal dysphagia. These tumors are submucosal sarcomas originating in the smooth muscle pacemaker cell of Cajal. The neoplastic behavior of a GIST is the result of mutations in the C-KIT gene. The

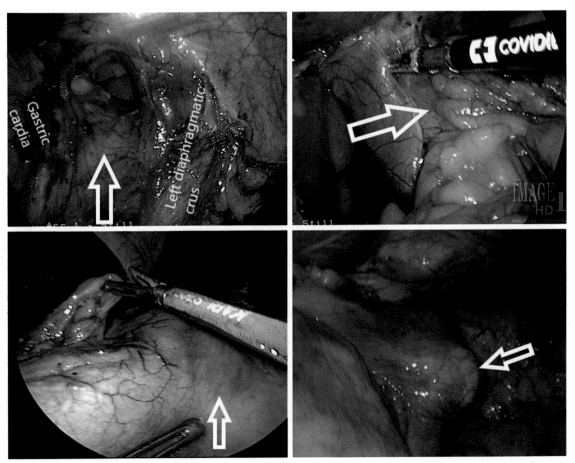

FIG. 22.4 Malignant etiologies of esophageal dysphagia, marked by *arrows*. Infiltrative gastroesophageal junction malignancy (*upper left*); distal esophageal and proximal gastric cardia metastatic adenopathy (*upper right*, instrument tip on right diaphragmatic crus); proximal gastric cancer (*lower left*); gastrointestinal stromal tumor at left cardia and fundus (*lower right*).

stomach is the most common location for GISTs, with only approximately 1% of GISTs occurring in the esophagus.[20]

SYMPTOMS

The hallmark of esophageal dysphagia is difficulty in swallowing that starts several seconds after initiating a swallow. It is this time course that distinguishes esophageal dysphagia from more proximal dysphagia. Additionally, patients classically describe a sensation of food becoming stuck in their chest or esophagus, though localization of symptoms may be more difficult than in patients with oropharyngeal dysphagia. Additional nonspecific associated symptoms consistent with esophageal dysphagia include reflux, regurgitation, nausea, vomiting, chest pain, respiratory symptoms, and weight loss.

Other symptoms vary by specific cause of esophageal dysphagia. Dysphagia to solids that later progresses to liquids is often associated with mechanical obstruction. Dysphagia to liquids but not solids is a finding more commonly seen in motility disorders. Spastic or hypercontractile dysmotility disorders (type III achalasia, DES, hypercontractile esophagus) are often associated with retrosternal chest pain. Infectious or inflammatory causes of esophageal dysphagia are often associated with odynophagia. These causes and neoplastic causes may be associated with hematemesis, melena, or other evidence of gastrointestinal bleeding.

DIAGNOSIS/EVALUATION

The evaluation of a patient with suspected esophageal dysphagia begins by taking a thorough history. The question most crucial to confirming an esophageal source of dysphagia is whether the patient has difficulty in the initial stages of swallowing or starting several seconds after successfully initiating a swallow, the latter being suggestive of esophageal dysphagia. Symptoms of coughing, nasal regurgitation, choking sensation, and proximal globus sensation are suggestive of oropharyngeal dysphagia and would not support a diagnosis of esophageal dysphagia. Patients should describe where they feel the food gets stuck, if possible. It is important to characterize the time course over which dysphagia has been present and the rate of progression of symptoms. Acute onset dysphagia is suggestive of food or foreign body impaction, while rapidly progressive dysphagia over days to weeks is suggestive of malignancy. Careful attention should be paid to whether dysphagia is present to liquids, solids, or both and whether this has changed over time. Associated symptoms as described above should be elicited. Additional symptoms suggestive of systemic illness including fevers, night sweats, weight loss, and dermatologic or neuromuscular symptoms should be explored. Relevant history also includes history of toxic ingestion, esophageal or gastrointestinal surgery, and radiation exposure. Concurrent medical problems should be examined including history or current evidence of scleroderma, systemic sclerosis, other connective tissue disorders, cancer, Chagas' disease, Allgrove syndrome, immune compromise, and neuromuscular disorders.

Physical exam findings may offer some suggestion of the cause of esophageal dysphagia in certain circumstances. Inspection of the oropharynx may reveal ulcers suggestive of HSV infection, or white plaques suggestive of candidiasis. The neck, chest, and abdomen should be inspected for surgical scars or signs of prior trauma. A careful lymph node exam may provide evidence of infection or malignancy. Skin should be examined for sclerotic lesions suggestive of scleroderma.

Upper endoscopy is the preferred initial diagnostic test for evaluation of esophageal dysphagia. Endoscopy allows for the accurate diagnosis of a wide range of pathologies including esophagitis, evidence of GERD, caustic injury, esophageal strictures and rings, hiatal hernias, and benign and malignant neoplasms. It can accurately assess the extent and severity of caustic injury. Achalasia or EGJ outflow obstruction may be suggested by difficulty in passing the scope through the EGJ. Endoscopic biopsy can be performed if esophagitis or a suspected neoplasm is identified. Certain conditions are also amenable to endoscopic treatment, as discussed below.

In the case of normal upper endoscopy, the next diagnostic test is typically either a barium esophagram or esophageal manometry, based on symptoms and the suspected etiology. In the context of dysphagia preferentially to solids, barium esophagram is likely to be of the highest utility. This may be pursued even prior to endoscopy in cases of known anatomic abnormality where passing an endoscope is likely to be risky, such as in cases of prior surgery, stricture, radiation exposure, or caustic injury (Fig. 22.5). Barium esophagram may detect lower esophageal rings or extrinsic compression not detected on endoscopy.[21]

Esophageal manometry should be considered after endoscopy in the case of dysphagia to liquids alone or liquids and solids equivalently. It should also be considered after any esophageal dysphagia with normal findings on endoscopy and barium esophagram. High-resolution manometry (HRM) with esophageal pressure topography offers several benefits over conventional manometry, specifically a greater number and concentration of pressure sensors along the length of

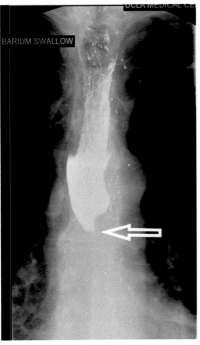

FIG. 22.5 Esophageal barium swallow with distal esophageal stricture (*arrow*).

the esophagus and output that allows comprehensive evaluation of anatomy and function along the esophagus (Fig. 22.6 and 22.7). The key measurements for diagnosis of motility disorders are the integrated relaxation pressure, a measure of relaxation at the LES, and the distal contractile integral, a calculated metric of distal esophageal contractile vigor (see Chapter 12). Diagnostic criteria are described in the Chicago Classification,[4] shown in Table 22.1.

Additional specialized tests are available for further workup of specific conditions. In the case of esophageal or proximal gastric mass or extrinsic compression causing esophageal dysphagia, cross-sectional imaging with CT or MRI may be useful in characterizing the mass. Any esophageal or gastric cancer without metastases warrants endoscopic ultrasound (Fig. 22.8) for further characterization and tumor staging. A nuclear medicine gastric emptying study can determine if *gastroparesis* or delayed gastric emptying is contributing to symptoms that have otherwise been attributed to esophageal dysphagia. Likewise, esophageal pH monitoring can document GERD, which may contribute to similar symptoms.

TREATMENT

The treatment of esophageal dysphagia is tailored to the specific cause. Management principles for each of the above causes will be discussed here.

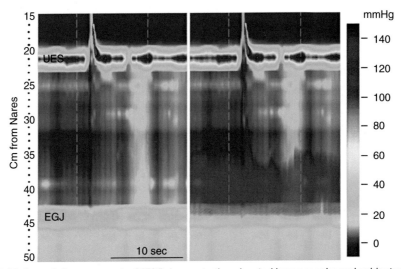

FIG. 22.6 High-resolution manometry (HRM) demonstrating elevated lower esophageal sphincter relaxation pressure, absence of esophageal pressurization, and aperistalsis (type 1 achalasia). Time is on horizontal axis; initiation of swallow seen as contraction in oropharynx, but no contractility present below upper esophageal sphincter (aperistalsis). EGJ, esophagogastric junction; UES, upper esophageal sphincter.

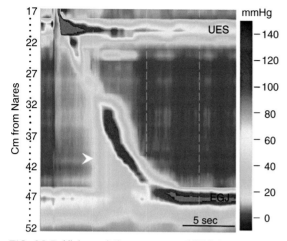

FIG. 22.7 High-resolution manometry (HRM) demonstrating peristaltic esophageal contraction with elevated lower esophageal sphincter (LES) pressures (esophageal outlet obstruction). In this instance, contractility propagates down length of esophagus (successful peristalsis), but LES pressure does not appropriately drop. Pressurization of distal esophagus is seen as green area under peristaltic curve *(arrowhead)*, caused by peristalsis pushing esophageal contents against obstructed LES. EGJ, esophagogastric junction; UES, upper esophageal sphincter.

Treatment for achalasia is aimed at relieving the obstruction at the LES caused by failed relaxation during swallowing. Currently available treatments cannot improve peristalsis, so swallowing may improve but does not return to normal after treatment. Results are typically best in type II achalasia. The obstruction at the LES is relieved by disrupting the esophageal muscle fibers at this level, either by stretching or surgically dividing them. The least invasive means of accomplishing this is by pneumatic dilation. This requires a skilled endoscopist and carries a risk of esophageal perforation, a complication which can require surgical repair. Graded pneumatic dilation refers to the practice of serially increasing dilations as required to obtain an adequate clinical response. Esophageal myotomy is the alternative means of obtaining durable improvements in achalasia. This may be accomplished by means of Heller myotomy (Fig. 22.9), which can be performed laparoscopically, and is often combined with a partial gastric fundoplication. Alternatively, it may be performed endoscopically via per-oral endoscopic myotomy (POEM). This relatively new alternative to surgical myotomy has not been

TABLE 22.1 The Chicago Classification of Esophageal Motility Disorders	
Motility Disorder	**Criteria**
ACHALASIA AND EGJ OUTFLOW OBSTRUCTION	
Type I achalasia (classic achalasia)	• Elevated median IRP (>15 mmHg) • 100% failed peristalsis • DCI <100 mmHg
Type II achalasia (with esophageal compression)	• Elevated median IRP (>15 mmHg) • 100% failed peristalsis • Panesophageal pressurization with ≥20% of swallows
Type III achalasia (spastic achalasia)	• Elevated median IRP (>15 mmHg) • No normal peristalsis • Premature (spastic) contractions with DCI >450 mmHg s cm with ≥20% of swallows • May be mixed with panesophageal pressurization
EGJ outflow obstruction	• Elevated median IRP (>15 mmHg) • Sufficient evidence of peristalsis such that criteria for types I–III achalasia are not met
MAJOR DISORDERS OF PERISTALSIS	
Absent contractility	• Normal median IRP • 100% failed peristalsis
Distal esophageal spasm	• Normal median IRP • ≥20% premature contractions with DCI >450 mmHg s cm • Some normal peristalsis may be present
Hypercontractile esophagus (jackhammer)	• At least two swallows with DCI >8000 mmHg s·cm • Hypercontractility may involve, or even be localized to, the LES
MINOR DISORDERS OF PERISTALSIS	
Ineffective esophageal motility	• ≥50% ineffective swallows • Ineffective swallows can be failed or weak (DCI <450 mmHg s cm)
Fragmented peristalsis	• ≥50% fragmented contractions with DCI > 50 mmHg s cm

DCI, distal contractile integral; *EGJ*, esophagogastric junction; *IRP*, integrated relaxation pressure; *LES*, lower esophageal sphincter.

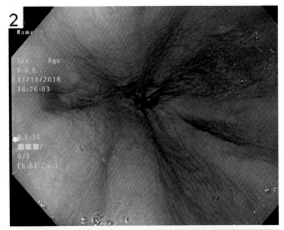

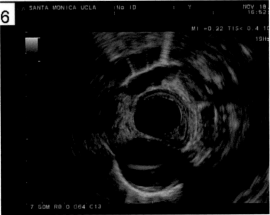

FIG. 22.8 Endoscopic ultrasound to assess for infiltrative, extrinsic, or mass lesions.

extensively studied, but initial results from its use are promising.[22,23] For patients who are not surgical candidates, less invasive means of managing achalasia include botulinum injection into the LES and pharmacological therapy with calcium channel blockers such as nifedipine and nitrates such as isosorbide dinitrate. Botulinum toxin interferes with the excitatory neurons in the LES, resulting in decreased baseline muscle tone in that region. Treatment effects may last 6–12 months. If botulinum toxin injection fails, calcium channel blockers and nitrates may still offer some benefit. When taken before meals, both work by relaxing the smooth muscle of the LES.

Treatment for hypercontractile esophagus and DES are primarily pharmacologic. First-line drugs include calcium channel blockers and tricyclic antidepressants (TCAs). Calcium channel blockers, including diltiazem, tend to be more effective for complaints of dysphagia, while TCAs such as trazodone or imipramine offer improved relief of chest pain. Second-line treatment options include botulinum toxin injection, nitrates, and the phosphodiesterase inhibitor sildenafil. Alternative treatments such as myotomy or peppermint oil have been described but are not well studied in these motility disorders.

Treatment of the esophageal effects of systemic disease consists of identifying the systemic disease (e.g., scleroderma, Chagas disease), treating it to the extent possible, and managing any residual esophageal conditions. Treatment for hypocontractile esophagus caused by scleroderma or other sclerosing conditions focuses on antireflux procedures and management of complications of chronic reflux such as pneumatic dilation or short segment esophagectomy for stricture. Treatment of esophagitis is similarly aimed at treating the underlying cause. Acid-reducing medications and procedures can improve esophagitis resulting from GERD, while the antiviral medications acyclovir, valacyclovir, and famciclovir are the treatment for HSV esophagitis. In cases of idiopathic eosinophilic esophagitis, treatment consists of dietary modification to avoid food allergens, acid suppression, and/or topical steroids.

Most benign mechanical causes of dysphagia occurring in the esophagus itself may be treated with pneumatic dilation. This is true of strictures (from GERD, caustic ingestion, etc.) and esophageal rings. In the presence of esophagitis, gradual serial dilations are necessary to minimize risk of perforation. The practice of injecting strictures with corticosteroids prior to dilation may reduce scar formation and need for repeat dilation.[24] For refractory strictures, esophageal stent placement (Fig. 22.10) is an option that can offer clinical improvements but carries a risk of stent migration and other complications. Short segment esophagectomy is rarely indicated for the treatment of benign strictures and rings but may be of benefit in certain refractory cases.

Symptomatic hiatal and paraesophageal hernias may be surgically repaired by a transabdominal or transthoracic approach. Laparoscopic repairs have demonstrated superior outcome,[25,26] though an

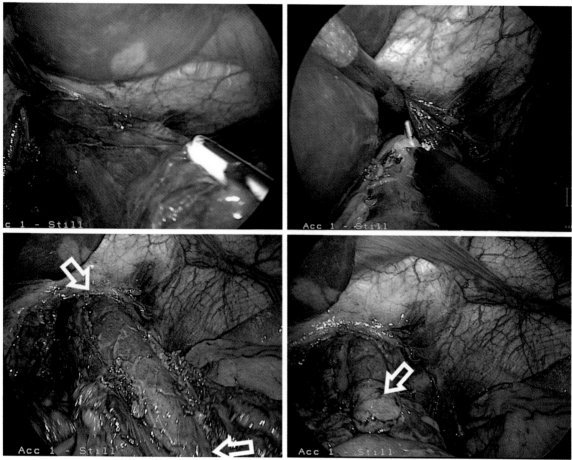

FIG. 22.9 Esophageal myotomy for achalasia. Esophageal muscularis longitudinal fibers (*upper left*); myotomy of the circular fibers (*upper right*); completed Heller myotomy (*lower left*, circular fibers between *arrows* divided); anterior Dor Fundoplication (*lower right*, gastric fundus marked by *arrow*).

alternative approach may be superior in cases of complex past abdominal surgery or prior failed transabdominal repair. Gastric volvulus can be approached surgically or endoscopically, with laparoscopic or open gastric fixation, or with endoscopic derotation and percutaneous endoscopic gastrostomy gastric fixation.

Benign neoplasms of the esophagus, most commonly leiomyomas, may be enucleated if symptomatic. These may be approached endoscopically, from an open surgical approach, or via video-assisted thoracoscopic surgery. The optimal approach depends on location, size, technical feasibility, and expertise.

Treatment of esophageal and EGJ cancer is complex and a complete discussion is beyond the scope of this chapter. Initial management consists of accurately assessing the primary tumor for local advancement and staging the cancer. Subsequent treatment is multimodal in most circumstances. Generally, nonmetastatic cancers that are resectable proceed directly to surgery or may receive neoadjuvant chemoradiation for locally advanced disease followed by resection. Metastatic disease or otherwise unresectable disease may be treated with chemotherapy, radiation therapy, and palliative procedures such as stenting for obstructive tumors.

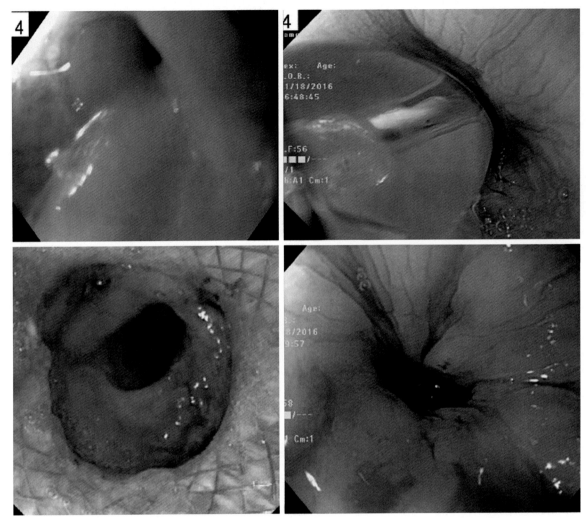

FIG. 22.10 Peptic stricture from gastroesophageal reflux disease and hiatal hernia (*upper left*); dilation (*upper right*); stenting (*lower left*); postendoscopic intervention and operative hiatal hernia repair and fundoplication (*lower right*).

CONCLUSIONS

The wide variety of pathophysiologic processes that may result in esophageal dysphagia underscores the importance of accurate diagnosis and appropriately selected management. A carefully performed history and physical guides the diagnostic process and the selection of appropriate diagnostic tests. Effective management of esophageal dysphagia requires a familiarity with the variety of its causes, the diagnostic studies that aid in making a final diagnosis, and the corresponding medical and surgical treatment modalities.

REFERENCES

1. Roden DF, Altman KW. Causes of dysphagia among different age groups: a systematic review of the literature. *Otolaryngol Clin North Am.* 2013;46(6):965–987.
2. Kraichely RE, Farrugia G. Achalasia: physiology and etiopathogenesis. *Dis Esophagus.* 2006;19(4):213–223.
3. Ates F, Vaezi MF. The pathogenesis and management of achalasia: current status and future directions. *Gut Liver.* 2015;9(4):449–463.
4. International High Resolution Manometry Working Group. The Chicago classification of esophageal motility disorders, v3.0. *Neurogastroenterol Motil.* 2015;27(2): 160–174.

5. Kahrilas PJ, Ghosh SK, Pandolfino JE. Esophageal motility disorders in terms of pressure topography: the Chicago classification. *J Clin Gastroenterol.* 2008;42(5):627–635.
6. Jung HY, Puckett JL, Bhalla V, et al. Asynchrony between the circular and the longitudinal muscle contraction in patients with nutcracker esophagus. *Gastroenterology.* 2005;128(5):1179–1186.
7. Sperandio M, Tutuian R, Gideon RM, Katz PO, Castell DO. Diffuse esophageal spasm: not diffuse but distal esophageal spasm (DES). *Dig Dis Sci.* 2003;48(7):1380–1384.
8. Roman S, Kahrilas PJ. Distal esophageal spasm. *Curr Opin Gastroenterol.* 2015;31(4):328–333.
9. Roman S, Kahrilas PJ. Distal esophageal spasm. *Dysphagia.* 2012;27(1):115–123.
10. Bassotti G, Battaglia E, Debernardi V, et al. Esophageal dysfunction in scleroderma: relationship with disease subsets. *Arthritis Rheum.* 1997;40(12):2252–2259.
11. Savarino E, Furnari M, de Bortoli N, et al. Gastrointestinal involvement in systemic sclerosis. *Presse Med.* 2014;43(10 Pt 2):e279–e291.
12. Zargar SA, Kochhar R, Nagi B, Mehta S, Mehta SK. Ingestion of strong corrosive alkalis: spectrum of injury to upper gastrointestinal tract and natural history. *Am J Gastroenterol.* 1992;87(3):337–341.
13. Havanond C. Is there a difference between the management of grade 2b and 3 corrosive gastric injuries? *J Med Assoc Thai.* 2002;85:340–344.
14. Fisher RA, Eckhauser ML, Radivoyevitch M. Acid ingestion in an experimental model. *Surg Gynecol Obstet.* 1985;161(1):91–99.
15. Engel LS, Chow WH, Vaughan TL, et al. Population attributable risks of esophageal and gastric cancers. *J Natl Cancer Inst.* 2003;95(18):1404.
16. Akhtar S, Sheikh AA, Qureshi HU. Chewing areca nut, betel quid, oral snuff, cigarette smoking and the risk of oesophageal squamous-cell carcinoma in South Asians: a multicentre case-control study. *Eur J Cancer.* 2012;48(5):655–661.
17. Enzinger PC, Mayer RJ. Esophageal cancer. *N Engl J Med.* 2003;349(23):2241–2252.
18. Zhai R, Chen F, Liu G, et al. Interactions among genetic variants in apoptosis pathway genes, reflux symptoms, body mass index, and smoking indicate two distinct etiologic patterns of esophageal adenocarcinoma. *J Clin Oncol.* 2010;28(14):2445–2451.
19. Buas MF, Vaughan TL. Epidemiology and risk factors for gastroesophageal junction tumors: understanding the rising incidence of this disease. *Semin Radiat Oncol.* 2013;23(1):3–9.
20. Tran T, Davila JA, El-Serag HB. The epidemiology of malignant gastrointestinal stromal tumors: an analysis of 1,458 cases from 1992 to 2000. *Am J Gastroenterol.* 2005;100(1):162–168.
21. Ott DJ. Radiographic techniques and efficacy in evaluating esophageal dysphagia. *Dysphagia.* 1990;5(4):192.
22. Talukdar R, Inoue H, Nageshwar Reddy D. Efficacy of peroral endoscopic myotomy (POEM) in the treatment of achalasia: a systematic review and meta-analysis. *Surg Endosc.* 2015;29(11):3030–3046.
23. Kumbhari V, Tieu AH, Onimaru M, et al. Peroral endoscopic myotomy (POEM) vs laparoscopic Heller myotomy (LHM) for the treatment of Type III achalasia in 75 patients: a multicenter comparative study. *Endosc Int Open.* 2015;3(3):E195–E201.
24. Kochhar R, Makharia GK. Usefulness of intralesional triamcinolone in treatment of benign esophageal strictures. *Gastrointest Endosc.* 2002;56(6):829.
25. Mungo B, Molena D, Stem M, Feinberg RL, Lidor AO. Thirty-day outcomes of paraesophageal hernia repair using the NSQIP database: should laparoscopy be the standard of care? *J Am Coll Surg.* 2014;219(2):229–236.
26. Kubasiak J, Hood KC, Daly S, et al. Improved patient outcomes in paraesophageal hernia repair using a laparoscopic approach: a study of the national surgical quality improvement program data. *Am Surg.* 2014;80(9):884–889.

CHAPTER 23

Eosinophilic Esophagitis

KEVIN GHASSEMI, MD

INTRODUCTION/HISTORICAL BACKGROUND

While our knowledge of eosinophilic esophagitis (EoE) has evolved tremendously over the past 3 decades, the heterogeneity in symptom presentation, disease severity, and treatment response have made it a challenging condition to address uniformly. It is a clinicopathologic diagnosis, taking into account symptoms of esophageal dysfunction and esophageal mucosal biopsies showing eosinophil-predominant inflammation, and a diagnosis of EoE should not be made on the basis of either component in isolation.[1] Decades ago, the finding of a "ringed esophagus" that did not respond to acid suppression therapy was treated with dilation in severe cases. Historically, esophageal eosinophilia was attributed to gastroesophageal reflux disease (GERD), and it wasn't until the 1990s that convincing data emerged to suggest an alternative, non-GERD, etiology for this eosinophilia.[2]

It was initially believed to be necessary to exclude GERD before making a diagnosis of EoE.[3] Subsequently, the thinking changed to accept that patients could have both GERD and EoE, but these were separate entities.[1] More recently, a significant subset of patients has been identified who meet diagnostic criteria for EoE but respond to proton pump inhibitor (PPI) therapy, suggesting that there is more of a continuum of disorders involving esophageal eosinophilia.[4] This evolving perspective in diagnosis has impacted recommendations on initial treatment approach in patients with suspected EoE. However, various factors (severity of disease, comorbidities, and patient preferences) will influence what therapeutic strategies clinicians employ in individual cases.

This chapter will review EoE with regard to pathophysiology, clinical manifestations, diagnostic evaluation, and approach to treatment. The reader can identify specific situations in which to employ one or a combination of interventions to achieve a successful response.

EPIDEMIOLOGY AND PATHOPHYSIOLOGY

The incidence of EoE is estimated to range between 6 and 13 cases per 100,000 person-years in North American and Europe, and the prevalence has increased from 10 (in 2000) to 43 (in 2014) per 100,000 persons.[5] While it can occur at any age, most cases occur in children, adolescents, and adults younger than 50 years. Males are affected more than females, at a ratio of about 3:1.[6] Patients with EoE are more likely to have atopic disorders such as asthma, eczema, and rhinitis, although it is unclear if atopy predisposes to EoE.[7]

EoE is a distinct form of food allergy. Many patients with EoE are sensitized to food or aeroallergens, identified by serum immunoglobulin E (IgE) measurements or skin prick testing.[8] However, a significant proportion do not have concomitant atopy, and IgE testing is negative.[9] It is likely characterized by Th2 lymphocytes with an impaired esophageal barrier function. Important molecular factors include interleukin-13, eotaxin-3, and transforming growth factor-β.[10]

SYMPTOMS

Symptoms of EoE vary with age. Younger children and infants commonly present with vomiting, reflux-like symptoms, abdominal pain, refusal of food, and even failure to thrive.[11] In adults, intermittent dysphagia to solid foods is the most common symptom, followed by food impaction, and less commonly heartburn, regurgitation, chest pain or discomfort, and globus sensation.[12] The most common foods that cause dysphagia or food impaction tend to be dense, dry, or rough-textured, such as meats, bread, and rice, although many other foods have been reported to cause symptoms. Patient localization of the bolus is not always reliable. Frequently, the impacted bolus is sensed at the level of the cricoid cartilage, even though at endoscopy significant pathology is identified only in the distal esophagus or at the esophagogastric junction. Typically, patients do not have dysphagia to liquids alone, but they might describe the feeling of choking if they try to wash down the impacted food bolus with liquid. Either the bolus eventually passes down (with or without the aid of liquid) or it needs to be "vomited" out of the mouth.

DIAGNOSIS/EVALUATION

Patients with symptoms of esophageal dysfunction or suspected EoE should undergo upper gastrointestinal endoscopy to visually inspect the esophagus and obtain mucosal biopsies from the esophagus to confirm the presence of eosinophilic infiltration. In most cases, a standard diagnostic endoscope can be used. However, in patients with known or suspected significant fibrostenotic disease (history of food impaction, very frequent/daily dysphagia, always having to "vomit" up the food bolus), it is worth having an ultraslim endoscope

available in case the standard endoscope does not allow for complete examination.

On endoscopic inspection, features of EoE include fixed esophageal rings (can also be described as trachealization), linear or longitudinal furrows, white exudates or plaques, edema (mucosal pallor or reduced vascularity), and diffuse esophageal narrowing/narrow-caliber esophagus (Fig. 23.1). A dominant esophageal ring/stricture, or multiple focal areas of narrowing might be present. None of these findings can be considered pathognomonic for EoE, as they have been described in other esophageal conditions.[13] Therefore, mucosal biopsies must be obtained.

Performing multiple biopsies from different locations in the esophagus is important to increase the diagnostic yield, as inflammatory changes in EoE are often patchy. At least six biopsies total across the distal and proximal esophagus should be taken to maximize

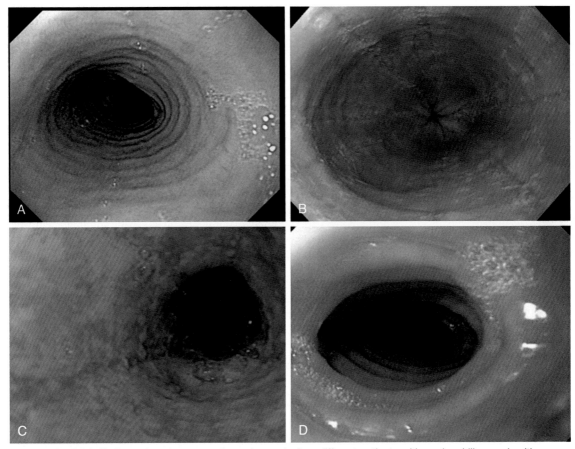

FIG. 23.1 Endoscopic appearance of esophagus in four different patients with eosinophilic esophagitis (EoE). **(A)** Concentric rings. **(B)** Linear/longitudinal furrows. **(C)** White plaques. **(D)** Diffuse esophageal narrowing.

sensitivity.[14] Targeting areas that have white exudates and longitudinal furrows are associated with higher peak eosinophil counts.[15] Even if the esophagus appears normal, biopsies should be obtained because EoE has been diagnosed in up to 32% of patients with an endoscopically normal-appearing esophagus.[16] It also has been recommended to obtain gastric and duodenal mucosal biopsies at the time of initial diagnostic evaluation to rule out eosinophilic gastroenteritis.[1]

The accepted threshold for eosinophil density to diagnose EoE is 15 eosinophils per high-power field (eos/hpf). It is the peak concentration that is used, not the mean density across several fields (Fig. 23.2). Using this threshold, there is a sensitivity of 100% and a specificity of 96% for the diagnosis of EoE.[17] While it is thought that GERD-related esophageal eosinophilia is much less (usually <5 eos/hpf), there can be considerable overlap between EoE and GERD. But because GERD tends to have more of an effect on the distal esophagus, whereas EoE is thought to involve the esophagus more diffusely, the finding of eosinophilia in both proximal and distal esophagus increases the likelihood that it is due to EoE. Other histologic findings that can be seen in EoE include eosinophil abscesses, basal zone hyperplasia, dilated intercellular spaces, eosinophil surface layering, and papillary elongation of the squamous epithelium.[18] None of these findings, however, are specific for EoE.

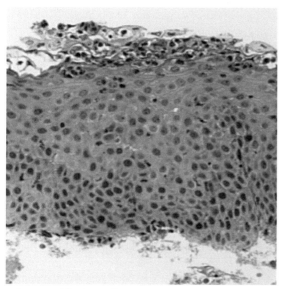

FIG. 23.2 Histologic findings in eosinophilic esophagitis (EoE). More than 15 eosinophils are seen in this high-power field. Additionally, there is superficial layering of eosinophils (top of specimen) and basal cell hyperplasia (bottom).

Other diagnostic modalities (serum biomarkers, high-resolution esophageal manometry, endoscopic ultrasonography, impedance planimetry, and esophagram) have not been shown to offer a clear clinical benefit.[1] Worth mentioning separately, however, is ambulatory pH testing. With the concept of PPI-responsive esophageal eosinophilia (PPI-REE, discussed in more detail in the Treatment section), a subset of patients meeting diagnostic criteria will respond to PPI. However, in the key study that highlighted the significance of PPI-REE, 33% of patients responded to PPI despite a lack of objective evidence for acid reflux.[4] This suggests that a negative pH study does not sufficiently predict that a patient will not respond to PPI if diagnostic criteria for EoE are met. Therefore, routine use of ambulatory pH testing in this situation is not warranted.

TREATMENT

Simplistically speaking, the choices for treating EoE are the three Ds: drugs, diet, and dilation. Of course, deciding which treatment option(s) to use will depend on several factors, including findings at endoscopy and their severity, symptom severity, patient comorbidities, and patient preference for treatment.

Proton pump inhibitors

PPIs have been shown in randomized controlled trials to provide a significant clinicopathologic response for patients diagnosed with EoE, with remission rates ranging from 33% to 57% depending on the threshold eosinophil count used to determine remission.[19] Response to PPI is more common in patients with documented GERD compared to those with negative pH testing.[20] Recommended starting dose, among available PPIs, in adults is 20–40 mg twice daily (in children, it is 1–2 mg/kg daily) for 8 weeks, continuing until the time of follow-up endoscopy and biopsy. If there is documented clinicopathologic remission, it is suggested to reduce to the lowest PPI dose that is effective to remain in remission.[13,21]

Topical Corticosteroids

Topical, swallowed corticosteroids have been shown consistently to induce histologic remission in EoE. There has been less consistency regarding symptom improvement.[22,23] Various formulations, doses, and delivery systems have been used, making it difficult to identify the best choice among the corticosteroid options. The most commonly used steroids are fluticasone via inhaler (440 mcg swallowed twice daily) and oral viscous budesonide (OVB, 1 mg swallowed twice daily). OVB has been prepared at home by mixing 1 mg of budesonide solution, designed for nebulizers, into five packets of sucralose. OVB also can be compounded at specialty pharmacies. It is important not to eat or drink for at least 30 min after administering the medication, so as to prolong contact time of the medication with the esophagus (typically, after breakfast and before bedtime are recommended). A small amount of water should be gargled, swished in the mouth, and then spit out to rinse off any residue in the oropharynx and reduce the risk of oral thrush. Patients typically will use the corticosteroid for 8–12 weeks. The decision to continue at the initial dose, reduce to a lower "maintenance" dose (usually once daily), or stop the medication completely might depend on several factors. Patients who should be considered for maintenance steroid therapy include those with narrow-caliber esophagus, prior esophageal stricture requiring repeated dilations, severe or ongoing symptoms, and patient preference.[13] Maintenance therapy has been shown to be effective and safe.[24] No serious side effects, such as clinical signs of adrenal insufficiency, have been reported. Esophageal candidiasis might occur in 10% of patients and is usually an incidental finding.[21]

Dietary Therapy

The rationale for approaching EoE through dietary elimination is that the condition is mediated by one or more food allergens, so removal of the allergen(s) should result in resolution of the inflammatory response. Three general strategies are available: total elimination of all allergens with elemental or amino acid-based formulas, specific food elimination guided by allergy testing, and empiric food-group elimination, highlighted by the *six-food elimination diet* (SFED).

Elemental diets have been shown to induce histologic remission in about 90% of patients,[25] there has been less consistency with regard to symptomatic improvement, especially among adults.[26] While it is effective, there are numerous disadvantages, including cost, poor palatability (usually requiring a feeding tube in children), lack of adherence, and social implications due to complete avoidance of table food.

The current thought is that EoE is primarily non-IgE mediated,[27] thus is it not surprising skin-prick testing for IgE-related allergic reactions is not very helpful for identifying EoE triggers.[9] Atopy patch testing assesses the presence of non-IgE and cell-mediated reactions, but has not been validated in food allergies.[28] A study in 2014 evaluating food-specific serum IgE-targeted elimination diet found that fewer foods needed to be eliminated (compared to the standard SFED) in order

to achieve histologic remission, although accuracy was significant only when milk was identified as the food trigger.[29] Taken together, allergy testing can be performed, but the results should be used with caution. A negative result does not mean that a particular food is not a trigger, and a positive result does not indicate that elimination of that specific food will lead to a symptomatic or histologic response.

As far as elimination diets go, the SFED has been the most popular because it is effective in achieving clinical and histologic remission in around 75% of patients[9,25] and does not involve elimination of all table food that would occur with an elemental diet. The six foods most commonly associated with food allergy (wheat, cow's milk protein, egg, soy, peanut/tree nuts, and seafood) are avoided for 6 weeks. After this duration, patients who achieve histologic response undergo reintroduction of one food group at a time until the triggers are identified. In the clinical trial setting, patients underwent individual food reintroduction and subsequent endoscopy every 2 weeks.[9] This might not be practical in clinical practice, not just from a cost standpoint but also because symptom frequency for some patients might not allow for identification of triggers with such a short interval of food reintroduction. Less restrictive approaches, including the four-food elimination diet (FFED) and two-food elimination diet (TFED) have emerged as feasible alternatives to the SFED. The FFED (cow's milk, wheat, eggs, and legumes) and the TFED (cow's milk and wheat) achieved remission in 54% and 43% of EoE patients, respectively.[30,31] This step-up approach might reduce the diagnostic time process and number of endoscopic procedures performed.

Esophageal Dilation

While it does not have an effect on the underlying inflammatory process, dilation improves dysphagia in up to 75% of adult EoE patients with a reduced esophageal caliber.[32] There is limited information in the pediatric population. Dilation can be employed in two general situations: (1) as an adjunct to medication/dietary therapy addressing stenotic disease and (2) as the sole treatment of stenotic disease in patients who either cannot or do not want to use medication or dietary elimination.

Dilation of EoE-related strictures can be performed using either wire-guided bougie or through-the-scope balloon. After identifying the area(s) of maximal narrowing and estimating the degree of stenosis, the dilation device is inserted. When using a bougie, the endoscopist should appreciate tactile resistance to passage and might see blood on the bougie when it is

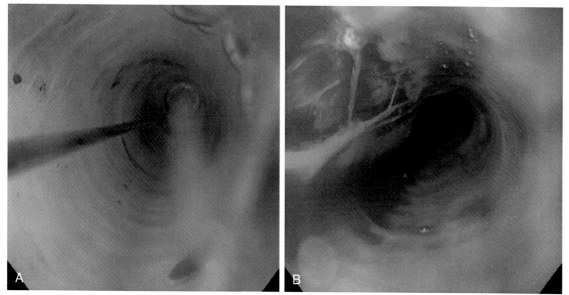

FIG. 23.3 Balloon dilation of stricture in the proximal esophagus. **(A)** View through the balloon. The concentric esophageal rings are seen being compressed by the expanding balloon, with focal erythema in the *upper left* corner indicating where mucosal tearing occurs. **(B)** Postdilation showing a large mucosa tear with underlying submucosal fibers.

withdrawn. This should prompt an endoscopic assessment before determining if further dilation is appropriate during the same procedure. With the balloon, the nurse or technician can inform the endoscopist if resistance is encountered during inflation. However, one advantage of the balloon is that the endoscopist can dynamically assess for mucosal tearing and degree of stenosis even while the balloon is inflated (Fig. 23.3). Unlike with peptic strictures, in which common thinking allows for increasing the esophageal diameter by three balloon sizes, once mucosal tearing has occurred in an EoE dilation, no further dilation should be performed that day to reduce the chances of perforation. When dilation is used as the sole treatment, a recommended goal esophageal caliber is 15–18 mm (45–54 French), and more than one treatment session might be necessary to reach this goal. With this goal diameter, symptom relief for 1–2 years is common before another dilation is required.[33,34] Dilation in EoE is safe, with a similar low rate of major complications compared with dilation in other esophageal diseases. The rate of perforation is 0.3% and of hemorrhage is 0.1%. Chest pain is common, experienced immediately postprocedurally in over half of patients, but typically is mild and resolves with 1–2 days.[34,35]

Choice of Therapy

Previous guidelines have recommended starting with a twice-daily PPI to determine if the patient has PPI-REE.[1,13] Due to ease of administration, this still can be considered first-line therapy. However, the most recent guideline suggests that PPI, dietary elimination, or topical steroids might be offered as the first-line anti-inflammatory treatment.[21] Choice of therapy should be individualized and might change over time. It is important to ensure that the patient understands what is involved with each option, such as the level and duration of commitment with food elimination diets, the potential adverse effects of short- and long-term medication therapy, and the lack of addressing underlying inflammation as well as the potential risks associated with esophageal dilation. Regardless of treatment, with a sound patient-provider relationship, EoE generally is a treatable chronic condition with a good long-term outcome.

REFERENCES

1. Liacouras CA, Furuta GT, Hirano I, et al. Eosinophilic esophagitis: updated consensus recommendations for children and adults. *J Allergy Clin Immunol.* 2011;128: 3–20.

2. Kelly KJ, Lazenby AJ, Rowe PC, et al. Eosinophilic esophagitis attributed to gastroesophageal reflux: improvement with an amino acid-based formula. *Gastroenterology.* 1995;109:1503–1512.

3. Furuta GT, Liacouras CA, Collins MH, et al. Eosinophilic esophagitis in children and adults: a systematic review and consensus recommendations for diagnosis and treatment. *Gastroenterology.* 2007;133:1342–1363.

4. Molina-Infante J, Ferrando-Lamana L, Ripoll C, et al. Esophageal eosinophilic infiltration responds to proton pump inhibition in most adults. *Clin Gastroenterol Hepatol.* 2011;9:110–117.

5. Dellon ES, Jensen ET, Martin CF, Shaheen NJ, Kappelman MD. Prevalence of eosinophilic esophagitis in the United States. *Clin Gastroenterol Hepatol.* 2014;12: 589–596.

6. Kapel RC, Miller JK, Torres C, Aksoy S, Lash R, Katzka DA. Eosinophilic esophagitis: a prevalent disease in the United States that affects all age groups. *Gastroenterology.* 2008; 134:1316–1321.

7. González-Cervera J, Arias Á, Redondo-González O, Cano-Mollinedo MM, Terreehorst I, Lucendo AJ. Association between atopic manifestations and eosinophilic esophagitis: a systematic review and meta-analysis. *Ann Allergy Asthma Immunol.* 2017;118:582–590.

8. Simon D, Marti H, Heer P, Simon HU, Braathen LR, Straumann A. Eosinophilic esophagitis is frequently associated with IgE-mediated allergic airway diseases. *J Allergy Clin Immunol.* 2005;115:1090–1092.

9. Gonsalves N, Yang GY, Doerfler B, Ritz S, Ditto AM, Hirano I. Elimination diet effective treats eosinophilic esophagitis in adults; food reintroduction identifies causative factors. *Gastroenterology.* 2012;142:1451–1459.

10. Clayton F, Peterson K. Eosinophilic esophagitis: pathophysiology and definition. *Gastrointest Endosc Clin N Am.* 2018;28:1–14.

11. Spergel JM, Brown-Whitehorn TF, Beausoleil JL, et al. 14 years of eosinophilic esophagitis: clinic features and prognosis. *J Pediatr Gastroenterol Nutr.* 2009;48:30–36.

12. Remedios M, Campbell C, Jones DM, Kerlin P. Eosinophilic esophagitis in adults: clinical, endoscopic, histologic findings, and response to treatment with fluticasone propionate. *Gastrointest Endosc.* 2006;63:3–12.

13. Dellon ES, Gonsalves N, Hirano I, Furuta GT, Liacouras MD, Katzka DA. ACG clinical guideline: evidenced based approach to the diagnosis and management of esophageal eosinophilia and eosinophilic esophagitis (EoE). *Am J Gastroenterol.* 2013;108: 679–692.

14. Nielsen JA, Lager DJ, Lewin M, Rendon G, Roberts CA. The optimal number of biopsy fragments to establish a morphologic diagnosis of eosinophilic esophagitis. *Am J Gastroenterol.* 2014;109:515–520.

15. Salek J, Clayton F, Vinson L, et al. Endoscopic appearance and location dictate diagnostic yield of biopsies in eosinophilic oesophagitis. *Aliment Pharmacol Ther.* 2015;41: 1288–1295.

16. Kim HP, Vance RB, Shaheen NJ, Dellon ES. The prevalence and diagnostic utility of endoscopic features of eosinophilic esophagitis: a meta-analysis. *Clin Gastroenterol Hepatol.* 2012;10:988–996.

17. Dellon ES, Speck O, Woodward K, et al. Distribution and variability of esophageal eosinophilia in patients undergoing upper endoscopy. *Mod Pathol.* 2015;28:383–390.

18. Collins MH. Histopathologic features of eosinophilic esophagitis and eosinophilic gastrointestinal diseases. *Gastroenterol Clin N Am.* 2014;43:257–268.

19. Moawad FJ, Veerappan GR, Dias JA, Baker TP, Maydonovitch CL, Wong RK. Randomized controlled trial comparing aerosolized swallowed fluticasone to esomeprazole for esophageal eosinophilia. *Am J Gastroenterol.* 2013;108:366–372.

20. Molina-Infante J, Katzka DA, Gisbert JP. Review article: proton pump inhibitor therapy for suspected eosinophilic oesophagitis. *Aliment Pharmacol Ther.* 2013;37:1157–1164.

21. Lucendo AJ, Molina-Infante J, Arias Á, et al. Guidelines on eosinophilic esophagitis: evidence-based statements and recommendations for diagnosis and management in children and adults. *United Eur Gastroenterol J.* 2017;5: 335–358.

22. Dellon ES, Sheikh A, Speck O, et al. Viscous topical is more effective than nebulized steroid therapy for patients with eosinophilic esophagitis. *Gastroenterology.* 2012;143: 321–324.

23. Tan ND, Xiao YL, Chen MH. Steroids therapy for eosinophilic esophagitis: systematic review and meta-analysis. *J Dig Dis.* 2015;16:431–442.

24. Straumann A, Conus S, Degen L, et al. Long-term budesonide maintenance treatment is partially effective for patients with eosinophilic esophagitis. *Clin Gastroenterol Hepatol.* 2011;9:400–409.

25. Arias A, Gonzalez-Cervera J, Tenias JM, Lucendo AJ. Efficacy of dietary interventions for inducing histologic remission in patients with eosinophilic esophagitis: a systematic review and meta-analysis. *Gastroenterology.* 2014;146: 1639–1648.

26. Peterson KA, Byrne KR, Vinson LA, et al. Elemental diet induces histologic response in adult eosinophilic esophagitis. *Am J Gastroenterol.* 2013;108:759–766.

27. Simon D, Cianferoni A, Spergel JM, et al. Eosinophilic esophagitis is characterized by a non-IgE-mediated food hypersensitivity. *Allergy.* 2016;71:611–620.

28. Hong S, Vogel NM. Food allergy and eosinophilic esophagitis: learning what to avoid. *Clevel Clin J Med.* 2010;77: 51–59.

29. Rodríguez-Sánchez J, Gómez Torrijos E, López Viedma B, et al. Efficacy of IgE-targeted vs empiric six-food elimination diets for adult eosinophilic oesophagitis. *Allergy.* 2014;69:936–942.

30. Molina-Infante J, Arias A, Barrio J, Rodriguez-Sanchez J, Sanchez-Cazalilla M, Lucendo AJ. Four-food group elimination diet for adult eosinophilic esophagitis: a prospective multicenter study. *J Allergy Clin Immunol.* 2014;134: 1093–1099.

31. Molina-Infante J, Arias A, Alcedo J, et al. Step-up empiric elimination diet for pediatric and adult eosinophilic esophagitis: the 2-4-6 study. *J Allergy Clin Immunol.* 2017 (Epub ahead of print).
32. Moawad FJ, Cheatham JG, DeZee KJ. Meta-analysis: the safety and efficacy of dilation in eosinophilic oesophagitis. *Aliment Pharmacol Ther.* 2013;38:713−720.
33. Prieto R, Richter JE. Eosinophilic esophagitis in adults: an update on medical management. *Curr Gastroenterol Rep.* 2013;15:324−326.
34. Schoepfer AM, Gonsalves N, Bussmann C, et al. Esophageal dilation in eosinophilic esophagitis: effectiveness, safety, and impact on the underlying inflammation. *Am J Gastroenterol.* 2010;105:1062−1070.
35. Jung KW, Gundersen N, Kopacova J, et al. Occurrence of and risk factors for complications after endoscopic dilation in eosinophilic esophagitis. *Gastrointest Endosc.* 2011;73: 15−21.

CHAPTER 24

Swallowing Therapy

PRATIK B. PATEL, MD • ANDREW ERMAN, MA, CCC-SLP •
DINESH K. CHHETRI, MD

INTRODUCTION

Speech language pathologists (SLPs) perform swallow therapy (ST), using exercises and/or behavioral maneuvers to reduce aspiration risk and/or improve swallow efficiency. Success in therapy can lead to improved health status and quality of life. This chapter will elucidate who may benefit from STs, exercises and compensations that are used in treatment, and technology that may be utilized to improve efficacy. By understanding these considerations, the otolaryngologist will be better equipped to make appropriate referrals for swallowing therapy. Common conditions causing dysphagia that an otolaryngologist might encounter are noted in this chapter. More unusual dysphagia etiologies are purposefully omitted.

SWALLOW THERAPY CANDIDACY

An instrumental swallowing assessment, such as modified barium swallow study (MBSS) and/or flexible endoscopic evaluation of swallowing (FEES) is required to understand a patient's swallowing to determine candidacy for ST and how to structure the therapy.

Patients with an obstructive etiology should have that condition treated before ST is considered. These conditions include pharyngeal or esophageal stricture or stenosis (see Chapter 15), epiglottic dysfunction (see Chapter 16), cricopharyngeal hypertrophy/bar (see Chapter 19), and Zenker's diverticulum (see Chapter 20).

In general, patients with mild dysphagia have a better prognosis for improved swallowing with therapy, compared to those with severe dysphagia. Patients with a new onset of dysphagia may expect greater improvement compared to those with a chronic condition. However, this may depend on the etiology of the swallowing problem. For example, new stroke patients are likely to experience some resolution of dysphagia symptoms (some without any ST at all), due to spontaneous post-stroke recovery over several months or more. Patients with certain neurodegenerative diseases, such

as Parkinson's disease, can experience some improvement temporarily with swallowing therapy, with eventual worsening of dysphagia as the underlying condition progresses. It is unclear if ST is helpful or harmful for people with amyotrophic lateral sclerosis (ALS). Some think that exercise is contraindicated in ALS because it may cause muscle fatigue and may promote motor neuron degeneration.[1] Plowman and colleagues reviewed 18 evidence-based studies that examined the impact of exercise on ALS.[2] These studies focused on respiration, speech or limb function. The authors did not find studies that examined the impact of exercise on dysphagia with ALS, concluding that there is inadequate data to determine if exercise is beneficial or detrimental for this patient population.

ST is often performed in the outpatient setting. However, the otolaryngologist may consider whether ST is appropriate for her/his inpatients. Elderly patients with an acute infection (such as a urinary tract infection or pneumonia) may experience a temporary dysphagia that tends to resolve after recovery from the illness—thus ST is typically not needed for these patients. Instead, periodic evaluation of swallowing is advised. Patients who are status-post anterior cervical discectomy and fusion (ACDF) will demonstrate a postsurgical decline in swallowing function as assessed with an MBSS. Specifically, reduced hyoid elevation, increased pharyngeal residue, and increased pharyngeal wall thickness is seen.[3] However, these symptoms are often temporary and ACDF patients usually require observation for expected improvement, rather than ST in the inpatient or immediate outpatient setting.

Otolaryngologists frequently encounter tracheotomized patients in the inpatient and outpatient settings. Therefore, a working understanding of dysphagia issues specific to this patient population is important. Previously, it was thought that tracheostomy tubes (especially with the cuff inflated) reduce hyolaryngeal elevation during the swallow. However, studies comparing pre- and post-decannulation measures concluded that the presence of a tracheostomy itself does not significantly alter kinematics of swallowing, pharyngeal phase function, or hyolaryngeal elevation.[4–6] Tracheostomy has been associated with aspiration in 69%–87% of patients studied.[7,8] Gross and colleagues demonstrated improved bolus transit times and better lower airway protection in four patients with occluded versus unoccluded tracheostomy tubes (occluded using one-way speaking valves).[9] The authors theorized that subglottal mechanoreceptors were activated during the swallow by the restored subglottal pressure. These receptors may stimulate recruitment of lower motor neurons important for swallowing. However, other researches have concluded that tracheostomy occlusion was beneficial for speaking purposes but did not reduce aspiration.[10,11] Occlusion or capping may be pursued, when tolerated from a respiratory standpoint, for possible improved airway protection, and for other benefits such as being able to speak without finger occluding the tracheostomy tube, improved lung recruitment, and as a bridge to decannulation. In patients who are likely to be tracheotomized temporarily (e.g., for airway protection during composite resection for cancer), ST is probably not necessary. Pending MBSS or FEES results, ST can be considered in chronically or newly tracheotomized patients who are likely to have the tracheostomy tube for some time.

Patients radiated in the head and neck region are at risk for progressive dysphagia due to associated muscle and nerve changes (see Chapter 15). However, symptom onset and the course of the swallow disorder are variable among patients.[12] Providing ST during radiation therapy (XRT) is becoming a more common practice. The goals of this service are to maintain swallow function and facilitate adequate oral intake during XRT, so that patients may avoid feeding tube placement. Maintaining oral intake and performing swallowing therapy exercises during XRT improves long-term swallowing outcomes, such as returning to regular texture diet or removal of gastrostomy tube.[13] Patients with dysphagia following XRT may also benefit from ST.

Patients with severe radiation fibrosis may benefit from postural changes and/or lower airway protective maneuvers; however, there is a lower likelihood that strengthening exercises will help this patient population. Prognosis for improved swallowing with therapy following surgery for head and neck cancer is often better for patients who have had smaller resections and did not require large tissue flap reconstruction. This is especially significant in the newer population of oral/oropharyngeal cancer patients undergoing transoral robotic surgery.[14] Patients with good sensation for aspiration and pharyngeal residue have a better prognosis to modify swallow behaviors—those who do not sense pharyngeal residue and/or aspiration may be less able and/or motivated to implement behavioral techniques designed to improve swallow efficiency or lower airway protection.

BARRIERS TO SWALLOW THERAPY NOT DIRECTLY RELATED TO A PATIENT'S DYSPHAGIA

Patients must have adequate cognition to participate in therapy. Those with cognitive impairments, for example, may have difficulty learning exercises or monitoring performance. Language impairment can also pose an obstacle. Patients with aphasia may have difficulty following instructions due to associated auditory comprehension deficits. Additionally, people with aphasia may have challenges asking questions or expressing difficulties with their exercises.

ST is physically demanding. Therefore, patients with reduced physical reserve will likely not be good treatment candidates. Also, poor motivation can limit progress, since it may influence the effort employed and consistency of practice.

FURTHER CONSIDERATIONS FOR SWALLOWING THERAPY

Should the Patient Swallow Liquid or Food During Therapy?

The physician and SLP should consult to determine if oral intake may be used during ST for those patients at high risk of aspiration. Aspiration in the absence of other risk factors is not highly associated with the development of aspiration pneumonia.[15,16] There are multiple benefits of swallowing food, liquid, or ice chips during therapy. Patients who are nil per os often have xerostomia, making it difficult to initiate a swallow (which is required for a number of swallow exercises). Additionally, brainstem control of swallow physiology alters contraction based on bolus size and consistency.[17,18] Therefore, increasing bolus size and the viscosity of a consistency can facilitate increased muscular effort.[19] Finally, greater gains may be made when an exercise resembles the activity one wishes to improve.[20] Therefore, swallowing food or liquid in a manner designed to strengthen swallow muscles (for example, using the effortful swallow) may be beneficial.

Rehabilitative Versus Compensatory Techniques

Rehabilitative swallow exercises seek to alter muscle physiology to improve strength and range of motion of swallow structures. Compensatory techniques are designed to improve swallow efficiency or decrease aspiration risk by applying techniques such as postural changes (e.g., lowering the chin or turning the head left or right while swallowing) or lower airway protective maneuvers (such as the supraglottic swallow). Compensatory techniques do not result in improved muscle strength or range of motion as may occur with exercise. The need to use compensatory maneuvers may be temporary, depending on how a patient's dysphagia improves over time. It is useful to perform an MBSS or FEES to determine the efficacy of compensatory maneuvers, to make sure these strategies do not cause more residue or aspiration.

COMMONLY PERFORMED REHABILITATIVE EXERCISES

Exercises Designed to Impact Oral Structures

Trismus therapy

Trismus, restricted mouth opening, is a well-documented complication of XRT used to treat head and neck cancer. Trismus may severely affect placing food in one's mouth, oral hygiene, and/or dental care. Trismus in posttreatment head and neck cancer patients may be treated with jaw-opening exercises. Devices to improve mandibular abduction have been demonstrated to be somewhat efficacious in postradiation patients with trismus.[21,22] Pauli and colleagues studied 50 head and neck cancer patients who were at least 3 months status-post XRT.[21] Subjects and controls had maximal interincisal opening (MIO) of <35 mm. The subjects' trismus was treated with two different mandibular abduction devices. The subject population demonstrated a mean MIO improvement of 6.4 mm. The control group, who received no treatment, showed an improved MIO of 0.7 mm. Starting trismus therapy early after detecting the problem can be helpful.[23] At our institution, head and neck cancer patients at risk of developing trismus during the course of their XRT are asked to perform prophylactic mandible-opening exercises using a mobilization device, during the period they are receiving radiation. In our experience, it appears that these patients are less likely to develop post-XRT trismus sufficient to interfere with function. However, we have yet to systematically study this effect.

Tongue press

The tongue plays a significant role in propelling a bolus from the oral cavity into the pharynx. Reduced oral tongue range of motion and strength is associated with oral and pharyngeal residue. Resistance exercises may improve oral tongue strength and can involve pushing the tongue against the hard palate. Biofeedback may be employed so that the amount of effort may be regulated, in keeping with the strength-building principles of exercise physiology.[20] Robbins and colleagues used the tongue press exercise with 10 stroke patients (6 had strokes within 3 months of the study and 4 subjects had had strokes for 3 or more months at the time the study was conducted).[24] Results showed significantly increased isometric pressure at the anterior tongue and maximum swallow pressures. Penetration–aspiration scale scores[25] were significantly improved.

Exercises Designed to Improve the Pharyngeal Swallow

Effortful swallow

The purpose of this maneuver is to facilitate greater pharyngeal pressure during the swallow. The patient is instructed to "swallow hard" or to increase tongue pressure against the palate when swallowing. Huckabee and colleagues used surface electromyography of the submental muscles and manometry to compare normal and effortful swallowing in normal subjects.[26] Electromyographic amplitudes with the effortful swallow were significantly greater compared to normal swallowing, indicating increased muscle contraction of the floor of mouth muscles. Additionally, upper esophageal sphincter (UES) pressure was significantly reduced and pressure in the lower pharynx was significantly increased. Hoffman and colleagues used high-resolution manometry with normal subjects to study pharyngeal pressures associated with the effortful swallow and the Mendelsohn maneuver compared to normal swallows.[27] The effortful swallow produced significantly lower UES pressure for longer time periods when compared to normal swallowing. Interestingly, maximum tongue base pressure was reduced compared to normal swallows.

Mendelsohn maneuver

The Mendelsohn maneuver is designed to facilitate better UES opening. The patient is instructed to maintain hyolaryngeal elevation for a prescribed time period. Feedback is beneficial to help the patient to understand if he/she is performing the exercise correctly—this either can be provided by tactile feedback of laryngeal elevation or surface electromyography.

McCullough et al. studied poststroke patients (mean of 9.5 months poststroke) using the Mendelsohn maneuver.[28] The authors noted significantly improved hyoid maximum elevation and hyoid maximum anterior excursion. UES opening duration improved but this was not statistically significant. Study participants also demonstrated improved scores on the Dysphagia Outcome and Severity Scale.[29] Hoffman et al. used high-resolution manometry to study the Mendelsohn maneuver compared to normal swallows.[27] The Mendelsohn maneuver resulted in significantly longer periods of lower UES pressure when compared to normal swallowing.

Masako maneuver

The Masako or tongue-hold maneuver is designed to improve pharyngeal wall contraction. This exercise is performed with the first quarter-inch of the tongue tip held between the teeth during swallowing. Improved contraction occurs near the level of C2. Because it increases vallecular residue (and possibly aspiration risk), it should only be used as an exercise, with small amounts of liquid or with saliva. However, the long-term benefit of this exercise is unknown.[30,31]

Shaker head lift

The Shaker head lift is for patients with reduced UES opening. This exercise focuses on improving strap muscle strength, to move the hyolaryngeal complex upward and forward, which together with cricopharyngeal relaxation, helps the UES open and protect the lower airway. Limited UES opening is associated with increased hypopharyngeal residue that the patient may aspirate. The exercise is performed with the patient lying supine. In the first part, the patient elevates her/his head to look at his/her toes while the shoulders remain down. The patient holds this position for 1 min and then rests for 1 min—this process is repeated two more times. In the second portion, the patient raises her/his head to view the toes and then completely lowers the head, 30 times in continuous movements. This exercise tends to place significant physical demands on patients, which may decrease their compliance. Shaker and colleagues used this exercise with 31 healthy, asymptomatic patients.[32] The magnitude of anterior laryngeal excursion and UES opening were significantly larger. In another study, Shaker et al. studied the impact of this exercise on patients with dysphagia related to central nervous system insults (including chronic and acute stroke patients), and head and neck cancer (the latter treated with XRT).[33] The treatment group demonstrated significantly improved UES opening and anterior

laryngeal elevation compared to the control group, who practiced a sham exercise.

Chin tuck against resistance

Chin tuck against resistance (CTAR) strengthens the suprahyoid musculature to improve UES opening. The seated participant tucks the chin to compress an inflated ball. While similar in purpose to the Shaker head lift exercise, the CTAR may be better tolerated by patients who experience too much sternocleidomastoid muscle fatigue or have difficulty fully elevating their head (e.g., patients who have had procedures for head and neck cancer that impact neck strength or range of motion). Further, surface electromyography of the suprahyoid muscles during CTAR were significantly higher than for Shaker exercise.[34]

Tongue press

As mentioned above, an isometric tongue press against the palate can improve swallow function. The tongue press has been associated with improved tongue base contraction (thus improving pharyngeal driving force). Robbins et al. described using the tongue press exercise while utilizing the Iowa Oral Pressure Instrument (IOPI) for biofeedback on 10 patients with swallowing problems who had strokes, some of whom were in the acute phase of recovery while others had chronic dysphagia.[24] Lower airway protection assessed using the penetration–aspiration scale scores[25] was significantly improved.

Expiratory muscle strength training

Expiratory muscle strength training (EMST) is performed to improve hyolaryngeal elevation and UES opening and to reduce aspiration. EMST is performed with a calibrated, one-way, spring-loaded valve that is utilized to "overload the expiratory and submental muscles."[35] Troche et al. studied Parkinson's patients in a prospective and randomized study.[36] Thirty-three percent of the treatment group demonstrated improved penetration–aspiration scores compared to 14% of the sham exercise group. This improvement was statistically significant. Pitts et al. used EMST to study the effects on voluntary coughing and swallowing with 10 Parkinson's patients.[35] Posttreatment scores on the penetration aspiration scale were significantly improved.

Thermal-tactile stimulation and sensory-motor integration

The pharyngeal swallow response is typically initiated when the head of the bolus passes the ramus of the mandible, though in older adults, the pharyngeal swallow may be triggered when the head of the bolus reaches the valleculae. Pharyngeal phase triggering results in lower airway closure at the level of the larynx and pharyngeal contraction for bolus transport. Some patients with sensory deficits demonstrate delayed triggering of the pharyngeal swallow. A common problem associated with delayed pharyngeal phase onset is thin liquid aspiration before the pharyngeal swallow is elicited, with associated lower airway closure at the level of the larynx. The aspiration occurs because thin liquid flows more quickly than food and thick liquids, and therefore is more likely to enter the larynx before that structure can close to protect the lower airway. Thermal tactile stimulation is a technique to quicken the triggering of the pharyngeal swallow, using a chilled laryngeal mirror to stimulate the anterior faucial arches prior to swallowing. Unfortunately, results are variable within and between patients.[25] Additionally, evidence of long-term benefit for this therapeutic technique demonstrates a weak effect.[37]

BIOFEEDBACK

Biofeedback is an adjunct to swallowing therapy that is typically used to help individuals alter behaviors that are thought of as involuntary. The majority of swallow structures and their movements are not visible during therapy, making it difficult for the patient or clinician to monitor performance. Biofeedback is employed during ST so the patient can gain insight into swallow behaviors, to modify those behaviors. There are a number of available biofeedback tools. For example, surface electromyography measures the electrical activity of muscles and provides auditory and/or visual representation of muscular effort and the duration of muscle contraction. Clinicians monitor surface electromyography feedback to measure patient performance. The patient uses the information to incentivize greater effort. However, surface electromyography cannot isolate individual muscles. Further, the surface electromyography measures are relative since the unit cannot be calibrated. Surface electromyography seems to correlate well to biomechanical events during the swallow, particularly in relation to hyolaryngeal elevation.[38] Surface electromyography can be utilized with the Mendelsohn maneuver, effortful swallow, CTAR, and tongue press. Videoendoscopy also can be useful to help patients learn the supraglottic swallow, or super supraglottic swallow, to protect the lower airway. Some clinicians have monitored oxygen saturation in the belief that a drop in oxygen values

may indicate aspiration. Unfortunately, studies of oxygen saturation and swallowing did not reveal a relationship.[39] Cervical auscultation has been utilized as a biofeedback tool, by using a speaker and microphone with the stethoscope bell. Regrettably, reliability of this technique has been poor.[40] The IOPI or the Madison Oral Strengthening Therapeutic (MOST) device provide quantitative data for tongue-to-palate pressure and can be used with the tongue press exercise.

ELECTRICAL STIMULATION

The goal of electrical stimulation in swallowing is to improve pharyngeal contraction and hyolaryngeal elevation. For purposes of dysphagia treatment, electrical stimulation is largely delivered transcutaneously. Patients can voluntarily contract the targeted muscles by swallowing or using the previously described swallow exercises designed to improve strength, with augmentation by electrical stimulation. Alternatively, the patient may remain at rest and allow the stimulation to cause muscle contraction. Placing electrodes to stimulate only the target muscles is challenging given that the muscles of the neck are short, span small distances, and are in close proximity to one another. Thus, transcutaneous electrical stimulation may inadvertently stimulate infrahyoid muscles and therefore restrict hyolaryngeal elevation. Studies show that electrical stimulation should not be used in patients who cannot overcome this resistive lowering of the hyolaryngeal complex due to an increased risk of penetration and aspiration.[41] Electrical stimulation has not been studied enough to draw conclusions on its effectiveness, side effects, and ideal patient population.[42]

COMPENSATORY TECHNIQUES
Head Postures

Postural techniques modify movement of the bolus through the oral cavity and/or pharynx in targeted ways to compensate for structural or functional deficits. Tilting the chin upward assists bolus transit through the oral cavity. This posture is used with patients with compromised ability to generate oral pressure to squeeze a bolus into the pharynx. Chin elevation can also be helpful for patients with labial incontinence. However, this chin-up maneuver can interfere with the timing of swallowing events, since material (especially liquid) can enter the pharynx prematurely and hence, increase aspiration risk. Tilting the head to the right or left may help reduce oral cavity residue or increase control of the bolus for patients who have ipsilateral oral control difficulties and pharyngeal weakness. These patients may benefit from tilting their head to the stronger side. The chin-down posture is employed to improve pharyngeal driving force, since the tongue base is positioned closer to the posterior pharyngeal wall. Additionally, this posture may help reduce aspiration by widening the valleculae—this can be helpful for some patients who have premature spillage of material from the oral cavity into the pharynx or who have delayed triggering of the pharyngeal swallow. Turning the head right or left (to the weak side, as determined during an instrumental swallow assessment) while swallowing may reduce pharyngeal residue. Some patients are able to greatly reduce pharyngeal residue by swallowing with their head turned either left or right and with the chin down. Best practice requires that the efficacy (or lack thereof) of a head posture be assessed instrumentally, as patients may be insensate to residue and aspiration.

Lower Airway Protective Maneuvers

Patients with coronary artery disease or a history of stroke should not perform the following two maneuvers without physician clearance since abnormal cardiac findings (including supraventricular tachycardia, premature atrial contractions, and premature ventricular contractions) have been associated with these compensatory maneuvers.[43]

Supraglottic Swallow

The supraglottic swallow is used to voluntarily close the glottis before and during the swallow to prevent aspiration. Specifically, the patient (1) takes a deep breath, (2) holds breath while swallowing, and (3) coughs immediately after each swallow. Patients with poor pharyngeal clearance of a bolus may need to maintain the breath-hold during and between multiple swallows to clear the residue while protecting the lower airway.

Super-Supraglottic Swallow

The super-supraglottic swallow is the same as the supraglottic swallow, with the addition of a Valsalva maneuver, to more completely close the laryngeal valve. Efficacy of the supraglottic swallow and super supraglottic swallow needs to be verified with an instrumental assessment before utilization is recommended. Extra effort is required to perform these techniques (this is especially true of the super supraglottic swallow), which may impact if the technique is consistently and correctly performed.

Bolus Clearance Maneuvers

Either of the following maneuvers can be useful for patients with xerostomia and/or reduced oral and pharyngeal driving force.

Liquid wash: A liquid wash is simply swallowing liquid to clear food residue already present in the oral cavity and/or pharynx.

Liquid assist: This technique requires the patient to swallow food and liquid simultaneously. We recommend instrumental assessment to determine the efficacy of both of these techniques, to ensure that aspiration does not increase with the use of these maneuvers.

CONCLUSION

Swallowing therapy offers a nonsurgical adjunct or primary treatment option for some patients suffering from dysphagia. This treatment modality requires commitment from the patient and caregivers. Depending on subjective and objective instrumental evaluation findings, specific deficits may be targeted to help the patient achieve a safe and efficient swallow. ST may be limited or even counterproductive when an untreated obstructive physiology exists. A broad understanding of these issues will guide the otolaryngologist in performing thorough evaluations, counseling patients and caregivers, and making appropriate referrals.

In general, swallow exercise efficacy has not been well studied. Observation shows that some patients have better swallowing after therapy while others do not. High quality research could improve treatment planning and outcomes. There are a number of opportunities for future research, such as determining how the combination of different swallow exercises may improve or impede progress and ascertaining the optimal frequency and intensity for the various swallow exercises.

REFERENCES

1. Jones HN, Rosenbek JC. *Dysphagia in Rare Conditions: An Encyclopedia*. Plural Pub. 2010;page 5.
2. Plowman E. Is there a role for exercise in the management of bulbar dysfunction in amyotrophic lateral sclerosis? *J Speech Lang Hear Res*. 2015;58:1151−1166.
3. Muss L, Wilmskoetter J, Richter K, et al. Changes in swallowing after anterior cervical discectomy and fusion with instrumentation: a presurgical versus postsurgical videofluoroscopic comparison. *J Speech Lang Hear Res*. 2017;60(4):785−793.
4. Kang JY, Choi KH, Yun GJ, Kim MY, Ryu JS. Does removal of tracheostomy affect dysphagia? A kinematic analysis. *Dysphagia*. 2012;27(4):498−503.

5. Terk AR, Leder SB, Burrell MI. Hyoid bone and laryngeal movement dependent upon presence of a tracheotomy tube. *Dysphagia.* 2007;22(2):89−93.

6. Ledl C, Ullrich YY. Occlusion of tracheostomy tubes does not alter pharyngeal phase kinematics but reduces penetration by enhancing pharyngeal clearance: a prospective study in patients with neurogenic dysphagia. *Am J Phys Med Rehabil.* 2017;96(4):268−272.

7. Cameron J, Reynolds J, Zuidema G. Aspiration in patients with tracheostomies. *Plast Reconstr Surg.* 1973;52(2):206.

8. Bone D, Davis J, Zuidema G, Cameron J. Aspiration pneumonia: prevention of aspiration in patients with tracheostomies. *Ann Thorac Surg.* July 1974:30−37.

9. Gross RD, Mahlmann J, Grayhack JP. Physiologic effects of open and closed tracheostomy tubes on the pharyngeal swallow. *Ann Otol Rhinol Laryngol.* 2003;112(2):143−152.

10. Leder SB, Joe JK, Hill SE, Traube M. Effect of tracheotomy tube occlusion on upper esophageal sphincter and pharyngeal pressures in aspirating and nonaspirating patients. *Dysphagia.* 2001 Spring;16(2):79−82.

11. Leder SB, Tarro JM, Burrell MI. Effect of occlusion of a tracheotomy tube on aspiration. *Dysphagia.* 1996 Fall;11(4):254−258.

12. Hutcheson KA, Lewin JS, Barringer DA, et al. Late dysphagia after radiotherapy-based treatment of head and neck cancer. *Cancer.* 2012;118(23):5793−5799.

13. Hutcheson KA, Bhayani MK, Beadle BM, et al. Eat and exercise during radiotherapy or chemoradiotherapy for pharyngeal cancers: use it or lose it. *JAMA Otolaryngol Head Neck Surg.* 2013;139(11):1127−1134.

14. Hutcheson KA, Holsinger FC, Kupferman ME, Lewin JS. Functional outcomes after TORS for oropharyngeal cancer: a systematic review. *Eur Arch Otorhinolaryngol.* 2015;272(2):463−471.

15. Langmore SE, Skarupski KA, Park PS, Fries BE. Predictors of aspiration pneumonia in nursing home residents. *Dysphagia.* 2002 Fall;17(4):298−307.

16. Kaneoka A, Pisegna JM, Saito H, et al. A systematic review and meta-analysis of pneumonia associated with thin liquid vs. thickened liquid intake in patients who aspirate. *Clin Rehabil.* 2017;31(8):1116−1125.

17. Nascimento WV, Cassiani RA, Santos CM, Dantas RO. Effect of bolus volume and consistency on swallowing events duration in healthy subjects. *J Neurogastroenterol Motil.* 2015;21(1):78−82.

18. Steele CM, Alsanei WA, Ayanikalath S, et al. The influence of food texture and liquid consistency modification on swallowing physiology and function: a systematic review. *Dysphagia.* 2015;30(1):2−26.

19. Newman R, Vilardell N, Clavé P, Speyer R. Effect of bolus viscosity on the safety and efficacy of swallowing and the kinematics of the swallow response in patients with oropharyngeal dysphagia: white paper by the European Society for Swallowing Disorders (ESSD). *Dysphagia.* 2016;31(2):232−249.

20. Burkhead LM, Sapienza CM, Rosenbek JC. Strength-training exercise in dysphagia rehabilitation: principles, procedures, and directions for future research. *Dysphagia.* 2007;22(3):251−265.

21. Pauli N, Svensson U, Karlsson T, Finizia C. Exercise intervention for the treatment of trismus in head and neck cancer. *Acta Oncol.* 2014;53:502−509.

22. Pauli N, Andréll P, Johansson M, Fagerberg-Mohlin B, Finizia C. Treating trismus: a prospective study on effect and compliance to jaw exercise therapy in head and neck cancer. *Head Neck.* 2015;37(12):1738−1744.

23. Kamstra JI, Roodenburg JL, Beurskens CH, Reintsema H, Dijkstra PU. TheraBite exercises to treat trismus secondary to head and neck cancer. *Support Care Cancer.* 2013;21(4):951−957.

24. Robbins J, Kays SA, Gangnon RE, et al. The effects of lingual exercise in stroke patients with dysphagia. *Arch Phys Med Rehabil.* 2007;88(2):150−158.

25. Rosenbek J, Robbins J, Roecker E, Coyle J, Wood J. A penetration aspiration scale. *Dysphagia.* 1996;11:93−98.

26. Huckabee ML, Butler SG, Barclay M, Jit S. Submental surface electromyographic measurement and pharyngeal pressures during normal and effortful swallowing. *Arch Phys Med Rehabil.* 2005;86(11):2144−2149.

27. Hoffman M, Mielens J, Ciucci M, Jones C, Jiang J, McCulloch T. High-resolution manometry of pharyngeal swallow pressure events associated with effortful swallow and the Mendelsohn maneuver. *Dysphagia.* 2010;27:418−426.

28. McCullough GH, Kim Y. Effects of the Mendelsohn maneuver on extent of hyoid movement and UES opening post-stroke. *Dysphagia.* 2013;28(4):511−519. https://doi.org/10.1007/s00455-013-9461-1. Epub 2013 Mar 14.

29. O'Neil K, Purdy M, Falk J, Gallo L. The dysphagia outcome and severity scale. *Dysphagia.* 1999;14:139−145.

30. Fujiu-Kurachi M. Developing the tongue holding maneuver. *Perspect Swallowing Swallowing Disord (Dysphagia).* 2002;11(1):9−11.

31. Fujiu M, Logemann JA. Effect of a tongue-holding maneuver on posterior pharyngeal wall movement during deglutition. *Am J Speech Lang Pathol.* 1996;5(1):23−30.

32. Shaker R, Kern M, Bardan E, et al. Augmentation of deglutitive upper esophageal sphincter opening in the elderly by exercise. *Am Physiol Soc.* 1997;272:G1518−G1522.

33. Shaker R, Easterling C, Kern M, et al. Rehabilitation of swallowing by exercise in tube-fed patients with pharyngeal dysphagiasecondary to abnormal UES opening. *Gastroenterology.* 2002;122(5):1314−1321.

34. Yoon WL, Khoo JK, Rickard Liow SJ. Chin tuck against resistance (CTAR): new method for enhancing suprahyoid muscle activity using a Shaker-type exercise. *Dysphagia.* 2014;29(2):243−248.

35. Pitts T, Bolser D, Rosenbek J, Troche M, Okun MS, Sapienza C. Impact of expiratory muscle strength training on voluntary cough and swallow function in Parkinson disease. *Chest.* 2009;135(5):1301−1308. https://doi.org/10.1378/chest.08-1389. Epub 2008 Nov 24.

36. Troche MS, Okun MS, Rosenbek JC, et al. Aspiration and swallowing in Parkinson disease and rehabilitation with EMST: a randomized trial. *Neurology*. 2010;75(21): 1912–1919.

37. Rosenbek JC, Robbins J, Fishback B, Levine RL. Effects of thermal application on dysphagia after stroke. *J Speech Hear Res*. 1991;34(6):1257–1268.

38. Crary MA, Carnaby Mann GD, Groher ME. Biomechanical correlates of surface electromyography signals obtained during swallowing by healthy adults. *J Speech Lang Hear Res*. 2006;49(1):186–193.

39. Colodny N. Comparison of dysphagics and nondysphagics on pulse oximetry during oral feeding. *Dysphagia*. 2000;15:68–73.

40. Leslie P, Drinnan M, Finn P, Ford G, Wilson J. Reliability and validity of cervical auscultation: a controlled comparison using videofluoroscopy. *Dysphagia*. 2004;19: 231–240.

41. Ludlow CL. Electrical neuromuscular stimulation in dysphagia: current status. *Curr Opin Otolaryngol Head Neck Surg*. 2010;18(3):159–164.

42. Humbert IA, Michou E, MacRae PR, Crujido L. Electrical stimulation and swallowing: how much do we know? *Semin Speech Lang*. 2012;33(3):203–216.

43. Chaudhuri G, Hildner C, Brady S, Hutchins B, Aliga N, Abadilla E. Cardiovascular effects of the supraglottic and super-supraglottic swallowing maneuvers in stroke patients with dysphagia. *Dysphagia*. 2002;17:19–23.

CHAPTER 25

Future Directions in Dysphagia Treatment

JENNIFER L. LONG, MD, PHD • DINESH K. CHHETRI, MD

INTRODUCTION

Appreciation of dysphagia as a significant public health problem is growing, and translational research has become more prevalent. Novel techniques and approaches are currently being evaluated and may reduce the impact of this disorder in the future. This chapter highlights recent advances and suggests other focus areas that could benefit from further research efforts.

ASSESSMENT

Dysphagia diagnosis remains largely subjective. Patient history and swallowing rating scales are rightfully key factors in assessment. Instrumental exams (flexible endoscopic evaluation of swallowing [FEES] and modified barium swallow study [MBSS]) are essential for diagnosis, but the current subjective nature of evaluating these exams leads to significant variability among raters and discrepancies between the two exam types.[1–3] FEES is clearly more sensitive to pharyngeal residue, which should be taken into consideration in evaluations. Quantitative measures for MBSS assessment have been developed but have not achieved widespread clinical application yet.[4–6] Barriers include lack of standardized software, clinician time requirements, and concerns about test reproducibility and variation. High-resolution manometry (HRM) does offer quantifiable data[7] but has been somewhat limited by invasiveness and lack of trained providers. In addition, application of HRM to assess the pharyngeal phase of swallow is early in development.[8] A widespread effort including software developers and large numbers of normal patients could produce benchmarks that would enhance the utility of current tests. Newer HRM systems are also capable of three-dimensional measurement, which should greatly enhance the spatiotemporal data that is currently generated in two-dimensional studies.

Radiologic assessment in four dimensions, such as dynamic MRI of swallowing, would reveal swallow physiology in high resolution; this image acquisition technology is still developing.[9,10] An additional limitation of MRI technology is the current requirement for supine positioning, which is difficult for many dysphagic patients.

New diagnostic measures that do not rely on radiologic imaging techniques would also be helpful to more directly assess function and could provide simpler in-office assessment. For example, pharyngeal motor strength is currently indirectly inferred by tongue base motion and degree of residue. A quantitative strength measure would be more precise. The Iowa Oral Performance Instrument may approach this goal with a manometer within a balloon in the oral cavity to measure pressures generated by the oral tongue. Validation studies are underway.[11,12] Similarly, upper esophageal sphincter (UES) function and dysfunction is currently assessed indirectly by visualization on an MBSS. Large-scale incorporation of HRM to quantitate both pharyngeal constrictor strength and UES function could improve the classification of those disorders.

Looking ahead, a single direct examination of multilevel swallow function would greatly advance the care of dysphagia patients. Other standard physiologic tests, such as pulmonary function tests and cardiac echocardiograms, have generated extensive quantitative parameters from complex systems. Each is noninvasive and is routinely performed. Software permits immediate comparison with normal benchmark values. Swallowing physiology deserves a similar comprehensive, quantitative, and direct examination of function. For example, combining high-resolution spatiotemporal imaging of swallowing with concurrent high-resolution manometric data would produce a paradigm shift in swallow assessment.

PREVENTION

Epidemiologic studies have clearly demonstrated several populations at risk for dysphagia, including those patients experiencing head and neck cancer, cerebrovascular accident, surgical procedures involving the lower cranial nerves, and certain genetic or congenital conditions. Previous approach was to observe these patients, then treat dysphagia if it arose. More recently, a shift toward personalized medicine seeks to identify those patients at the highest risk for either dysphagia or its complications and to employ preventive strategies to maintain function. Dysphagia outcomes after chemoradiation have already improved from this preventive strategy. Multidisciplinary head and neck cancer care now screens patients for dysphagia, and institutes swallow preservation exercises for all patients at risk, even before clinical symptoms arise. Swallow preservation protocols successfully improve outcomes, confirming that it is easier to maintain function than restore it.[13–15]

The success of swallow preservation for cancer patients should be extended to other at-risk patients. Increasing public and professional awareness of dysphagia will increase the fruitful referrals of early-stage patients. Ultimately, better prevention should reduce the burden of advanced dysphagia.

More precise identification of those patients at risk will further refine targeting for preventive treatment. For example, chemoradiation does not equally impact all patients' swallowing. As tumor markers are now influencing choice of chemotherapy, perhaps patient-specific gene markers could identify those patients at the highest risk for dysphagia. Understanding of the genetic underpinnings might also suggest specific preventive strategies for swallowing preservation, perhaps by introducing specific pharmaceuticals in addition to exercises. Prevention is thus closely aligned with bioinformatics, discussed next.

BIOINFORMATICS

The emergence of "Omics," including studies of the genome, transcriptome, proteome, secretome, and microbiome, has introduced previously unimagined detail into our understanding of molecular pathophysiology. Bioinformatics assessments may help distinguish causes and features of dysphagia much more precisely than is currently understood. The promise of "omics" is to extrapolate from massive amounts of population data to allow individualized therapeutics. For example, omics data could stratify individual persons' risk of developing radiation fibrosis, which may influence treatment choice in head and neck cancer. Such

applications of big data to dysphagia are thus far limited. One example is a molecular panel for diagnosing eosinophilic esophagitis from random esophageal biopsies. This panel examines the transcriptome of 1610 genes for a more definitive test than the traditional eosinophil counts. It could also be used to select treatments and examine treatment effects in affected patients.[16]

PHARMACEUTICALS

Widespread marketing and adoption of proton-pump inhibitors in the last three decades has led to the use of these drugs in massive numbers of patients with complaints of globus sensation and dysphagia. Yet, relatively few pharmaceuticals have been developed specifically for dysphagia. With the popularity of proton-pump inhibitors waning, as treatment failures and adverse effects become more apparent, there is an appetite for new medicines in dysphagia treatment. Esophageal dysmotility and xerostomia would be excellent disease targets, because they affect a large population of patients, causing significant distress and without adequate treatments currently. Ironically, both dysmotility and xerostomia can result as adverse effects of other drugs. Better recognition of the impact of these side effects could eventually result in reduced occurrence through patient advocacy for better drugs overall. Similarly, numerous neuromodulating drugs developed for other purposes have actions in the gut as well and may serve as springboards for the identification of new, better targeted agents. Examples include the GABA agonist baclofen to increase lower esophageal sphincter (LES) tone[17] and the serotonin receptor agonist buspirone to promote esophageal peristalsis.[18]

SURGICAL TECHNIQUES

Several new techniques are growing in popularity among gastroenterologists and general surgeons. As otolaryngologists, some understanding of these techniques will be valuable in counseling and referring those patients with multilevel swallowing dysfunction. Among them, longitudinal per-oral endoscopic myotomy (POEM) offers a new treatment for achalasia[19–21] and could expand the number of patients selected for treatment. New implantable devices are in trials for LES augmentation to reduce reflux.[22] Laparoscopic magnetic sphincter augmentation (the LINX device) has had good efficacy and safety results thus far, although dysphagia prompted device removal in 52 of 3283 patients.[23] An implantable electrical stimulator for the LES (the EndoStim device) is less advanced in development, but all of the reported 25 patients had excellent patient satisfaction.[24]

In the otolaryngology sphere, creative methods are needed to treat esophageal stricture, for example, after radiation therapy. Currently the norm is repeated pneumatic dilation, sometimes with the addition of antistenotic pharmaceuticals. A more durable result is needed, either with better targeted drugs, physical stents, or perhaps a biodegradable drug-eluting stent similar to that now introduced for endoscopic sinus surgery.[25] Esophageal stents in general have been a mainstay for patients with malignant esophageal obstruction, yet they are prone to complications.[26] Newer manufactured stent materials incorporating novel polymers or extracellular matrix molecules may improve the safety of this technique.[27,28]

Treatment of UES is another challenge in patients with radiation fibrosis. The decreased compliance of the UES is often unresponsive to dilation. Laryngohyoid suspension is sometimes performed but may be technically difficult, especially in radiated necks, and results have been less than satisfactory. A dynamic surgical technique to improve hyolaryngeal elevation and UES opening would be valuable. In the most severe manifestation of oropharyngeal dysphagia, secretions alone are aspirated even in the setting of complete nonoral feeding. These profoundly affected patients risk recurrent life-threatening pneumonia. A small number elect to undergo the radical procedures of laryngectomy or laryngotracheal separation in hopes of improving life expectancy. As an alternative, some surgeons have proposed intermediate measures including laryngohyoid suspension. A cadaveric ovine study reported that combining laryngohyoid suspension with cricopharyngeal (CP) myotomy greatly reduced bolus aspiration, in a model of complete neuromuscular inactivity.[29] Clinical experience has been limited and results mixed.

NEUROSTIMULATION

Much dysphagia can be attributed to neurologic deficits. Stroke, traumatic brain injury, iatrogenic injury of lower cranial nerves or the pharyngeal plexus, recurrent laryngeal nerve (RLN) impairment—all these can impair swallowing to varying degrees. The only treatment currently available is swallow therapy, with the hope of recovering some function over time. Those persons with RLN weakness among their symptoms can undergo vocal fold medialization for some protection against aspiration, but medialization alone cannot be expected to restore normal swallowing if other nerves or global coordination are affected.

Reinnervation strategies could provide meaningful improvement for these patients. Vocal fold reinnervation with ansa cervicalis for unilateral vocal fold paralysis and selective reinnervation for bilateral vocal fold abductor paralysis have both been successful in selected patients.[30,31] It is reasonable therefore to reach beyond current practice to investigate alternative surgical reinnervation approaches for swallowing as well. Implanted cranial nerve stimulators are in phase III clinical trials for obstructive sleep apnea,[32,33] and deep brain stimulators are widespread in Parkinson's disease and seizure disorders. Perhaps direct nerve stimulation could promote pharyngeal constriction, esophageal peristalsis, or the timed coordination of swallowing movements. Skilled research teams, including swallowing experts, could have significant patient impact in this area.

REGENERATIVE MEDICINE

Regenerative medicine uses implanted or native cells to control repair processes in the body. Implanted cells may engraft and become a long-lasting part of the host, or may simply supply paracrine signals temporarily to alter the host's own cellular activity. It can also be a platform for gene therapy or tailored drug delivery. This new realm of medicine has produced creative research projects in all areas of health. A number of projects have advanced to human trials, and a few to Food and Drug Administration approval.

Cell-based therapies for dysphagia are generally earlier along the development pipeline but could address some of the challenges noted above. For example, a tissue-engineered esophageal graft or stent that heals without stricture or erosion could provide valuable palliation or long-term luminal patency.[34] A cell-based therapy to improve tongue or pharyngeal constrictor muscle strength would fill a significant treatment gap for patients affected by radiation fibrosis or neurodegenerative atrophy.[35,36] Restoring salivary gland function would be a boon for many patients.[37]

Oculopharyngeal muscular dystrophy (OPMD), a rare autosomal dominant genetic disorder producing progressive pharyngeal weakness, has been a target of innovative cell-based therapies. Its standard care with CP myotomy is inadequate, with high recurrence rate of dysphagia and aspiration.[38] A clinical trial of autologous myoblast transplantation along with CP myotomy did improve function in 12 humans for up to 2 years.[39] In another strategy, genetically affected mice treated with gene transfer therapy to eliminate toxic accumulating proteins and replace normal proteins have shown improved muscle strength.[40] While OPMD is uncommon, its homogeneity and severity make it attractive for research which could eventually be adapted to other disorders as well.

CONCLUSIONS

Several aspects of dysphagia would benefit from novel approaches. Emerging technologies, such as bioinformatics, neurostimulation, and regenerative medicine, should be applied to this difficult disorder. Progress will require broad understanding of the clinical aspects of disease and the research methodologies.

REFERENCES

1. Lee JW, Randall DR, Evangelista LM, Kuhn MA, Belafsky PC. Subjective assessment of videofluoroscopic swallow studies. *Otolaryngol Head Neck Surg.* 2017;156(5):901–905.
2. Pisegna JM, Langmore SE. Parameters of instrumental swallowing evaluations: describing a diagnostic dilemma. *Dysphagia.* 2016;31(3):462–472.
3. Giraldo-Cadavid LF, Leal-Leaño LR, Leon-Basantes GA, et al. Accuracy of endoscopic and videofluoroscopic evaluations of swallowing for oropharyngeal dysphagia. *Laryngoscope.* 2017;127(9):2002–2010.
4. Ellerston JK, Heller AC, Houtz DR, Kendall KA. Quantitative measures of swallowing deficits in patients with Parkinson's disease. *Ann Otol Rhinol Laryngol.* 2016;125(5):385–392.
5. Kendall KA. Evaluation of airway protection: quantitative timing measures versus penetration/aspiration score. *Laryngoscope.* 2017;127(10):2314–2318.
6. Leonard R, Rees CJ, Belafsky P, Allen J. Fluoroscopic surrogate for pharyngeal strength: the pharyngeal constriction ratio (PCR). *Dysphagia.* 2011;26(1):13–17.
7. Hoffman MR, Jones CA, Geng Z, et al. Classification of high-resolution manometry data according to videofluoroscopic parameters using pattern recognition. *Otolaryngol Head Neck Surg.* 2013;149(1):126–133.
8. Rosen SP, Jones CA, McCulloch TM. Pharyngeal swallowing pressures in the base-of-tongue and hypopharynx regions identified with three-dimensional manometry. *Laryngoscope.* 2017;127(9):1989–1995.
9. Lee E, Xing F, Ahn S, et al. Magnetic resonance imaging based anatomical assessment of tongue impairment due to amyotrophic lateral sclerosis: a preliminary study. *J Acoust Soc Am.* 2018;143(4):EL248.
10. Olthoff A, Joseph AA, Weidenmüller M, Riley B, Frahm J. Real-time MRI of swallowing: intraoral pressure reduction supports larynx elevation. *NMR Biomed.* 2016;29(11):1618–1623.
11. Adams V, Mathisen B, Baines S, Lazarus C, Callister R. A systematic review and meta-analysis of measurements of tongue and hand strength and endurance using the Iowa Oral Performance Instrument (IOPI). *Dysphagia.* 2013;28(3):350–369.
12. Van den Steen L, Vanderveken O, Vanderwegen J, et al. Feasibility of tongue strength measurements during (chemo)radiotherapy in head and neck cancer patients. *Support Care Cancer.* 2017;25(11):3417–3423.
13. Peng KA, Kuan EC, Unger L, Lorentz WC, Wang MB, Long JL. A swallow preservation protocol improves function for veterans receiving chemoradiation for head and neck cancer. *Otolaryngol Head Neck Surg.* 2015;152(5):863–867.
14. Duarte VM, Chhetri DK, Liu YF, Erman AA, Wang MB. Swallow preservation exercises during chemoradiation therapy maintains swallow function. *Otolaryngol Head Neck Surg.* 2013;149(6):878–884.
15. Virani A, Kunduk M, Fink DS, McWhorter AJ. Effects of 2 different swallowing exercise regimens during organ-preservation therapies for head and neck cancers on swallowing function. *Head Neck.* 2015;37(2):162–170.
16. Wen T, Rothenberg ME. Clinical applications of the eosinophilic esophagitis diagnostic panel. *Front Med.* 2017;4:108.
17. Scarpellini E, Ang D, Pauwels A, De Santis A, Vanuytsel T, Tack J. Management of refractory typical GERD symptoms. *Nat Rev Gastroenterol Hepatol.* 2016;13(5):281–294.
18. Aggarwal N, Thota PN, Lopez R, Gabbard S. A randomized double-blind placebo-controlled crossover-style trial of buspirone in functional dysphagia and ineffective esophageal motility. *Neurogastroenterol Motil.* 2018;30(2).
19. Kahrilas PJ, Katzka D, Richter JE. Clinical practice update: the use of per-oral endoscopic myotomy in achalasia: expert review and best practice advice from the AGA Institute. *Gastroenterology.* 2017;153(5):1205–1211.
20. Kahrilas PJ, Bredenoord AJ, Fox M, et al. Expert consensus document: advances in the management of oesophageal motility disorders in the era of high-resolution manometry: a focus on achalasia syndromes. *Nat Rev Gastroenterol Hepatol.* 2017;14(11):677–688.
21. Vaezi MF, Felix VN, Penagini R, et al. Achalasia: from diagnosis to management. *Ann NY Acad Sci.* 2016;1381(1):34–44.
22. Chiu J, Soffer E. Novel surgical options for gastroesophageal reflux disease. *Expert Rev Gastroenterol Hepatol.* 2015;9(7):943–951.
23. Smith CD, Ganz RA, Lipham JC, Bell RC, Rattner DW. Lower esophageal sphincter augmentation for gastroesophageal reflux disease: the safety of a modern implant. *J Laparoendosc Adv Surg Tech A.* 2017;27(6):586–591.
24. Rodríguez L, Rodriguez P, Gómez B, et al. Two-year results of intermittent electrical stimulation of the lower esophageal sphincter treatment of gastroesophageal reflux disease. *Surgery.* 2015;157(3):556–567.

25. Huang Z, Hwang P, Sun Y, Zhou B. Steroid-eluting sinus stents for improving symptoms in chronic rhinosinusitis patients undergoing functional endoscopic sinus surgery. *Cochrane Database Syst Rev.* 2015;(6):CD010436.
26. Doosti-Irani A, Mansournia MA, Rahimi-Foroushani A, Haddad P, Holakouie-Naieni K. Complications of stent placement in patients with esophageal cancer: a systematic review and network meta-analysis. *PLoS One.* 2017; 12(10):e0184784.
27. Dua KS. History of the use of esophageal stent in management of dysphagia and its improvement over the years. *Dysphagia.* 2017;32(1):39—49.
28. Dua KS, Hogan WJ, Aadam AA, Gasparri M. In-vivo oesophageal regeneration in a human being by use of a non-biological scaffold and extracellular matrix. *Lancet.* 2016. https://doi.org/10.1016/S0140-6736(15)01036-3.
29. Johnson C, Venkatesan N, Siddiqui T, et al. Outcomes of laryngohyoid suspension techniques in an ovine model of profound oropharyngeal dysphagia. *Laryngoscope.* 2017;127:E422—E427.
30. Paniello RC, Edgar JD, Kallogjeri D, Piccirillo JF. Medialization versus reinnervation for unilateral vocal fold paralysis: a multicenter randomized clinical trial. *Laryngoscope.* 2011;121(10):2172—2179.
31. Marina MB, Marie JP, Birchall MA. Laryngeal reinnervation for bilateral vocal fold paralysis. *Curr Opin Otolaryngol Head Neck Surg.* 2011;19(6):434—438.
32. Kezirian EJ, Goding Jr GS, Malhotra A, et al. Hypoglossal nerve stimulation improves obstructive sleep apnea: 12-month outcomes. *J Sleep Res.* 2014;23(1):77—83.
33. Woodson BT, Soose RJ, Gillespie MB, et al. Three-year outcomes of cranial nerve stimulation for obstructive sleep apnea: the STAR trial. *Otolaryngol Head Neck Surg.* 2016; 154(1):181—188.
34. Catry J, Luong-Nguyen M, Arakelian L, et al. Circumferential esophageal replacement by a tissue-engineered substitute using mesenchymal stem cells: an experimental study in mini pigs. *Cell Transplant.* 2017;26(12):1831—1839.
35. Kuhn MA, Black AB, Siddiqui MT, Nolta JA, Belafsky PC. Novel murine xenograft model for the evaluation of stem cell therapy for profound dysphagia. *Laryngoscope.* 2017;127(10):E359—E363.
36. Plowman EK, Bijangi-Vishehsaraei K, Halum S, et al. Autologous myoblasts attenuate atrophy and improve tongue force in a denervated tongue model: a pilot study. *Laryngoscope.* 2014;124(2):E20—E26.
37. Chibly AM, Nguyen T, Limesand KH. Palliative care for salivary gland dysfunction highlights the need for regenerative therapies: a review on radiation and salivary gland stem cells. *J Palliat Care Med.* 2014;4(4).
38. Coiffier L, Périé S, Laforêt P, Eymard B, St Guily JL. Long-term results of cricopharyngeal myotomy in oculopharyngeal muscular dystrophy. *Otolaryngol Head Neck Surg.* 2006;135(2):218—222.
39. Perie S, Trollet C, Mouly V. Autologous myoblast transplantation for oculopharyngeal muscular dystrophy: a phase I/IIa clinical study. *Mol Ther.* 2013;22:219—225.
40. Malerba A, Klein P, Bachtarzi H, et al. PABPN1 gene therapy for oculopharyngeal muscular dystrophy. *Nat Commun.* 2017;8:14848.

Index

Note: Page numbers followed by "f" indicate figures, "t" indicate tables.

Printed in the United States
By Bookmasters